HIV and the Eye

HIV and the Eye

Editor

Susan Lightman

Department of Clinical Ophthalmology
Institute of Ophthalmology and Moorfields Eye Hospital
London, UK

ICP

Imperial College Press

Published by

Imperial College Press
57 Shelton Street
Covent Garden
London WC2H 9HE

Distributed by

World Scientific Publishing Co. Pte. Ltd.
P O Box 128, Farrer Road, Singapore 912805
USA office: Suite 1B, 1060 Main Street, River Edge, NJ 07661
UK office: 57 Shelton Street, Covent Garden, London WC2H 9HE

Library of Congress Cataloging-in-Publication Data
HIV and the eye / editor, Susan Lightman.
     p.   cm.
  Includes bibliographical references.
  ISBN 1-86094-084-6
  1. Ocular manifestations of general diseases. 2. AIDS (Disease) -
-Complications. 3. Eye--Infections.   I. Lightman, Susan.
  RE65.H58   1999
  617.7'1--dc21   99-29629
                                                        CIP

British Library Cataloguing-in-Publication Data
A catalogue record for this book is available from the British Library.

For photocopying of material in this volume, please pay a copying fee through the Copyright Clearance Center, Inc., 222 Rosewood Drive, Danvers, MA 01923, USA. In this case permission to photocopy is not required from the publisher.

Printed in Singapore.

PREFACE

The aim of this book is to cover all aspects of involvement of the eye in HIV infection although HIV patients can also develop eye problems which are not associated with HIV infection. These people are looked after by various types of attendants, and it is therefore very likely that eye problems may first present to the non-ophthalmologist before referral to the ophthalmologist.

To address this, the first three chapters in this book are overview chapters: the first updates the reader on current management issues in HIV in these changing times while the second and third provide an overview of the different types of eye problems that can occur in both the pre-AIDS and AIDS phase of HIV infection. Chapters four, five, six and seven cover different types of ocular involvement in detail, and are particularly written for the ophthalmologist. Chapter eight details surgical procedures which are carried out by ophthalmologists and the safety issues which arise from intervention. Lastly, chapter nine discusses the ocular problems in developing countries, where the greatest number of HIV-infected patients live and where the patterns of ocular disease may be different.

Some disease entities appear in several chapters and this has been done in order to ensure that each chapter is relatively self-contained and the reader does not have to browse through other chapters in order to cover the topic. In addition, the chapters are cross-referenced to guide the reader to another chapter where the same topic is also covered, usually in more detail. The text is illustrated with colour pictures with appropriate radiolology to complete the topic.

I would like to thank all the contributors of this book who have so readily shared their expertise and the other experts in the field who have carried out the studies on which our current practice is based.

Susan Lightman

LIST OF CONTRIBUTORS

Stephen A Ash, FRCP
Consultant Physician
Ealing Hospital NHS Trust
London, UK

Peter J McCluskey, MD FRACO
Consultant Ophthalmologist
St. Vincents' Hospital and
Royal Prince Alfred Hospital
Sydney, Australia

Douglas A Jabs, MD
Professor of Ophthalmology
The Johns Hopkins University
School of Medicine
Baltimore, USA

Andrew B Tullo, MD FRCOphth
Consultant Ophthalmic Surgeon
Honorary Senior Lecturer
Manchester Royal Eye Hospital
UK

Baljean Dhillon, BMedSci FRCS
(Glasg. & Ed.) FRCOphth
Consultant Ophthalmic Surgeon
Princess Alexandra Eye Pavilion
Edinburgh, UK

Ahmed Kamal, MS FRCS (Ed.)
Specialist Registrar
Princess Alexandra Eye Pavilion
Edinburgh, UK

Thomas Kuriakose, FRCS (Ed.)
Specialist Registrar
Princess Alexandra Eye Pavilion
Edinburgh, UK

Anthony J Hall, MD FRACO FRACS
Consultant Ophthalmologist
The Alfred Hospital and
Royal Melbourne Hospital
Australia

Rosalyn M Stanbury, MRCP FRCOphth
Senior Registrar in Medical Ophthalmology
St. Thomas' Hospital
London, UK

Elizabeth M Graham, FRCP FRCOphth
Consultant Medical Ophthalmologist
St. Thomas' Hospital
London, UK

Steven D Schwartz, MD
Consultant Ophthalmologist
Jules Stein Eye Institute
Los Angeles, USA

Adnan Tufail, FRCOphth
Specialist Registrar
Moorfields Eye Hospital
London, UK

Philippe Kestelyn, MD
Professor of Ophthalmology
University Clinic
Gent, Belgium

CONTENTS

CONTENTS

ABBREVIATIONS

ACV	Aciclovir
AIDS	Aquired Immunodeficiency Disease Syndrome
ARN	Acute Retinal Necrosis
AZT	Zidovudine
CAR	Cancer Associated Retinopathy
CD4/CD8	T-lymphocyte subgroups as defined by surface markers (phenotype)
CM	Cryptococcal Meningitis
CMV	Cytomegalovirus
CMVR	Cytomegalovirus Retinitis
CNS	Central Nervous System
CSF	Cerebrospinal Fluid
CT	Computerised Tomography
CTP	Cerebral Toxoplasmosis
DNA	Deoxyribonucleic acid
EEG	Electroencephalogram
ESR	Erythrocyte Sedimentation Rate
FTA-ABS	Fluorescent Treponemal Antibody - Absorbed
GBS	Guillain-Barre Syndrome
MHATP	MicroHaemagglutination Assay for antibody to *T. Pallidum*
HAART	Highly Active Antiretroviral Therapy
HHV-8	Human Herpes Virus-8
HIV	Human Immunodeficiency Virus
HSK	Herpes Simplex Keratitis
HSV	Herpes Simplex Virus
HZO	Herpes Zoster Ophthalmicus
HZV	Herpes Zoster Virus
KS	Kaposi's Sarcoma
LIP	Lymphoid interstitial pneumonitis
MAC	Mycobacterium Avium Complex
MAI	Mycobacterium Avium Intracellulare
MDRTB	Multi-Drug Resistant Tuberculosis
MRI	Magnetic Resonance Imaging
NHL	Non-Hodgkin's Lymphoma
ON	Optic Neuritis
PCP	Pneumocystis Carinii Pneumonia
PCR	Polymerase Chain Reaction
PI	Protease Inhibitor
PML	Progressive Multifocal Leucoencephalopathy

PORN	Progressive Outer Retinal Necrosis
RD	Retinal Detachment
RES	Reticuloendothelial System
RNA	Ribonucleic Acid
RPR	Rapid Plasma Reagin
RSV	Respiratory Syncitial Virus
RTI	Reverse Transcriptase Inhibitor
SJS	Stevens Johnson Syndrome
TB	Tuberculosis
TG	Toxoplasma Gondii
VDRL	Venereal Disease Research Laboratory
VEP	Visual Evoked Potential
VZV	Varicella-Zoster Virus

CHAPTER 1

CURRENT MANAGEMENT APPROACHES IN HIV INFECTION

Stephen A Ash

Introduction

The modern management of patients with HIV infection has improved greatly over the past year or so. The old strategies of using prophylaxis against opportunistic infections to which an individual may be vulnerable are still important. The use of triple combination antiretroviral therapy with agents inhibiting different HIV enzymes involved in viral replication, has produced improvements in immune function as well as improved quality and length of life of people, even those with quite advanced AIDS. The full potential of these therapies for patients with AIDS, those with lesser symptoms, and asymptomatic HIV-infected patients is not yet known.

There has been an immense and rapid change in the clinical management of people with HIV over the last two years or so, and further developments are likely to occur at a similar to pace in the next few years. The most profound new events centre around the use of plasma HIV viral quantitation ("viral load") and the prescribing of a new group of antiretroviral drugs — the protease inhibitors — as part of a combination of drugs with reverse transcriptase inhibitors. As far as one can tell, these advances are set to substantially improve the prognosis for people with HIV. As might be expected with new innovations, the full potential of these new treatments will not be realised for some years yet. The use of combination antiretroviral therapy for adult patients with early, asymptomatic HIV disease is currently controversial, and its use in paediatric practice is poorly developed at present. However, the future appears much brighter for people with HIV than ever before. Sadly, these new developments are expensive and unlikely to be available in underdeveloped countries where, in fact, most of the global HIV-infected population live. Nevertheless, much has been learnt about HIV and the effects it has on both the immune system and the neurological system — knowledge which can be used to advantage in clinical practice even in the absence of the availability of these new drugs.

Natural History of HIV Infection, Surrogate Markers, and Viral Load

Adults who are infected with HIV may experience a very varied pattern and time-course of progression of their illness. After the initial infection, whether it be blood borne or transmitted by sex, seroconversion with the production of antibodies, and thus a positive blood test, may take from two to six weeks, and occasionally three months to occur. Just prior to the appearance of antibodies in the circulation, a proportion of infected individuals may experience a self-limiting "seroconversion illness", lasting for about two to three weeks.[1] The usual manifestations of this illness are mild and their significance easily overlooked: headache, fever, lymphadenopathy, sore throat and a rash[2,3] (see Table 1.1). Occasionally, the illness may have quite severe neurological symptoms of meningitis, encephalitis,[4] myelitis, and Guillain-Barre syndrome, which all seem to resolve spontaneously. Ocular features are uncommon. For a few, there may be a transient, but substantial, fall in CD4 T-lymphocyte numbers for a week or two at the time of seroconversion,[5] and this can lead to quite severe opportunistic infections such as pneumocystis pneumonia and oesophageal candidiasis. Lymphocyte numbers recover afterwards, but not usually to a level as high as that prior to infection. Those individuals who experience a severe seroconversion illness seem more likely to have a worse long-term prognosis.[6,7] Complete recovery is the rule, and the infected individual may remain without symptoms for many years.

Table 1.1 Features of HIV seroconverison illness.

- rash
- sore throat
- fever
- lymphadenopathy
- headache

occasionally:
- meningitis
- encephalitis
- transverse myelitis
- Guillain-Barre syndrome
- acute opportunistic infections, eg. candida

Original data collected from a large cohort of gay men in California in the 1980s showed that it took an average of ten years from infection to death or developing AIDS.[8] However, there is a wide spread around this average, some people developing AIDS within just a year or two of primary infection. A small percentage, probably about 10%, seem to progress very much slower than others, many having HIV infection for over 14 years without developing AIDS or severe immunodeficiency.[9] It is thought that many of these individuals may have a heterozygous condition whereby they have a deficiency of a cell membrane receptor termed CKR-5. This is a chemokine receptor and about 1% of the Caucasian population are in a homozygous state with a complete absence of the genes coding for this receptor, and do not seem to suffer ill health as a result. Curiously, these individuals seem unable to get infected with HIV. It is now known that HIV requires two cell membrane receptors in order to infect a cell: the CD4 and the CKR-5 receptor.[10]

The natural history of HIV infection in a particular patient usually proceeds through a number of phases. The asymptomatic stage, which may last several years, may be followed by a period during which CD4 lymphocyte numbers start to fall and patients may experience repeated minor illnesses usually of an infective nature, and related to a subtle disturbance of immune function. It has been found that this stage is preceded by an upregulation of HIV viral activity, perhaps due to a failure of the immune system to keep it in check. Measurement of levels of plasma HIV-RNA (often referred to as viral load) have proved to be useful in determining which individuals are likely to be at risk of progression. Those patients with high plasma HIV-RNA levels in the first few months of infection are more likely to progress over the subsequent year than those with lower viral loads, in terms of a fall in CD4 lymphocyte numbers and the development of immunodeficiency and its consequences.[11,12]

CD4 T-lymphocyte numbers in blood samples have provided a clinically useful marker of the level of immunodeficiency in an individual at a given time point.[13,14] Although absolute numbers in the circulation may fluctuate due to migration in and out of the reticulo endothelial system, CD4 lymphocyte counts in the blood persistently below a value of 500/µl are considered abnormal. CD4 counts may be low due to the cells leaving the circulation and entering lymph nodes in numerous other infective illnesses such as TB, and common viral infections. In these cases, when unassociated with HIV, the percentage of CD4 cells to total T-cell numbers is preserved as is the ratio of CD4 to CD8 T-cells.

It is usually only when CD4 counts fall below 200/µl that patients become vulnerable to the more severe and AIDS-defining opportunistic infections. CD8 T-cell lymphocyte numbers do show changes with progression of HIV-associated immunodeficiency, but interpreting results is usually clinically unhelpful.

The measurement of plasma levels of HIV-RNA or viral load, has become a standard procedure in the clinical management of patients with HIV. The quantitative measurement of plasma levels of HIV-RNA, has been shown to have prognostic value in determining the probability of progression of HIV-associated disease as judged by a fall in CD4 T-lymphocyte numbers and the incidence of AIDS-defining illness. In a study of patients recently infected with HIV, the level of HIV-RNA in the plasma correlated closely with subsequent progression: the higher the viral load the greater the probability of progression, and that this feature is a graded one when the viral load is plotted in a logarithmic fashion.[11] There is growing evidence that a similar situation exists for people at other stages of HIV infection and that this phenomenon is not just present at the time around primary infection. Some studies have shown that the plasma HIV-RNA level parallels the viral load level in biopsied tonsillar tissue, but it may be several log values higher in the reticuloendothelial (RE) tissue. Much work has been done to show very convincingly that the main focus of HIV infection is within the RE system and that viral replication continues actively even at the early, asymptomatic stage of HIV infection and before any obvious fall in CD4 T-lymphocyte numbers has occurred,[15] although there may be minor and subtle functional immune changes at this time. More obvious immunodeficiency seems to occur when the balance between the rate of viral replication upsets both the destruction and production of CD4 T-lymphocytes.[16]

If this hypothesis is correct, then lowering HIV replication rates should preserve CD4 cells and immune function, and be reflected in improved health and survival. This forms the basis for antiretroviral therapy discussed later in this chapter, where viral load levels may help identify when an individual may be advised to start therapy. It is also of value in determining the efficacy of therapy.

The results are reported in copies of RNA per millilitre, and are plotted on a logarithmic scale. The test has an inherent variation of about 0.3 of a log value, and, according to what type of assay is being used, may have a sensitivity that can detect down to 20, 50, 200, or 400 copies per ml. Monitoring viral load is now routine and the result is useful in making clinical management decisions. It is important to remember that viral load may be temporarily elevated by intercurrent coincidental infection in an individual.

Counselling, Testing and Confidentiality

There is still a large degree of stigma and fear attached to the diagnosis of HIV infection and AIDS. Patients feel reassured by the demonstration that their diagnosis and details are to be dealt with sensitively and confidentially.

Testing for HIV infection involves a blood test to detect antibodies to HIV-1 (and usually HIV-2, the variant affecting parts of West Africa). This test will only become positive after seroconversion, which takes anywhere between two weeks to three months after infection. Diagnosing HIV infection before seroconversion is difficult to do, although the use of plasma viral RNA detection may prove useful in doing this, but as yet, is not fully validated. It has become traditional now to provide counselling before and after proceeding to HIV-antibody testing, because of the many issues that have developed around testing over the last two decades. Many of these issues relate to non-medical matters such as subsequently obtaining life insurance or a property mortgage. The impact of a positive HIV-antibody test result on an individual may be devastating, and they may need considerable professional support. Sensitive discussion should take place about who else might have been at risk of acquiring HIV infection, eg. sexual partners. A negative test result is usually of great reassurance to an individual, but the opportunity should be taken to inform patients of future safe practices in terms of sexual intercourse, drug use etc.

Screening and Prophylaxis

It may be helpful when seeing a newly diagnosed HIV-seropositive patient for the first time, to undertake some screening tests to assess their vulnerability to certain infections if they should develop immunodeficiency. These tests might include serological tests for syphilis, hepatitis B, hepatitis C, toxoplasma, and CMV (as IgG).

In the US, skin reactivity to tuberculin antigen is important, but in countries such as the UK where BCG vaccinations are given routinely to the population around the age of 13 years, this skin test is difficult to evaluate. Women with HIV should have regular cervical smear screening tests, perhaps every six months, because of their increased risk.[17]

When an individual's CD4 lymphocyte count falls below 200/µl, this is a major milestone in terms of vulnerability to severe opportunistic infections. It is standard practice to advise patients with counts below 200/µl to undertake prophylactic measures in order to protect them from many of these infections. Chemoprophylaxis against pneumocystis and toxoplasmosis (see Table 1.2) has had a big impact on the frequency of these infections. The risk of cryptosporidial infections (and perhaps microsporidial infections) can be reduced by boiling or filtering drinking water. Once the CD4 count has fallen below 75/µl there is a significant risk of mycobacterium avium intracellulare infection. Chemoprophylaxis is then recommended with either weekly azithromycin

(1200 mg), daily rifabutin (300 mg), or daily clarithromycin (250 mg bd). Patients with recurrent herpes virus infections may take continuous secondary prophylaxis with aciclovir.

Table 1.2 Prophylactic regimens against pneumocystis.

- cotrimoxazole: daily or thrice weekly*
- pyrimethamine + dapsone: thrice weekly*
- nebulised pentamidine
- atovaquone: thrice daily*

* These regimens also have prophylactic value against toxoplasma.

Early Manifestations of HIV Infection and Associated Skin Conditions

Patients may experience several years of minor ill health before progressing to develop conditions associated with AIDS, and many of these conditions are quite common in the population as a whole. The astute clinician may be presented with the opportunity to diagnose someone with HIV who may have a history of several of these disorders occurring over a period of one year, or if their symptoms seem unusually severe, recurrent or difficult to treat. Some of the more common conditions are listed in Table 1.3. Dermatological disorders are extremely common and sometimes effect the eyelids and conjunctiva.[18]

Table 1.3 Early manifestations of HIV infection.

- oral ulceration
- oral and genital candidiasis
- persistent generalised lymphadenopathy
- sinusitis
- perianal sepsis
- herpes simplex virus infection: peri-oral and genital
- genital warts
- recurrent lower respiratory infections
- dermatological disorders:
  eczema
  seborrhoeic dermatitis
  pruritis
  molluscum contagiosum
  dry skin
  psoriasis
  folliculitis, both bacterial and eosinophilic

Management of the Major Opportunistic Infections Associated with AIDS

A wide variety of organisms can cause opportunistic infections in those vulnerable due to a low number of, or poorly functioning, CD4 T-cell lymphocytes (see Table 1.4). There may be some geographical variation in the incidence of some infections, for example, pneumocystis infections are uncommon in the tropics and histoplasmosis, coccidioidomycosis and blastomycosis fungal infections have distinct distributions around the world. Just about all tissues and organs of the body can be involved. Occasionally, more than one opportunistic infection may exist simultaneously.

Table 1.4 Common opportunistic pathogens in AIDS.

- VIRAL: herpes simplex, varicella-zoster, CMV, parvovirus, JC virus, RSV
- BACTERIAL: pneumococcus, salmonella
- MYCOBACTERIAL: tuberculosis, *Mycobacterium avium intracellulare*
- FUNGAL: candida, *Cryptococcus neoformans*
- PROTOZOAL: *Pneumocystis carinii, Toxoplasma gondii*, cryptosporidium, microsporidium

Pneumocystis Pneumonia

The commonest opportunistic infection at first presentation of AIDS in Europe and the US is still pneumocystis carinii pneumonia (PCP). This is despite a decrease in the incidence of PCP due to the widespread practice of prescribing primary prophylaxis against PCP to people with HIV and those CD4 T-cell lymphocyte counts below 200/μl.

PCP presents in an insidious manner with increasing breathlessness and dry cough over some two or three weeks. Fever and sweats are common, but sputum production and pleurisy are uncommon with PCP and should make one think of tuberculosis or PCP with tuberculosis as diagnoses. Apart from a fever there may be little to find on examination. Desaturation, using a pulse oximeter and particularly on exercise, is often present even in early PCP infections when the chest X-ray may be relatively normal. Diagnosis can be confirmed by bronchio-alveolar lavage at bronchoscopy, or by examination of a sample of induced sputum. Staining with fluorescent monoclonal antibodies to pneumocystis is probably the most sensitive test with which to detect the organism within samples. It is, however, an accepted practice to treat on an empirical basis cases of presumptive PCP where the history, examination, and radiology all point to this being the likely diagnosis.

Many antimicrobial agents have been used to treat PCP (see Table 1.5), but the gold standard remains high-dose cotrimoxazole for 21 days.[19] The numerous alternatives have developed importance because of the high probability of intolerance to cotrimoxazole at these doses, where nausea, bone marrow suppression, and skin rash (erythema multiforme and Stevens-Johnson syndrome) may all limit its use.

Table 1.5 Treatment alternatives for acute pneumocystis pneumonia.

- high dose cotrimoxazole (with folinic acid)
- trimethoprim and dapsone
- clindamycin and primaquine
- intravenous pentamidine
- trimetrexate (with folinic acid)
- atovaquone

Steroid therapy should be used for patients with moderate to severe pneumocystis pneumonia for the first five days of treatment.

Many patients with moderate to severe PCP will deteriorate 48 to 72 hours after starting effective anti-PCP treatment. Worsening lung function and chest X-ray are characteristic features of what appears to be a reaction to the destruction of pneumocystis organisms within the lung. It is now standard practice to treat all such cases of PCP from the outset with high doses of glucocorticosteroids for the first five to seven days of therapy in order to avoid this occurrence.[20] Some patients will, however, require a period of ventilation during this worst phase of the illness. With these improvement in management skills it has become much less common for people to die of PCP. Secondary prophylaxis is advised once the treatment course has been completed.

Pneumocystis infections can occasionally occur outside the lung, such as in the skin, lymph nodes, and in the eye. A patient receiving inhaled nebulised pentamidine as a sole form of PCP prophylaxis will have no effective extra-pulmonary anti-pneumocystis prophylaxis. In most cases, pneumocystis infections occur as a reactivation of organisms present within the body for years. Very occasionally, a susceptible individual may acquire PCP by direct transmission from another patient, and for this reason isolation procedures may be wise.

Tuberculosis

Tuberculosis is the most common presenting feature of AIDS in the developing parts of the world (see chapter 9). It is also becoming more common in the developed world.[21] Worryingly, there have been reports of cases of multi-drug resistant tuberculosis (MDRTB) which may be very much more likely to affect the immunocompromised host.[22]

Pulmonary TB presents with a cough, usually productive, fever and night sweats, occasionally pleurisy, breathlessness and weight loss. Chest radiology may show apical cavitating lesions, but quite often, particularly in the very immunodeficient individual, any part of the lung may be affected and the lesions may not cavitate at all. However, tuberculosis may also infect numerous other sites within the body of someone with AIDS, eg. liver, spleen, bone, lymph nodes, skin (see Fig. 1.1), eyes, kidney, brain, and meninges.[23] Infection of multiple sites by TB is common in people with low CD4 T-lymphocyte counts.

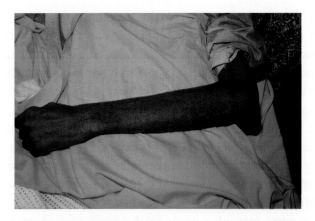

Fig. 1.1 Widespread tuberculous infection of the skin in a man with AIDS who had additional sites of infection in the lungs, lymph nodes, and liver. Skin biopsy showed large numbers of organisms present, with little surrounding inflammation.

Diagnosis is confirmed on finding the organism within appropriate samples stained with auramine or Zeil-Neilsen stain. It is important to attempt to culture all organisms in order to verify the type of mycobacterial infection and specific antimicrobial sensitivities. Unfortunately, because mycobacteria grow only slowly, this may take several weeks. Several new diagnostic techniques are presently starting to prove useful in the diagnosis of TB. PCR-based techniques are able to detect and identify the DNA of the tubercle organism as well as which mutations it may have conferring antimicrobial resistance.

The therapy of TB in people with HIV is the same as for all patients.[23] Triple or quadruple antimicrobial regimens are employed and modified after two or three months to a dual regimen according to culture and sensitivity results. Pulmonary TB may be treated for a total of six months, lymphadenitis for nine months, TB of the bone and nervous system for at least 12 months. A few centres may continue secondary prophylaxis for a period of time afterwards. Despite the immunodeficiency, the response to standard antituberculous therapy is good. Many of the drugs employed in the treatment of TB may have toxicities, including those affecting the eye, as well as interactions with other drugs such as some protease inhibitors.

A patient with possible or proven pulmonary TB should be managed according to appropriate infection control measures. Public health strategies should be engaged in order to undertake contact tracing.

Toxoplasmosis

Primary toxoplasma infections are usually acquired following exposure to the organism as a result of eating poorly cooked meat, and occasionally from cats and other human beings with acute toxoplasmosis. The organism subsequently remains dormant only to reactivate if CD4 T-cell lymphocyte dysfunction occurs. Such patients will usually be serologically positive at screening. Opportunistic infections usually occur in the brain, presenting as a space-occupying lesion, often multiple.[24] Symptoms and signs may be of raised intracranial pressure, convulsions, focal neurological deficits, or diminished consciousness.[25] CT scanning of the head may show single or multiple ring-enhancing lesions. A similar appearance may occur with cerebral lymphoma, and only a stereotactic brain biopsy may be able to differentiate between the two (see chapter 7).

Toxoplasma cysts may also occur in the eye[26] (see chapter 5) and lung[27] and occasionally in other tissues. Many of the prophylactic regimens used to prevent PCP also effectively prevent toxoplasmosis. There are two commonly used drug regimens for the initial treatment of cerebral toxoplasmosis: pyrimethamine + sulphadiazine (+ folinic acid)[28]; or pyrimethamine + clindamycin (+ folinic acid).[29] A period of around six weeks therapy should be followed by life-long secondary prophylaxis. Bone marrow suppression and skin rashes, including Stevens-Johnson syndrome, may complicate these drug regimens. Repeat CT scans should show a diminution in the size of lesions after two weeks of therapy.

Candida

Oral and genital candidal infections are common at all stages of HIV infection. However, once CD4 T-cell lymphocyte numbers fall below about 150/µl, more deep-seated candidal infections may occur, including those of the eye especially if intravenous lines have been used. The most common though is oesophageal candidiasis.[30] This presents as a retrosternal pain on swallowing, although a number of patients may have oesophageal candidiasis with little or no specific symptoms. Oral candidiasis is not always present at the same time. The definitive diagnosis is made upon endoscopy. Most patients will respond within two or three days of starting oral systemic antifungal therapy with fluconazole or itraconazole, or clotrimazole troches may be used. Local treatments with nystatin or amphotericin lozenges or mouth washes are usually ineffective. The development of resistant strains of candida associated with prolonged use of systemic antifungals, has led many physicians to avoid suggesting secondary prophylaxis as a routine, but rather to treat recurrences as and when they occur.

Cryptococcus

Meningitis is the commonest presentation of cryptococcal opportunistic infection in AIDS, and is associated with a CD4 T-cell lymphocyte count of less than 200/μl.[31] It often presents with mild symptoms of a headache and slight fever, building up over several days or weeks. Initially, the individual may not look too unwell. Signs of meningism such as neck rigidity and Kernig's sign may be absent. If left untreated, the condition worsens with a rise in intracranial pressure which may be complicated by visual loss. Death may ensue. All patients with low CD4 T-cell counts and a headache should be fully investigated with a CT head scan and followed, only if this is safe, by a lumbar puncture. The CSF pressure may be substantially raised,[32] and withdrawal of fluid may relieve headache. Routine examination of the CSF may fail to reveal any abnormality, but specific testing for cryptococcal antigen should be undertaken to confirm the diagnosis.

Treatment is with intravenous amphotericin and 5-flucytosine for at least two weeks.[33] Repeat lumbar punctures may help reduce headache and might also prevent sight loss. This initial period of induction therapy should be followed by long-term maintenance therapy with high dose, oral fluconazole to prevent relapses which are common.

Cryptosporidium

Cryptosporidial infections are acquired from drinking contaminated tap water. Those patients with CD4 T-cell counts below 200/μl should be warned of this risk, and instructed to boil or filter their drinking water prior to consumption. Untreated bottled water may not be safe either. The protozoa can cause infections of the gut and biliary tree. In the former case, the organism does not invade the tissue, but attaches itself to the brush border of the enterocytes lining the small bowel. It causes a defect in absorption from this surface as well as a hyper-secretory state. Both these effects result in watery diarrhoea, often very severe, with resulting dehydration and malnutrition. Diagnosis is best made from biopsy samples from the duodenum taken at endoscopy as stool examination for cysts is less sensitive.

Antimicrobial treatment is unsatisfactory. The best agent is probably paromomycin, which is unlicensed in many countries, but available on a "named-patient" basis in some. Treatment failures and relapses are common. Antidiarrhoeal agents assume importance in symptom control. Octreotide can be used to try and reduce the secretory diarrhoea. Cryptosporidial infections may also cause sclerosing cholangitis. Dual infections with CMV are common. Treatment is difficult although intravenous paromomycin may work for some patients. Occasionally, pain from distension of the biliary tract can only be relieved by surgical decompression.

Microsporidium

Microsporidial infections of the gastrointestinal tract have been incriminated as a cause of diarrhoea in some patients with AIDS.[34] However, the organism has also been found in HIV-antibody positive patients without diarrhoea. Careful examination of endoscopically obtained biopsy material is necessary to make the diagnosis. Albendazole has shown promise in treating this condition.[35]

Mycobacterium Avium Intracellulare

MAI is an organism found widely in the environment and is very difficult to effect isolation. Patients with CD4 T-cell counts less than about 70/μl may be at risk of infection with this organism.[36] It is usually very slow growing, and by the time of presentation, there may be a vast number of organisms within the affected tissues.[37] Infection of the gastrointestinal tract is common and may cause diarrhoea, fever and weight loss. Infection of the bone marrow may cause anaemia or pancytopenia. Lymph node infection is common. Infected deep lymph nodes in the thorax and abdomen may give rise to fever, malaise and weight loss, but be very difficult to diagnose.

Isolation of the organism can be achieved by direct sampling of the affected tissue. Blood cultures and bone marrow cultures using specific culture medium are often helpful.[38] The sensitivities for the MAI organisms grown are not clinically helpful, however. Treatment consists of multiple drug therapy with three or four agents simultaneously.[39] A combination will usually consist of rifabutin and ethambutol with ciprofloxacin and clarithromycin, for example.[40] Parenteral amikacin for the first ten to 14 days may be helpful in those patients with severe symptoms. Drug interactions and effects on the eye are common with many of the regimens used.

Modern combination antiretroviral therapy has allowed some patients to enjoy a sustained improvement in immune function. Some have been noted to produce florid reactions to previously established, but symptomless, MAI infections as a result of their improved immunological competence (see Figs. 1.2(a) and 1.2(b)). This phenomenon, which can also be seen with CMV infection, has been called "immune restoration disease".

(a)

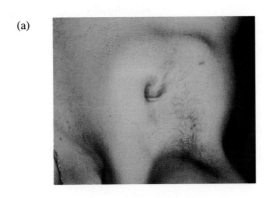

(b)

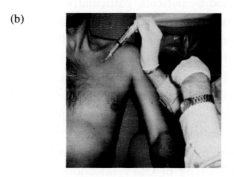

Fig. 1.2 (a) Fluctuant abscesses in the axilla of a man with AIDS appearing a month after starting HAART; (b) aspiration of an abscess in the same patient from a lymph node on the anterior chest wall grew MAI in culture.

Cytomegalovirus

CMV infections are common opportunists in patients with CD4 T-cell lymphocyte counts below 100/μl. These infections are usually reactivations of CMV acquired earlier in life, and therefore occur in those who have positive screening tests for IgG to CMV. CMV can present in many sites of the body (see Table 1.6). CMV retinitis is the commonest manifestation and is dealt with in greater detail in chapter 6.

Table 1.6 Common sites of CMV disease in AIDS.

- retinitis
- neurological:
    encephalitis
    myelopathy
    radiculopathy
- bone marrow
- gastrointestinal tract
    mouth ulcers
    oesophageal ulcers
    gastric ulcers
    colitis
- hepatobiliary
    hepatitis
    cholangitis
    pancreatitis
- pneumonitis
- adrenalitis

CMV may be excreted by patients, particularly in the urine and saliva, even though the virus is not causing disease. The diagnosis of clinically relevant CMV disease is based upon either finding owl's eye inclusion bodies on histologically examined tissue samples or the positive detection of early antigen foci within samples of buffy coat or bronchoalveolar lavage, for example.

There are now several agents to choose from which have anti-CMV effects (see also chapter 6). Intravenous ganciclovir is, perhaps, the gold standard and the one that most clinicians have the greatest experience with. Parenteral foscarnet and cidofovir have also been used with success. Intravenous ganciclovir or foscarnet are used for induction therapy of CMV infections. The frequency of doses is reduced to a maintenance frequency after induction therapy. This is commonly reached with doses three or five times a week. Specific regimens depend on individual patients and their site of CMV disease. Oral ganciclovir or fortnightly intravenous cidofovir may be used as maintenance therapy for selected patients.

Failure of maintenance therapy is common, particularly with oral ganciclovir, possibly due to its poor pharmacokinetics. An individual's strain of CMV may develop resistance to the antiviral used as maintenance therapy, so a switch may be necessary. For the same reasons, the use of two agents alternating, for example IV ganciclovir and IV foscarnet, may be advantageous for both therapy and maintenance in patients after multiple relapses. Many of these drugs have considerable problems in practical terms in relation to side effects and interactions with other drugs (see Table 1.7).

Table 1.7 Common side effects of anti-CMV drugs.

Ganciclovir
- nausea/vomiting
- abdominal discomfort
- fatigue
- bone marrow suppression

Foscarnet
- nephrotoxicity
- hypocalcaemia
- balanitis/vulvitis — can be avoided by washing after micturition

Cidofovir
- nephrotoxicity
- uveitis which may be associated with hypotony

Varicella-zoster Virus

Although the occurrence of episodes varicella-zoster virus infection is not an AIDS-defining event, frequent and severe attacks of shingles are common in patients with low or falling CD4 lymphocyte numbers. Sometimes several dermatomes may be affected simultaneously, or the lesions may disseminate outside a dermatomal distribution. Infections of the ophthalmic division of the trigeminal nerve may occur (see chapter 2) as well as a necrotising retinitis (see chapter 5). Early treatment with high oral doses of aciclovir or valaciclovir usually moderate the rash and symptoms.

Herpes Simplex Virus

HSV infections both genital and non-genital, are common. Occasionally, a condition of chronic mucocutaneous HSV infection may occur. Aciclovir or valaciclovir treatment is usually effective, but relapses are common and may necessitate long-term maintenance antiviral therapy. HSV can cause oesophageal ulcers and ulceration within the oral cavity. HSV may also cause a retinitis (see chapter 5).

JC Virus

JC virus infection may give rise to the condition of progressive multifocal leucoencephalopathy (PML) in patients with AIDS and CD4 lymphocyte counts generally below 200/µl. The lesions, as the name suggests, progress with time and also with the occurrence of new neurological deficits. The symptoms and signs depend very much on the sites within the brain affected. Visual symptoms are quite common (see chapter 7). The diagnosis is often suggested by the appearances of MRI scan pictures of the brain. Examination of the CSF should reveal antibodies to the JC virus in titres higher than those that might be present in the serum. The natural outcome of this condition before the advent of combination antiretroviral therapy, was such as to lead to death within a few months. No good specific treatment has been found. There have been some small trials suggesting some benefit from courses of cytarabine and alpha-interferon, and more recently cidofovir.

Management of HIV-associated Neoplasia

The immunodeficiency accompanying advancing HIV-disease seems to allow or promote the emergence of certain tumours (see Table 1.8). Some of these tumours also have associations with co-infecting viruses: Kaposi's sarcoma and human herpes virus-8 infection; and cervical neoplasia and human papilloma virus infection.

Table 1.8 Common neoplasms associated with HIV.

- Kaposi's sarcoma
- Non-Hodgkins lymphoma
- Cerebral lymphoma
- Cervical neoplasia
- Anal neoplasia
- Conjunctival neoplasia

Kaposi's Sarcoma

KS occurs as a purple or brown lesion usually on a visible site on the skin (see Fig. 1.3(a)), buccal mucosa, or palate. It has a bumpy feeling to it, but is not painful or pruritic. It is dry, and only ulcerates or bleeds if traumatised. Superficial lesions on the skin can be treated with superficial radiotherapy. Recurrence elsewhere is the norm. Patients with very poor immune function may experience particularly aggressive forms of KS. Lymph node involvement

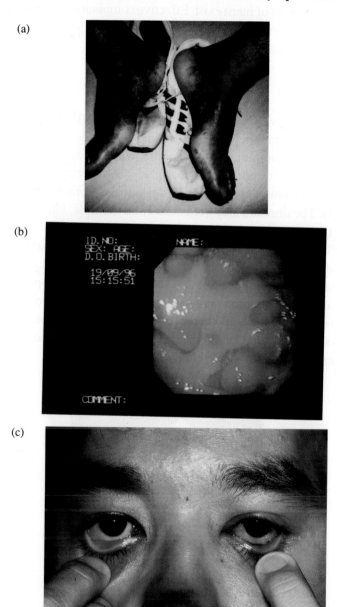

Fig. 1.3 (a) Widespread Kaposi's sarcoma affecting both feet; (b) multiple gastric lesions are seen on endoscopy in a man with AIDS. Following chemotherapy and the introduction of HAART, complete remission was achieved; (c) KS affecting both eyes and nose in a man with AIDS.

is common and spreads to the lungs and gastrointestinal tract (see Fig. 1.3(b)) occurs not infrequently. KS may affect the eye (see Fig. 1.3(c)) (see chapter 4). Chemotherapy may be useful, but is usually only palliative.[41] The preferred agents are currently liposomal daunorubicin and liposomal doxorubicin, but many other regimens of merit exist. Effective combination antiretroviral therapy has been reported to bring about an improvement in KS and occasionally what appears to be complete resolution.

Lymphoma

Lymphomas are relatively common in patients with AIDS, particularly those with very low CD4 lymphocyte counts, i.e. below 50/µl. Although opportunistic infections are less common following the widespread use of combination antiretroviral therapy, it appears that the incidence of lymphoma has not fallen. Lymphomas in the brain may present as would any other tumour in this site (see chapter 7). The tumours may occasionally be multiple. No effective treatment is available. Lymphoma outside the brain of the non-Hodgkins type may present in a number of ways. It may give rise to a period of fever, malaise, and weight loss before declaring a more obvious sign (see Fig. 1.4). Lymphoma of the gut may present with diarrhoea and weight loss. Lymphadenopathy is common, as are skin lesions. The orbit and eye may be involved too (see chapters 4 and 5). There are a few chemotherapeutic regimens that have been tried with some success for this type of lymphoma. The success of therapy is better in those patients with higher CD4 lymphocyte counts.

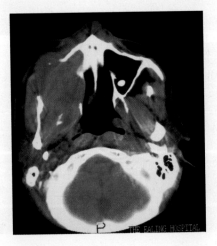

Fig. 1.4 CT scan of the head showing a mass occupying one maxillary sinus and eroding through the maxilla. Biopsy showed this to be a poorly-differentiated non-Hodgkin's lymphoma.

Management of HIV-associated Neuropathology

The neurological system may be affected directly by HIV or by opportunistic infections (see Table 1.9). Acute meningitis and encephalitis due to HIV occurs as a complication of a seroconversion illness at the time of primary infection. A form of encephalopathy due to HIV which can infect and destroy glial cells within the brain may lead to a variety of slowly progressing signs. These often present with intellectual deterioration and memory loss, leading to self neglect and loss of independence.[42] More severe psychiatric manifestations can occur with depression and paranoia. For neurophthalmic features, see chapter 7. The use of antiretroviral agents that penetrate to the nervous system may lead to a general reduction in the incidence and severity of HIV-encephalopathy.

Table 1.9 HIV-associated neuropathology.

- HIV encephalopathy and dementia
- acute HIV encephalitis/meningitis
- CMV
- lymphoma
- toxoplasma
- *Cryptococcus neoformans*
- JC virus (progressive multifocal leucoencephalopathy)

Nutrition, Weight Loss, and Wasting

Weakness, weight loss, and wasting are common problems with considerable morbidity in a number of people with AIDS or pre-AIDS. Sometimes this is due to diarrhoea caused by an opportunistic pathogen within the gut. Occasionally, HIV seems able to induce a form of enteropathy with loss of villous architecture in the small bowel leading to malabsorbtion. Some patients, however, lose weight solely due to poor nutritional intake. This may on some occasions be due to specific oral or dental conditions. Assessment and advice from a dietitian may be invaluable.

Prescribed drugs that patients may receive may also depress the appetite, or cause nausea and diarrhoea. Antidiarrhoeals may be tried for some, and many patients, after careful assessment, may benefit from anabolic steroids. Many wasted patients on combination antiretroviral therapy are experiencing weight gain. However, much of the weight put on in these circumstances seems to be fat and not muscle.

Antiretroviral Therapies, Toxicities and Interactions

Over the last two years or so, there have been great advances in antiretroviral therapy. Since the use of AZT (zidovudine), there have been a number of additions to the pharmacological armamentarium. The first few antiretroviral drugs available were inhibitors of the HIV-specific reverse transcriptase (RTI) enzyme, and chemically were nucleoside analogues either of thymidine or non-thymidine structures. These drugs were joined by RTIs that were non-nucleoside analogues. During the last few years, drug development was undertaken to produce an inhibitor of another HIV-specific enzyme, a protease (PI). Because of the pressure to produce these drugs and make them available to clinicians treating patients with HIV and AIDS, many of these new drugs were "fast-tracked" through the licensing system. For this reason, only a bare minimum is known about the long-term efficacy and toxicity of these drugs, or rarer and idiosyncratic reactions to them.

The use of a single antiretroviral drug is now an obsolete practice because the efficacy is poor and short lived due to the development of resistance by the HIV, which is often rapid because of its high inherent rate of mutation during replication. The use of two drugs, or dual therapy, was shown to be an improvement over monotherapy, but still resistance developed to one or both agents often within a year of treatment. The use of three drugs together in combination has been shown to have a far greater effect as judged by falls in viral load values,[43] and these effects can be maintained for long periods, quite often over two years.[44] Such combination therapy is often referred to as "highly active antiretroviral therapy" or "HAART" for short. Much knowledge is still to be gleaned about the use and efficacy of HAART, particularly the long-term effects and toxicities and also about when precisely to start combination therapy. Certain principles of therapy have, however, been established already, although there are some slight differences in practice between specialist centres and different countries. Guidelines have been drawn up by bodies of experts within various countries which are updated and modified according to new knowledge and experience, e.g. "BHIVA" guidelines in the UK,[45] and US.[44]

Table 1.10 lists the various drugs currently licensed or about to be licensed within the UK. For an individual starting HAART who has not received previous antiretroviral therapy, most clinicians would choose to advise the patient to take a combination of three agents consisting of two RTIs — one thymidine analogues and one non-thymidine analogue — and a PI.[46,47] If a patient has previously received antiretroviral therapy, those particular drugs are best avoided because of the possibility of resistance having developed in the past. Some permutations of drugs do not go well together for pharmacological reasons (e.g. ddC and 3TC combination may be antagonistic) or because of promotion of side effects (e.g. ddI and ddC causing neuropathy). Choosing a regimen of tablets (Table 1.11) also has other considerations in terms of the patients' ability to take tablets at a particular time of day, in relation to meals, and in terms of interactions with other tablets he or she may need to take.

Table 1.10 Antiretroviral agents: licensed or about to be licensed.

Nucleoside Analogue Reverse Transcriptase Inhibitors

Thymidine analogues (active mostly in dividing lymphocytes):
- AZT (zidovudine)
- D4T (stauvudine)

Non-thymidine analogues (active mostly in resting lymphocytes):
- 3TC (lamivudine)
- ddC (zalcitabine)
- ddI (didanosine)

Non-Nucleoside Reverse Transcriptase Inhibitors

- delavirdine
- nevirapine
- efavirenz

Protease Inhibitors

- saquinavir
- ritonavir
- indinavir
- nelfinavir
- abacavir

An effective regimen has value and benefits for most patients with symptoms, even those with very advanced disease. It is assumed that people who start HAART who have no symptoms, but whose viral load is high or CD4 counts are low, are doing so on the basis that it improves prognosis. Strong evidence that this is so is currently lacking and will take some time to accrue.[48] When to start therapy in certain situations may be quite controversial[49] (see Table 1.12).

After some weeks on HAART there is usually a rise in CD4 counts; sometimes this is quite dramatic and in other cases it is only modest. The rise may continue, albeit slowly for more than a year, perhaps longer. There is evidence that indicates that there is a functional improvement in the immune system to parallel this.[46] Occasionally this can manifest as an adverse event: allergies, especially those of the skin, may develop as a result of improved immune reactivity, and a more powerful immune response may develop a profound inflammatory response to infections within body tissues that were previously unnoticed. Examples of this

Table 1.11 Antiretroviral therapy: choosing a regimen.

- Ideal regimen close to 1 thymidine nucleoside analogue reverse transcriptase inhibitor + 1 non-thymidine nucleoside analogue reverse transcriptase inhibitor + 1 protease inhibitor.
- Previous use of antivirals may not allow this. Antiretrovirals that a patient has had previous exposure to are best avoided where possible because resistance may have developed.
- Viral resistance: genotypic and phenotypic methods of determing antiviral drug resistance are in research use at present. There are problems interpreting the clinical value of the results. However, demonstration of a person's viral resistance may be of help in the future, when considering which drugs with which to start therapy.
- Avoid antagonistic drug combinations.
- Choose a regimen that is the simplest in terms of frequency of pill taking, etc., and is therefore more likely to be adhered to.
- Avoid a regimen where interactions may take place with other drugs a patient may already be on, e.g. ritonavir and rifabutin.
- Nausea and diarrhoea are common side effects in the first few weeks of therapy with many protease inhibitors. Many clinicians suggest taking antiemetics and antidiarrhoeals routinely in the first week or two of therapy to prevent this happening and improve compliance. If ritonavir has been chosen as the protease inhibitor in the regimen, then it may be started in a low dose, building up to the full does over the first few weeks. This may reduce the severity of side effects.
- Regimens need to be tailored to individual requirements according to a number of factors including previous exposure, resistance, intolerance, etc. Combinations using four drugs may be needed to achieve satisfactory and durable low levels of viral load. Some regimens may include two protease inhibitors or a non-nucleoside reverse transcriptase inhibitor. These latter groups of drugs are usually reserved for second line therapy.

Table 1.12 Combination antiretroviral therapy: when to start?

- High viral load: the precise threshold upon which it becomes wise to advise starting therapy is not known. Those with levels above 50000 copies per ml probably should be started, and those with levels less than 5000 copies per ml without symptoms and a normal CD4 lymphocyte count probably should not. There is a large "grey" area between these values of viral load where the decision to start therapy is debatable.
- Low or falling CD4 lymphocyte count: a CD4 count persistently less than 350/µl or one that is falling progressively over time should prompt commencement of therapy. It may be advantageous to start antiretroviral therapy before the CD4 count has deteriorated too much, in order to preserve the maximum amount of immune function as possible.
- Symptoms: most patients with symptoms related to HIV will have high viral loads or low CD4 counts or both. A few, however, may not have startlingly deranged blood test results, and yet their symptoms may improve after starting antiviral therapy.
- Pregnancy: there is now clear evidence that antiretroviral therapy reduces the vertical transmission rate of HIV. Most authorities would advise combination therapy for the mother at least from the beginning of the second trimester .
- Seroconversion/primary infection: it has been suggested that there may be some advantage to start antiretroviral therapy soon after primary infection, i.e. within a few months, in order to limit the viral "burden" and the reservoir or number of cells infected in the body on the basis this may improve subsequent progression.[51]

---

latter response include flare-ups of MAI infection after starting HAART,[50] and also the very different inflammatory appearances seen on fundoscopy of CMV retinitis after starting HAART.

The benefits of HAART can be measured both in terms of longevity and also quality-of-life measures.[52] There are many reports of a substantial reduction in hospital admission rates in HIV centres the in US[53] and UK. This parallels a reduction in the frequency of opportunistic infections in patients taking HAART.[46] There are accumulating reports of remissions of CMV infections, KS, PML, chronic cryptosporidial infections, and MAI infections in people taking HAART, presumably as a result of improved immune function. There also appears to be an improved sense of well being, energy levels, weight-gain, etc., although many of these parameters are difficult to measure objectively.

Some basic principles of monitoring HAART have been established (see Table 1.13).[54] Monitoring of efficacy by routine measurement of plasma HIV-RNA levels (viral load) is an essential part of optimising HAART.[55] However, there may be benefits to recipients of HAART even if the viral load cannot be maintained below undetectable levels.[56]

Table 1.13 Antiretroviral therapy: monitoring efficacy.

- Establish a pre-treatment plasma HIV-RNA level (viral load) and CD4 lymphocyte count as baseline.
- Repeat viral load assay after five to six weeks after starting therapy. The level should have fallen at least 1 log value from the baseline measurement, and more desirably 2 log values. If the fall is more modest than 1 log drop, then two of the drugs in the regimen should be changed and the process started all over again.
- Repeat viral load and CD4 count after four months of therapy. The viral load should now be under 200/μl (often called undetectable[*]). The CD4 count should have risen. If the viral load has not been fully suppressed, consider changing two of the drugs.
- Repeat viral load assays about four times a year in order to reaffirm full efficacy of the regimen, and change two drugs if the viral load rises.
- Failure of the therapy can be due to viral resistance, poor adherence on the part of the patient, an antagonistic drug regimen, or poor absorbtion of the medication from the gut. Patients should be encouraged and informed of the importance of taking their tablets at every dose and at the right time, not to run out of tablets, and to seek immediate expert guidance if there are problems with the regimen or intolerable side effects occur. If a side effect occurs from one drug contained within the combination in a regimen that is otherwise successful (ie. with viral load drops) one need only change the one, incriminated drug.

[*]There are various tests available for testing HIV- RNA levels in the plasma. They may have different sensitivities and therefore an "undetectable" means different things according to which test is being used. The different tests do not always have good agreement between themselves even at higher values. Some, for example, may give quite low values for certain African strains of HIV. More sensitive tests are becoming available that can detect RNA levels down to 50 or even 20 copies per ml. It has been suggested that those patients on therapy who achieve viral load levels less than 50 copies per ml have a better and more durable long-term response. However, these newer tests have not been fully evaluated yet, and early experience suggests they have quite a degree of variability.

It is not possible, however, to know how long these benefits are likely to last. It has been speculated that HAART may be able to eradicate HIV from an individual if it can suppress viral replication in tissues for a period of around three years. Current indications suggest that this is unlikely, possibly due to the persistence of long-lived chronically infected but dormant lymphocyte or macrophage cells.[57–59]

As time goes by and more experience is gained about the benefits of HAART, so too will the knowledge of an increasing number of problems and toxicities of therapy (see Table 1.14).[60,61]

Table 1.14 Combination antiretroviral therapy: long-term problems.

- Failure of therapy due to drug resistance
- Cross resistance to other antiretroviral drugs
- Hyperglycaemia
- Hyperlipidaemia
- Cushingoid appearance (lipodystrophy), breast enlargement in women, buffalo hump, muscle wasting, abdominal adipose accumulation
- Haemolytic anaemia
- Hypertension
- Abnormal liver function tests
- Low serum testosterone levels in men

Table 1.15 Strategies that may reduce the vertical transmission of HIV from mother to baby.

- Good antenatal care: avoid invasive procedures, amniocentesis, and chorionic villous sampling
- Antiretroviral therapy: combination therapy from the second trimester onwards and for the baby for two weeks after birth[62, 63]
- At delivery: avoid foetal scalp electrodes, avoid foetal blood sampling, encourage delivery within four hours of the rupture of membranes, possible Caesarian section if delivery delayed beyond four hours post membrane rupture.
- Post-natal: avoid breast feeding
- Passive hyperimmune therapy: anti-HIV-Ig to mother during pregnancy

Pregnancy

Vertical transmission of HIV from mother to baby forms one of the commonest worldwide routes of transmission. All babies of HIV-seropositive mothers will be HIV-antibody positive, but not all will be infected. European studies suggest a transmission rate of around 12% to 15%. In the US this is higher at around 25%, and in Africa it may be as high as 40% or 50%. Mothers with a high viral load and low CD4 counts may be more likely to transmit HIV to their babies. There are various strategies that may reduce the rate of vertical transmission (see Table 1.15).

Pregnancy does not seem to accelerate HIV, and HIV does not seem to affect foetal development.

The Future

New developments are likely to continue to occur over the next few years and improve the clinical management of people with HIV. However, the discovery of a cure and the production of an effective vaccine seem a long way off still. New antiretroviral drugs will continue to be introduced, offering alternatives for those who cannot tolerate those currently available or for whom they have lost efficacy. Inhibitors of other HIV-specific enzymes are being developed, e.g. integrase inhibitors. Other antiviral modes of action may be explored further, e.g. CKR5 receptor blockers.

Making effective antiviral drugs easier to take will be important in improving adherence to therapy, which is an important cause of drug failure. New drugs active as treatment or prophylaxis against opportunistic infections are also likely to be introduced.

Lastly, therapeutic modalities to reconstitute the immune system in people starting HAART at an advanced stage of immunodeficiency are being explored. Sadly, most of the effective treatments available or in development are likely to be too expensive to be made accessible for the vast population of people with HIV infection in the less economically well-developed countries in the world.

References

1. Tindall B., Barker S., Donovan B. *et al.* "Characterisation of the acute clinical illness associated with human immunodeficiency virus infection," *Arch. Intern. Med.* **148** (1988), 945–949.

2. Tindall B., Cooper D.A. "Primary HIV infection: Host responses and intervention strategies," *AIDS* **5** (1991), 1–14.

3. Fox R., Eldred L.J., Fuchs E.J. *et al.* "Clinical manifestations of acute infection with human immunodeficiency virus in a cohort of gay men," *AIDS* **1** (1987), 35–38.

4. Hardy W.D., Daar E.S., Sokolov R.T. *et al.* "Acute neurologic deterioration in a young man," *Rev. Infect. Dis.* **13** (1991), 745–750

5. Cooper D.A., Tindall B., Wilson E.J. *et al.* "Characterisation of T-lymphocyte responses during primary HIV infection," *J. Infect. Dis.* **157** (1988), 889–896.

6. Keet I.P., Krijnen P., Koot M. *et al.* "Predictors of rapid progression to AIDS in HIV-1 seroconverters," *AIDS* **7** (1993), 51–57.

7. Sinicco A., Fora R., Sciandra M. *et al.* "Risk of developing AIDS after primary acute HIV-1 infection," *J. Acquir. Immune Defic. Syndr.* **6** (1993), 575–581.

8. Rutherford G.W., Lifson A.R., Hessol N.A. *et al.* "Course of HIV-1 infection in a cohort of homosexual and bisexual men: An 11 year follow-up study," *Brit. Med. J.* **301** (1990), 1183–1188.

9. Lifson A.R., Buchbinder S.P., Sheppard H.W. *et al.* "Long-term human immunodeficiency virus infection in asymptomatic homosexual and bisexual men with normal CD4+ lymphocyte counts: Immunologic and virologic characteristics," *J. Infect. Dis.* **163** (1991), 959–965.

10. Michael N.L., Louie L.G., Rohrbaugh A.L. *et al.* The role of CCR5 and CCR2 polymorphisms in HIV-1 transmission and disease progression. *Nat. Med.* 1997 10: 1160–1162.

11. Mellors J.W., Kingsley L.A., Rinaldo C.R *et al.* "Quantitation of HIV-1 RNA in plasma predicts outcome after seroconversion," *Ann. Intern. Med.* **122** (1995), 573–579.

12. Mellors J.W., Rinaldo C.R., Gupta P. *et al.* "Prognosis in HIV-1 infection predicted by the quantity of virus in the plasma," *Science* **272** (1996), 1167–1170.

13. Goedert J.J., Biggar R.J., Melbye M. *et al.* "Effect of T4 count and cofactors on the incidence of AIDS in homosexual men infected with human immunodeficiency virus," *JAMA* **257** (1987), 331–334.

14. Polk B.F., Fox R., Brookmeyer R. *et al.* "Predictors of the acquired immunodeficiency syndrome developing in a cohort of seropositive homosexual men," *N. Engl. J. Med.* **362** (1988), 61–66.

15. Pantaleo G., Graziosi C., Damarest J.F. *et al.* "HIV infection is active and progressive in lymphoid tissue during the clinically latent stage of disease," *Nature* **362** (1993), 355–358.

16. Pantaleo G., Graziosi C., Fauci A.S. "New concepts in the immunopathogenesis of human immunodeficiency virus infection," *N. Engl. J. Med.* **328** (1993), 327–335.

17. "Centres for Disease Control: Risk of cervical disease in HIV-infected women, New York City," *MMWR* **39** (1990), 826–849.

18. Coldiron B.M., Bergstresser P.R. "Prevalence and clinical spectrum of skin disease in patients infected with human immunodeficiency virus," *Arch. Dermatol.* **125** (1989), 357–361.

19. Masur H. "Prevention and treatment of *Pneumocystis* pnuemonia," *N. Engl. J. Med.* **327** (1992), p. 1853.

20. Montaner J.S.G., Lawson L.M., Levitt N. *et al.* "Oral corticosteroids prevent early deterioration in patients with moderately severe AIDS-related *Pneumocystis carinii* pneumonia," *Ann. Intern. Med.* **113** (1990), p. 14.

21. De Cock K.M., Jovo B., Coulibody I.M. *et al.* "Tuberculosis and HIV infection in Sub-Saharan Africa," *JAMA* **268** (1992), 1581–1587.

22. Edlin B.R., Tokaras J.I., Grieco M.H. *et al.* "An outbreak of multiple-drug-resistant tuberculosis among hospitalised patients with acquired immunodeficiency syndrome," *N. Engl. J. Med.* **326** (1997), 514–521.

23. Chaisson R.E., Schecter G.F., Theuer C.P. *et al.* "Tuberculosis in patients with the acquired immunodeficiency syndrome," *Am. Rev. Respir. Dis.* **136** (1987), 570–574.

24. Wong S.Y., Remington J.S. "Toxoplasmosis in the setting of AIDS, in: Broder S., Marigan T.C. Jr., Bologneo D. (Eds.), *Textbook of AIDS Medicine*, Williams & Wilkins, Baltimore (1994), 223–258.

25. Navia B.A., Petito C.K., Gold J.W.M. *et al.* "Cerebral toxoplasmosis complicating AIDS: Clinical and neuropathological findings in 27 patients," *Ann. Neurol.* **19** (1986), 224–238.

26. Cochereau-Massin I., LeHoang P., Lautier-Frau M. "Ocular toxoplasmosis in human immunodeficiency virus-infected patients," *Am. J. Ophthalmol.* **114** (1992), 130–135.

27. Schnapp L., Geaghan S., Campagna A. *et al.* "*Toxoplasma gondii* pneumonitis in patients infected with the human immunodeficiency virus," *Arch. Intern. Med.* **152** (1992), 1073–1076.

28. Luft B.J., Remington J.S. "Toxoplasmic encephalitis," *J. Infect. Dis.* **157** (1988), 1–6.

29. Danneman B.R., McCutchan J.A., Israelski D.M. *et al.* "Treatment of toxoplasma encephalitis patients with AIDS: A randomised trial comparing pyrimethamine plus clindamycin to pyrimethamine plus sulphonamides," *Ann. Intern. Med.* **116** (1992), 33–43.

30. Tavitian A., Ranfluan J.P., Rosenthal L.E. "Oral candidiasis as a marker for oesophageal candidiasis in the acquired immunodeficiency syndrome," *Ann. Intern. Med.* **104** (1986), p. 54.

31. Dismukes W.E. "Cryptococcal meningitis in patients with AIDS," *J. Infect. Dis.* **157** (1988), 624–628.

32. Denning D.W., Armstrong R.W., Lewis B.H. *et al.* "Elevated cerebrospinal fluid pressures in patients with cryptococcal meningitis and acquired immunodeficiency syndrome," *Am. J. Med.* **91** (1991), 267–272.

33. Dismukes W.E., Cloud G., Gallis H. *et al.* "Treatment of cryptococcal meningitis with combination of amphotericin B and flucytosine for four as compared with six weeks," *N. Engl. J. Med.* **317** (1087), 334–341.

34.   Molina J.M., Sarfati C., Beauvais B. *et al.* "Intestinal microsporidiosis in human immunodeficiency virus-infected patients with chronic unexplained diarrhoea: Prevalence and clinical and biologic features," *J. Infect. Dis.* **167** (1993), p. 217.

35.   Blanchard C., Ellis D.S., Tovey D.G. *et al.* "Treatment of intestinal microsporidiosis with albendazole in patients with AIDS," *AIDS* **6** (1992), p. 311.

36.   Jacobson M.A., Hopewell P.C., Yajko D.M. *et al.* "Natural history of disseminated mycobacterium avium complex infections in AIDS," *J. Infect. Dis.* **164** (1991), 994–998.

37.   Jacomet C., Rolla V., Salanje B. *et al.* "Mycobacteriosis and AIDS, a retrospective study of 58 cases," *International Conference on AIDS* (1993) **9** 328 (abs) PO-B07-1156.

38.   Nightingale S.D., Boyd L.T., Southern P.M. *et al.* "Incidence of mycobacterium avium complex bacteraemia in human immunodeficiency virus-positive patients," *J. Infect. Dis.* **165** (1992), 1082–1085.

39.   Kemper C.A., Meng T.C., Nissbaum J. *et al.* "Treatment of mycobacterium avium complex bacteraemia in AIDS with a four-drug oral regimen," *Ann. Intern. Med.* **116** (1992), 466–472.

40.   Masur H. "Public Health Service Task Force on prophylaxis and therapy for mycobacterium avium complex: Special Report; Recommendations on prophylaxis and therapy for disseminated mycobacterium avium complex disease in patients infected with the human immunodeficiency virus," *N. Engl. J. Med.* **329** (1993), 893–904.

41.   Volberding P.A., Kusick P., Feigal D. "Effects of chemotherapy for HIV-associated Kaposi's sarcoma on long-term survival," *Proc. Am. Soc. Clin. Oncol.* (1989) 3, San Francisco, CA.

42.   Price R.W., Brew B.J., Rosenblum M. "The AIDS dementia complex and HIV-1 brain infection: A pathogenetic model of virus-immune interaction," in: Waksman B.H. (Ed.), *Immunologic Mechanisms in Neurologic and Psychiatric Disease*, Raven Press, New York. (1990), 269–290.

43.   Markowitz M., Winslow D., Cao Y. *et al.* "Triple therapy with nelfinavir in combination with AZT and 3TC in 12 antiretroviral-naive subjects chronically infected with HIV-1," *11th International Conference on AIDS* (1996), Vancouver, (abs) LB-B1-6031.

44.   Carpenter C.C.J., Fischl M.A., Hammer S.M. *et al.* "Antiretroviral therapy for HIV-infection in 1997," *JAMA* **277** (1997), 1962–1969.

45.   BHIVA Guidelines Coordinating Committee, various authors., "British HIV Association guidelines for antiretroviral treatment of HIV seropositive individuals," *Lancet* **349** (1997), 1086–1095.

46.   Hammer S.M., Squires K.E., Hughes M.D. *et al.* "A controlled trial of two nucleoside analogues plus indinavir in persons with human immunodeficiency virus infection

and CD4 cell counts of 200 per cubic millimeter or less," *N. Engl. J. Med.* **337** (1997), 725–733.

47. Gazzard B. and Moyle G. "The role of proteinase inhibitors," *Genitourin. Med.* **72** (1996), 233–236.

48. DeMasi R., Staszewski S., Dawson D. *et al. International Workshop on HIV Drug Resistance, Treatment Strategies and Eradication.* St Petersburg, Florida (1997), Abstr. 128

49. Ho D.D. "Time to hit HIV, early and hard," *N. Engl. J. Med.* **333** (1995), 450–451.

50. Race E.M., Adebon-Mitty J., Kriegel G.R. *et al.* "Focal mycobacterial lymphadentis following initiation of protease-inhibitor therapy in patients with advanced HIV-1 disease," *Lancet* **351** (1998), 252–255.

51. Jolles S., Kinloch-de Loes S., Johnson M.A. *et al.* "Primary HIV-1 infection: A new medical emergency?" *Brit. Med. J.* **312** (1996), 1243–1244.

52. Mouton Y., Alfandari G., Valette M. *et al.* "Impact of protease inhibitors on AIDS-defining events and hospitalisations in 10 French AIDS reference centres," *AIDS* **11** (1997), 101–105.

53. Michael S., Clark R., Kissinger P. "Differences in the incidence rates of opportunistic processes before and after the availability of protease inhibitors," *5th International Conference on Retrovirus and Opportunistic Infections, Chicago* (1998), (abs) 180.

54. Rhone S.A., Hogg R.S., Yip B. *et al.* "Antiviral effect of double and triple combinations among HIV infected adults: Lessons from viral load driven antiretroviral therapy," *37th Interscience Conference on Antimicrobial Agents and Chemotherapy (ICAAC),* Toronto (1997), (abs) I-103.

55. Marschmer I.C., Collier A.C., Coombs R.W. *et al.* "Use of changes in plasma levels of human immunodeficiency virus type 1 RNA to assess the clinical benefit of antiretroviral therapy," *J. Infect. Dis.* **177** (1988), 40–48.

56. Kaufmann D, Pantaleo G., Sudre P. *et al.* "CD4-cell count in HIV-1-infected individuals remaining viraemic with highly active antiretroviral therapy (HAART)," *Lancet* **351** (1998), 723–724.

57. Wong J.K., Hezareh M., Gunthard H.F. *et al.* "Recovery of replication-competent HIV despite prolonged suppression of plasma viraemia," *Science* **278** (1997), 1291–1295.

58. Finzi D., Hermankova M., Pierson T. *et al.* "Identification of a reservoir for HIV-1 in patients on highly active antiretroviral therapy," *Science* **278** (1997), 1295–1300.

59. Lafeuillade A., Chollet L. Hittinger G. *et al.* "Residual human immunodeficiency virus type 1 RNA in lymphoid tissue of patients with sustained plasma RNA of <200 copies/ml," *J. Infect. Dis.* **177** (1998), 235–238.

60.   Dube M.P., Johnson D.C., Currier J.S., Leedom J.M. "Protease-inhibitor induced hyperglycaemia," *Lancet* **350** (1997), 713–714.

61.   Hengel R.L., Watts N.B., Lennox J.L. "Benign symmetric lipomatosis associated with protease inhibitors," *Lancet* **350** (1997), p. 1596.

62.   Connor E.M., Sperling R.S., Gelber R. *et al.* "Reduction of maternal-infant transmission of human immunodeficiency virus type 1 with zidovudine," *N. Engl. J. Med.* **331** (1994), 1173–1180.

63.   Cooper E.R., Nugent R.P., Diaz C. *et al.* "After AIDS Clinical Trial 076: The changing pattern of zidovudine use during pregancy, and the subsequent reduction in vertical transmission of human immunodeficiency virus in a cohort of infected women and their infants," *J. Infect. Dis.* **174** (1997), 1207–1211.

CHAPTER 2

OVERVIEW OF HIV INFECTION AND PRE-AIDS OCULAR MANIFESTATIONS

Peter J McCluskey

Introduction

The human immunodeficiency virus is a retrovirus that targets the immune system and infects a number of cell types within it including CD4 lymphocytes, macrophages, dendritic cells and other antigen presenting cells. The predominant cell population infected is the helper T-lymphocyte or CD4 cell, and the virus uses the CD4 receptor as its principal ligand to bind to cells.[1] Following infection there is widespread dissemination of HIV throughout the lymphoid system and the body including the central nervous system. There are persistent high rates of viral replication within lymph nodes following infection despite clinical well-being following infection.[1] An immune response is generated against the virus, which rarely, if ever, overcomes HIV infection. Slowly progressive destruction of the host immune system occurs over the ensuing ten to 15 years, with death as the final outcome.

HIV infection has been conceptualised as having a number of phases, each characterised by recognisable pathogenic mechanisms and clinical signs (see Tables 2.1 and 2.2).[1] These phases of HIV infection represent a convenient framework upon which the clinician can base his investigation and management of patients with HIV infection and its manifestations within the eye.

Up to 80 % of patients develop a recognisable seroconversion illness lasting ten to 14 days about two weeks after exposure to HIV (see also chapter 1). A wide variety of clinical manifestations may occur with fever, lethargy, malaise, skin rash, diarrhoea, transient peripheral neurological changes, headache, and painful eye movements being prominent. HIV spreads widely through the host immune system and proliferates rapidly. The CD4 count falls and then returns to near normal.[2]

Table 2.1 Ocular manifestations according to the stage of HIV infection.

	Seroconversion	Early	Intermediate
External	Injection of the conjunctiva	Sjogren's syndrome	Dry eye syndromes
		Allergic conjunctivitis	Blepharitis Bacterial conjunctivitis Follicular conjunctivitis Accelerated actinic neoplasia growth Kaposi's sarcoma Molluscum contagiosum
Anterior Segment		Reiter's syndrome	Herpes zoster Herpes simplex
Posterior Segment		HIV retinopathy Intermediate uveitis Retinal vasculitis	HIV retinopathy Tuberculous uveitis
Neuro-ophthalmic	Headache Retro-orbital pain	Optic neuropathy	Orbital aspergillosis Optic neuropathy

The early phase of HIV infection lasts several years and is characterised by a well individual who develops episodes of illness, some of which may involve the eye. The CD4 count slowly falls during this period but remains above 500/μl. Clinical manifestations of HIV infection in this early phase reflect dysregulation of the immune system and are expressions of allergic diathesis and autoimmunity rather than immunodeficiency. In the eye, allergic conjunctivitis and contact sensitivity reactions are common. Autoimmune eye disease is not uncommon and Sjogren's syndrome, Reiter's syndrome, intermediate uveitis and retinal vasculitis have each been described in patients with HIV infection.[3-6] Demyelinating optic neuropathy may also occur.[7]

As more CD4 cells are lost and the count falls below 500 cells/μl, the patient enters the intermediate phase of infection where in addition to immune dysregulation, early signs of immunodeficiency such as impaired mucosal defence, mild opportunistic infections and malignancies, begin to appear. In the eye, bacterial lid and conjunctival infections, seborrheic blepharitis, herpetic infection, and malignancies can develop. Tuberculosis is very common and often fatal in areas where TB is endemic and antituberculous drugs are not widely available.

Once the CD4 count falls below 200 cells/μl, severe immunodeficiency ensues with AIDS-defining illnesses such as CMV infections, cryptococcal meningitis and Kaposi's sarcoma being common events with ocular manifestations. Death usually occurs from overwhelming infection or malignancy.

Until recently the best surrogate marker of the stage of HIV infection in an individual was the CD4 cell count and the classification scheme for staging HIV infection has relied heavily on this parameter (see Table 2.2). Recent advances in molecular biology have resulted in the widespread availability of commercial quantitative assays of the amount of HIV in the plasma. The result is expressed as the number of copies of HIV detectable in the plasma by the assay system. The HIV viral load has emerged as the most accurate available marker of HIV infection and is now used routinely to monitor the effectiveness of anti-retroviral therapy (see chapter 1). The viral load and the CD4 count are used together to assess the progress of HIV infection within an individual. An excellent metaphor describes the relationship between HIV infection, CD4 count and viral load as a HIV-infected train travelling towards a chasm with no bridge; the distance from the train to the chasm is the CD4 count and the speed of the train is the viral load.[8]

Table 2.2 Ocular manifestations of HIV infection correlated with immune status.

HIV Stage	CD4 count/μl	Immunity/Eye Disease
Seroconversion	1000	Normal immune function
Early	500–1000	• Sporadic autoimmune disease
		• Allergic eye disease
Intermediate	200–500	• Sporadic autoimmune disease
		• Allergic eye disease
		• Reduced mucosal defence
		• "Milder" opportunistic infection
		• Neoplasia
		• Direct HIV mediated
Late	0–200	• AIDS
		• Direct HIV mediated
		• Severe opportunistic infections
		• Aggressive neoplasms

At this time there is an incomplete understanding of the relationship between viral load and various ocular manifestations of HIV infection. Currently, the CD4 cell count, its nadir within a patient, and the HIV viral load are used to determine the risk of an individual patient developing particular HIV manifestations. This is a rapidly evolving area and firm guidelines are not yet established at the time of this writing.

Pathogenesis of HIV-related Eye Disease

There have been several studies looking at the distribution of HIV within the eye using viral culture, immunohistochemistry and polymerase chain reaction (PCR) techniques. These studies have shown that HIV is recoverable from the tear film, aqueous and vitreous.[9–11] The viral load in the tear film is low and up to this time, no cases of HIV infection have been ascribed to transmission by tears.

HIV is found in resident ocular CD4 positive T-cells, Langerhans cells, and macrophages within the cornea, retinal endothelium, retinal tissue and optic nerve. The commonest cell type harbouring HIV within the eye is the macrophage/monocyte cell population.[12] The direct pathological effects of HIV within the eye are yet to be clearly determined. HIV infection of retinal vascular endothelium is thought to be a factor contributing to the development of HIV microvasculopathy.[12]

Ocular manifestations of HIV infection can be conveniently classified into groups based on their pathogenic mechanism (see Table 2.3). As discussed earlier, allergic disease and autoimmune-mediated eye disease tend to occur early in the course of HIV infection when there is a relatively intact immune system, while opportunistic infection and neoplasms occur later in the course of infection when there more advanced immune suppression.

Table 2.3 Classification of ocular manifestations of HIV infection.

Mechanism	Ocular Manifestation
Allergic	• Allergic conjunctivitis • Stevens-Johnson syndrome
Autoimmune	• Reiter's syndrome • Intermediate uveitis • Retinal vasculitis
Opportunistic infection	• Tuberculous eye disease • Toxoplasmosis • Aspergillosis
Neoplasia	• Lymphoma • Actinic-related neoplasms
HIV related	• HIV retinopathy • Conjunctival retinopathy
Treatment related and drug toxicity	• Rifabutin associated uveitis • Cidofovir associated uveitis • ddI retinopathy

A further mechanism of ocular disease recognised in patients with HIV infection is related to drug toxicity. Several years ago a pigmentary retinopathy was described in children taking the antiretroviral drug Didanosine (ddI).[13] More recently, the antimicrobial drugs rifabutin and cidofovir have been associated with an acute hypopyon uveitis in 15%–40% of patients taking these drugs.[14,15] Rifabutin uveitis has also been seen in non-HIV-infected patients.[16] The mechanism producing uveitis remains obscure at this time. Antituberculous drugs such as ethambutol can produce an acute optic neuropathy, and clofazamine can produce a vortex keratopathy.

Specific Ocular Manifestations at Different Disease Stages

Ocular manifestations of HIV infection are among its commonest clinical features and occur throughout the course of this disease. Early after seroconversion, ocular manifestations are episodic and not specific to HIV infection. In the later stages, opportunistic infections and neoplasms develop. The ocular manifestations represent opportunities to make the diagnosis of HIV infection, which should always be considered when a patient presents with unusual clinical features of a common ocular disease or when the history or review of systems suggests that HIV infection is possible.

Seroconversion and the Eye

There is a recognisable systemic illness commonly associated with acquiring infection from HIV.[2] Headache is a prominent feature of this seroconversion illness and is often accompanied by pain on eye movement. There can be a significant meningoencephalitis and other neurological involvement. The ocular features are not of sufficient severity to warrant involvement by an ophthalmologist or specific therapy.

Ocular Involvement in Early HIV-induced Immune Deficiency

Hypersensitivity and Allergic Eye Disease

Drug hypersensitivity is far commoner in patients with HIV infection than in other immunocompromised individuals. Its precise cause in HIV infection is unclear, but may be related to immune-mediated hypersensitivity mechanisms or direct drug toxicity.[17] Given the profound anergy present in patients with HIV infection, the high incidence of allergic disease and hypersensitivity is perplexing and unexplained. The eye is commonly involved in such reactions, with Stevens-Johnson syndrome (SJS) being the most severe form of involvement. The most common drugs involved are sulphonamides, β-lactam antibiotics and phenytoin.[18,19]

There are two phases to the ocular involvement of SJS. Initially, patients develop an acute non-specific conjunctivitis which may be associated with severe mucous over-production and pseudomembrane formation.[20] Corneal epithelial defects and anterior uveitis may also occur. Extensive conjunctival cicatrisation develops with healing of the acute lesions. This results in the development of severe ocular dryness from tear gland and duct obliteration, as well as goblet cell destruction. Significant eyelid and corneal changes also ensue.

The ophthalmologist is critically involved in the management of the chronic phase of the disease to deal with the permanent structural changes that are the major morbidity in survivors of severe disease.[21] Trichiasis, distichiasis, chronic meibomianitis, cicatrical entropion, and corneal epithelial defects are common and difficult to treat.[20,22] A range of surgical procedures such as eyelash cryotherapy, entropion surgery, mucous membrane grafting, tarsorrhaphy, or allogeneic limbal stem cell grafting may be necessary.[22,23]

Allergic eye disease is common in patients with HIV infection. This may take the form of the new onset of seasonal or perennial conjunctivitis or the development of a chronic papillary conjunctivitis similar to that seen in vernal keratoconjunctivitis. Allergic eye disease in patients with HIV infection is treated in the same manner as in other patients with topical antihistamines, judicious use of topical corticosteroids, a trial of sodium cromoglycate, and control of secondary lid margin disease.

Dry Eye Syndromes and Sjogren's Syndrome

Dry eye syndromes (sicca syndrome) are frequent in patients with HIV infection and are among the commonest ocular manifestations seen in clinical practice.[3,24] Patients with dry eyes complain of irritable, burning uncomfortable red eyes that typically get worse as the day progresses. The clinical signs vary depending on the layer of the tear film involved. The tear film may be obviously deficient and there may be positive Schirmer's tests. There may also be excess mucous in the tear film, and there may be rose bengal and fluorescein staining of the inferior cornea and exposed areas of conjunctiva. There are multiple causes of a dry eye in HIV infection and these are easiest when considered according to the layer of the tear film that they predominantly involve.

Abnormalities involving the lipid layer of the tear film are usually caused by blepharitis, which is common in HIV infection and may also have multiple aetiologies. A major clinical consequence of blepharitis is the development of a dry eye syndrome from lipid abnormalities within the tear film leading to a reduced tear break-up time.

Aqueous tear deficiency may occur as a result of cicatrising conjunctival disease from SJS or as a result of a Sjogren's syndrome-like condition.[22,24] The clinical features are similar to that of Sjogren's syndrome with a poor tear film, mucous over-production and rose bengal staining. The cellular infiltrate is a CD8 population in patients with HIV infection in distinction to the CD4 cell infiltrate of classical Sjogren's syndrome.[25] Autoantibodies to extractable nuclear antigens such as SS-A and SS-B are not seen. The aetiology of the sicca syndrome remains obscure, but may be related to Epstein-Barr virus infection.

SJS may result in severe ocular surface changes leading to aqueous, lipid and mucin abnormalities in the tear film and a resultant dry eye. Mucin deficiency may be severe as a result of widespread goblet cell destruction in the conjunctiva.

Treatment of dry eye syndromes in patients with HIV infection is similar to that of other patients with dry eyes. Elimination of exacerbating factors such as systemic medications known to reduce tear secretion, blepharitis, and allergic disease is essential. Tear supplements are the initial form of therapy and are adequate in most patients. An occasional patient will require other forms of therapy such as punctal occlusion.

Blepharitis

Blepharitis is a very common ocular manifestation of HIV infection and is usually caused by staphylococcal infection, seborrheic diathesis, or both processes. The typical signs and symptoms are those of anterior blepharitis with burning, irritable and uncomfortable red eyes that are worse in the mornings. There are collarettes around the lashes, erythematous lid margins, irregular eyelashes, and loss of lashes. There is often ulceration of the lid margin and around the bases of the eyelashes. There may be a mucopurulent discharge and a moderate papillary conjunctival reaction. Staphylococci can be cultured from the eyelids. There can be associated peripheral corneal ulceration and infiltrates that are sterile and are the result of an antibody-mediated response to staphylococcal exotoxin. Phlyctenular disease is rare as it is a delayed hypersensitivity response to staphylococcal antigens.

Seborrheic blepharitis (see Fig. 2.1) is a more indolent form of anterior blepharitis and in HIV infection is most often seen in association with widespread seborrheic dermatitis. Patients typically have seborrheic dermatitis involving the central chest, back, face, ears, scalp, and eyebrows. The aetiology of seborrheic blepharitis is unknown, but there is evidence it may be related to fungal infection.[26] Affected individuals complain of burning, watery red eyes. The blepharitis involves predominantly the glands of Zeiss and results in red eyelids and greasy yellowish-gray scales on the lid margin and eyelashes called "scurf". There is no ulceration of the eyelids and the posterior eyelid margin is normal. There is often secondary staphylococcal infection and the clinical picture becomes mixed with signs of both seborrheic and staphylococcal blepharitis.

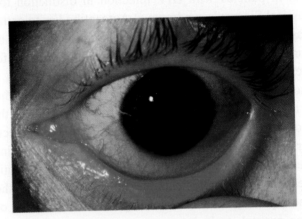

Fig. 2.1 The external eye of a patient with seborrheic blepharoconjunctivitis, staphylococcal infection, and associated sicca syndrome. Note the prominent scaling around the lashes and conjunctival reaction.

Treatment involves aggressive lid hygiene to remove collarettes and scurf, a course of topical antibiotics to treat staphylococcal infection, and systemic tetracycline or doxycycline to improve meibomian gland function. A short course of topical corticosteroids may be necessary.

Staphylococcal blepharitis, seborrhea, and dry eyes occur together very frequently as the pathogenesis and clinical effects of the conditions are complimentary. This combination is often designated the "triple S syndrome" (Staph, Seborrhea, Sicca) and should always be considered in patients with irritable, red, uncomfortable eyes and HIV infection.

Reiter's Syndrome

Reiter's syndrome is a well-recognised syndrome seen not uncommonly in HIV-infected patients.[24] It can occur at any time during the course of HIV infection but is more often an early event. Reiter's syndrome is presumed to be autoimmune in origin and is triggered by either enteric or genitourinary infection.[27] In HIV patients enteric infection by gram negative bacteria such as Campylobacter, Yersinia, Shigella and Salmonella species is the most common mechanism.[24,28] Clinically the patients may present following an acute diarrhoeal illness, or with chronic diarrhoea and manifestations of Reiter's syndrome. Chlamydial urethretis or bacterial prostatitis may lead to the development of Reiter's syndrome. Reiter's syndrome produces a range of clinical features including spondyloarthritis, peripheral arthritis, conjunctivitis, uveitis, oral ulceration, nail changes, and keratodermia.[29] Incomplete clinical forms are common in patients with HIV infection. About 60% of patients with Reiter's syndrome carry the HLA B27 phenotype.[30]

Conjunctivitis is a hallmark feature of Reiter's syndrome. It occurs at the onset of the disease and is usually bilateral, mild and self limiting. It does not generally require specific therapy. Anterior uveitis occurs commonly, some time after the onset of the illness is acute in onset, and severe in nature. Uveitis may persist and may be the major morbidity of the disease.[31] This is treated initially with intensive topical corticosteroids and cycloplegic agents. Severe disease may require the use of systemic corticosteroids. It is important to treat the uveitis aggressively in order to minimise the risk of developing into a chronic state. It is also important to look carefully for an underlying enteric or genitourinary infection and to treat this with appropriate systemic antibiotics. Ciprofloxacin is usually the antibiotic of choice.

Intermediate Uveitis

Intermediate uveitis is another common form of ocular inflammatory disease seen in patients with HIV infection, the aetiology of which is uncertain and is presumed to be autoimmune in nature.[5,24] It is a chronic bilateral indolent uveitis, which presents with floaters and blurred vision and which is characterised by pan vitreous cellular infiltration, vitreous degenerative changes, and low-grade anterior chamber cellular infiltration. There are no retinal or choroidal lesions except for macular oedema and/or optic disc swelling. Patients may develop cataracts and elevated intraocular pressure from their chronic inflammation.

Intermediate uveitis may be associated with a range of systemic and ocular diseases.[5] In patients with HIV infection, a differential diagnosis which includes syphilis, lymphoma, metastatic endophthalmitis, viral retinitis, toxoplasmic retinochoroiditis, and ocular ischaemia should be considered.[32] Fuchs heterochromic uveitis should always be considered as a differential in intermediate uveitis. Many of these diseases are clinical diagnoses with the principal differentiating clinical features being the presence of focal retinal or choroidal lesions. Selected patients may require vitreous biopsy for cytology and microbiological evaluation.

Treatment of intermediate uveitis is dependent on the presence of a threat to vision, usually macular oedema associated with reduced visual acuity. In general, patients with uniocular vision threatening inflammation are treated with local corticosteroid therapy such as topical and periocular corticosteroids while patients with bilateral vision-threatening disease are treated with systemic corticosteroids and other immunosuppressive drugs. In patients with HIV infection, there are additional considerations related to the stage and control of the HIV. This is best measured by the viral load and the CD4 cell count. Patients who are untreated or who have high viral loads need therapy to decrease the viral load as much as possible, preferably to undetectable levels. This improves control of the ocular inflammation by improving immune function and competence. There is often an increase in the CD4 cell count as well.

Intermediate uveitis is usually a mild disease in patients with HIV infection and improves rapidly with antiretroviral therapy. Local and systemic corticosteroids may be needed initially, but can usually be tapered as immune function improves. Additional immunosuppressive drugs should not be used. Patients having cataract or other intraocular surgery require systemic corticosteroid prophylaxis perioperatively.

Retinal Vasculitis

Retinal vasculitis is another ocular manifestation of HIV-associated autoimmunity. It shares many clinical features with intermediate uveitis, but is far less common.[6,24] In retinal vasculitis the predominant clinical signs involve the retina with retinal vascular sheathing (see Fig. 2.2), retinal haemorrhages, cotton wool spots, retinal and macular oedema, and optic disc swelling. There is an associated low-grade vitreous cellular infiltration. There is no retinal opacification. Fluorescein angiography is important to confirm the clinical diagnosis and to determine whether there is retinal capillary closure. Most retinal vasculitis in HIV-infected patients results in a leaky retinal capillary bed without vascular closure. This form responds well to treatment. Some patients develop widespread capillary closure either peripherally or centrally, and retinal or iris neovascularisation may occur. Occlusive, ischaemic retinal vasculitis is much more difficult to manage and has a poorer visual prognosis.

Retinal vasculitis is associated with a range of systemic inflammatory and infective diseases as well as a number of ocular disorders. In the setting of HIV infection, infective processes including syphilis, tuberculosis, herpetic retinitis, and ocular toxoplasmosis need to be considered and excluded by clinical examination and serological or other microbiological testing. Retinal vasculitis associated with systemic tuberculosis typically results in widespread capillary closure. Retinal vasculitis associated with systemic vasculitis such as Wegener's granulomatosis and polyarteritis nodosa is associated with the presence of antineutrophil cytoplasmic antibodies, anticardiolipin antibodies, and other autoreactive antibodies. These autoantibodies have been found in the sera of patients with HIV infection, however, their relationship to diseases such as retinal vasculitis remains unclear at this time.[17]

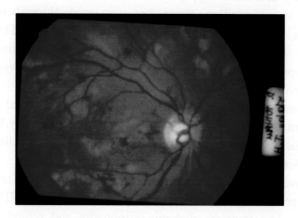

Fig. 2.2 Fundus photo of widespread retinal vasculitis with scattered retinal haemorrhages and numerous cotton wool spots. Vitreous cellular infiltration, decreased vision and the pattern of cotton wool spots allow differentiation from HIV microvasculopathy.

Retinal vasculitis is managed in a similar manner to intermediate uveitis with appropriate antiretroviral therapy and judicious use of periocular and systemic corticosteroids. Areas of the capillary bed occluded from retinal vasculitis need scatter retinal photocoagulation to control ischaemia. Topical medications are of no use in the treatment of this disease.

Ocular Involvement in Intermediate HIV-induced Immune Deficiency

HIV Microvasculopathy

HIV microvasculopathy is the most common ocular manifestation of HIV infection and occurs in 50% to 70 % of patients at some time during the course of the disease.[33] It occurs more commonly with increasing immunodeficiency.[34] The cause is unknown and is almost certainly multifactorial. There is evidence that immune complex deposition, direct HIV infection of vascular endothelium, abnormal blood rheology, and abnormal red cell deformability, are all factors contributing to the development of microvasculopathy.[35,36] With the advent of combination antiretroviral therapy using protease inhibitors, there has been a marked decrease in the incidence and severity of HIV microvasculopathy.[37]

Retinal involvement most commonly consists of cotton wool spots, which are areas of retinal opacification in the nerve fibre layer of the retina from stasis of axoplasmic flow in the nerve fibre layer secondary to blockage of the pre-capillary arterioles supplying the inner retina. Cotton wool spots are typically seen in peripapillary retina, but may occur throughout the posterior pole. They are white in colour and have ill-defined edges. They obscure the retinal vessels. Except for those located in the perifoveal retina, cotton wool spots are asymptomatic. Cotton wool spots gradually resolve over a six-to eight-week period without treatment and without sequelae.

Retinal haemorrhages, microaneurysms, and intraretinal microvascular abnormalities may also be seen as part of HIV microvasculopathy. With fluorescein angiography, such changes are nearly always present, even if not clinically apparent. Rarely, significant areas of capillary closure can develop.

HIV microvasculopathy needs to be considered in the differential diagnosis of any patient presenting with cotton wool spots and other non-HIV-related causes such as severe hypertension, diabetic retinopathy and retinal vasculitis. HIV microvasculopathy may also be confused with early CMV retinitis. Observation over time will resolve this, as CMV lesions will increase in size, whereas cotton wool spots will remain the same or break up.

The conjunctival circulation may also be affected by HIV microvasculopathy.[38] Changes include microaneurysms, telangiectatic vessels, and vascular occlusions. Studies have shown that although conjunctival changes are common, they do not have a high specificity for HIV infection. They are of no clinical significance.

Bacterial Conjunctivitis and Keratitis

As immunodeficiency progresses during HIV infection, the affected individual develops impaired mucosal immunity and becomes susceptible to infections such as recurrent bacterial conjunctivitis and chronic staphylococcal blepharitis. Bacterial conjunctivitis begins unilaterally and is characterised by red sticky eyes with mucopurulent discharge. Staphylococci and streptococcal species are the commonest pathogens, although a wide range of bacteria can infect the conjunctiva. In patients with HIV infection progression to involve the cornea can occur and is characterised by epithelial defects, stromal opacification and thinning. With virulent bacteria such as gonococci, rapidly progressive infection with corneal involvement and perforation can occur.

Treatment of bacterial conjunctivitis involves the frequent use of broad-spectrum topical antibiotics. Hyperacute conjunctivitis or corneal involvement requires corneal scraping and conjunctival smears for gram stain and cultures. Organisms such as *Neisseria gonorrhoeae* should be suspected and treated with systemic and topical antibiotics.

A small number of HIV-infected patients may spontaneously develop microbial keratitis in the absence of a predisposing cause.[39] This is most common in intravenous drug abusers and may be related to corneal exposure due to altered levels of consciousness from drug abuse.[40] Usually, there are factors such as severe conjunctival infection, corneal exposure secondary to seventh cranial nerve lesions, dry eye syndromes, reduced corneal sensation following herpetic infection, or contact lens wear that predispose to corneal infection. Microbial keratitis is managed along standard lines with corneal scrapings for microbiological investigations, intensive broad-spectrum topical antibiotics and close follow-up. A wide range of bacteria and fungi has been isolated from the corneas of patients with microbial keratitis and close liaison with the microbiology laboratory is essential.[41] Given the altered immune function in HIV-infected patients, a high level of suspicion for unusual organisms should be maintained. Highly pathogenic organisms such as pseudomonas can display a very aggressive clinical course.

Follicular Conjunctivitis

Follicular conjunctivitis may result from several different disease processes. A mild follicular response can be seen in patients with chronic staphylococcal or moraxella blepharoconjunctivitis. Molluscum contagiosum infection of the eyelid or conjunctiva produces a chronic follicular conjunctivitis. Chlamydial infection is the other common cause of a chronic follicular conjunctivitis. Management involves careful clinical and microbiological assessment to determine the aetiology. A chronic idiopathic non-infectious follicular conjunctivitis has been described in HIV infection.[42]

Molluscum Contagiosum

Molluscum contagiosum skin infection is common in patients with HIV infection and lesions are often widespread, persistent and recurrent despite treatment. Molluscum contagiosum is caused by a DNA pox virus infection of the epithelium. Eyelid involvement is common (see Fig. 2.3) and is usually seen in patients with multiple facial mollusca.

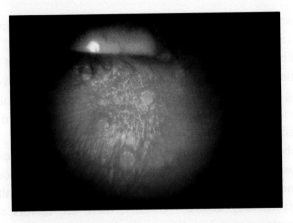

Fig. 2.3 Typical molluscum contagiosum lesions involving the eyelid skin. These may be associated with eyelid margin and conjunctival mollusca.

Mollusca present as pale, waxy, circular, elevated, superficial skin lesions with a central darker umbilication. Mollusca involving the eyelid are often multiple and tend to occur along the lid margin. Rarely isolated conjunctival and limbal mollusca have been reported.[43] A persistent follicular conjunctivitis develops with eyelid or conjunctival mollusca and toxic corneal epithelial changes may also occur.

Ocular mollusca are best treated by either excision or curettage. Multiple skin lesions can be a difficult management problem and combination antiretroviral therapy may result in regression of lesions. Mollusca may also regress following cidofovir therapy.

Herpes Zoster

Clinical manifestations of infection by Herpes group viruses are hallmark features of HIV infection. The commonest Herpes group viral infection involving the eye is CMV retinitis and infection commonly results in loss of vision. Varicella-zoster infection involving the eye is less common and infrequently results in severe visual loss. Herpes simplex infection uncommonly involves the eye and rarely causes severe visual loss. All herpes group viruses share the property of latency following primary infection. The site of latency is different for each virus; for varicella-zoster it is the satellite cells within the sensory ganglia and within the sensory neurones for herpes simplex.[44]

In patients with HIV infection, varicella-zoster infection is common and may have a prolonged clinical course.[45] Multiple episodes of zoster infection are not uncommon and disseminated infection may develop. In the developed world, HIV infection is the commonest systemic association of herpes zoster ophthalmicus and should always be considered in any patient presenting with this infection.[46] Atypical clinical features or clinical course should increase suspicion of the presence of HIV infection.[24]

Herpes zoster is the clinical syndrome that results from the reactivation of latent varicella zoster virus within satellite cells of the sensory ganglia.[44] Herpes zoster involving the trigeminal nerve is the second most common site of clinical involvement following the thoracic dermatomes and is potentially its most devastating form. The ophthalmic division is the commonest affected site and is termed Herpes Zoster Ophthalmicus (HZO).[47]

There is a prodrome of tingling, burning parasthesiae and lancinating pain in the distribution of the ophthalmic nerve which may develop up to 72 hours before the onset of the rash, and which may be accompanied by headache, fever and malaise. The skin rash consists of multiple-grouped vesicles in the distribution of the ophthalmic nerve.[48] Any or all three branches of the nerve (frontal, nasociliary, lacrimal) may be involved with the frontal branch being the most commonly affected (see Fig. 2.4). The rash is accompanied by severe pain and hyperasthesia. The vesicles initially contain clear fluid, which becomes turbid and haemorrhagic after four to six days. The vesicles then slowly crust over and heal.[48] Varicella zoster is present in the vesicles for the first three to six days of the rash in immunocompetent individuals, but may be cultured from vesicles for ten to 14

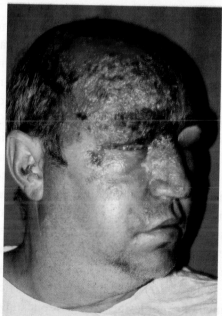

Fig. 2.4 Severe herpes zoster ophthalmicus that has become disseminated and involves all three divisions of the Trigeminal nerve.

days in HIV-infected patients. The acute inflammatory response and vasculitis that accompanies the vesicles involves the dermis and subcutaneous tissues as well as the epidermis and areas of deep ulceration and necrosis may occur. The healing phase may be prolonged and result in prominent scarring and pigmentary disturbance. There can be significant structural damage to the eyelids from varicella zoster infection and severe involvement may result in ischaemic necrosis of the eyelid.[48] There may be cicatrical ectropion or entropion, lid retraction, trichiasis, eyelash loss, and cutaneous pigmentary disturbance.

Treatment of HZO involves the use of high-dose oral aciclovir, famciclovir or valaciclovir for seven to ten days.[49] Severe disease may require the use of intravenous aciclovir. The role of systemic corticosteroids in patients with zoster infections is debated and in HIV-infected patients they should only be used for specific ocular complications where a clear benefit has been shown.[50,51] Post-herpetic neuralgia is a common sequel of infection and is commoner in middle-aged and older patients. In HIV-infected patients, neuralgia should be managed with appropriate analgesics, tricyclic antidepressants, and anticonvulsants such as carbamazepine and valproic acid.

The eye is involved in up to 50% of cases of HZO and a wide range of signs may develop involving either the anterior or posterior segment of the eye.[48] This review will focus on anterior segment complications as zoster retinitis is discussed in chapter 5.

A non-specific conjunctivitis is very common and consists of conjunctival injection and follicular reaction. Involvement of the superficial episcleral capillaries by zoster-induced vasculitis results in episcleritis. Involvement of the deep episcleral vascular plexus produces diffuse or nodular scleritis.[52] Rarely severe ischaemic vasculitis can result in severe necrotising scleritis or delayed onset anterior segment ischaemia and necrosis.[53]

Treatment with topical aciclovir and corticosteroids is sufficient for conjunctivitis and episcleritis, but scleritis requires the use of systemic non-steroidal anti-inflammatory drugs (naproxen, ibuprofen) or systemic corticosteroids.

Corneal involvement occurs in up to two thirds of patients and ranges in severity from mild infectious epithelial erosions to severe necrotising immune mediated keratitis (see Table 2.4).[54] The most frequent epithelial lesion is a punctate epithelial keratitis with underlying stromal infiltrates. This may resolve or progress to more severe forms of stromal disease and may be associated with other epithelial lesions. Pseudodendrites are superficial, gray, dendriform, opaque, poorly staining epithelial lesions due to replicating varicella-zoster virus and occur within the first two to three weeks following infection.[54] Pseudodendrites respond well to topical aciclovir, but will resolve without treatment. Delayed mucous plaque lesions are transient, opaque, raised, epithelial dendriform lesions that develop eight to 12 weeks after the onset of the rash. They also resolve without treatment.[54]

Table 2.4. Forms and incidence of zoster keratitis.*

Clinical Presentation	Incidence (%)
Pseudodendrites	51
Punctate epithelial keratitis	51
Anterior stromal infiltrates	41
Keratouveitis – endotheliitis	34
Neurotrophic keratitis	25
Delayed mucous plaques	13
Exposure keratitis	11
Disciform keratitis	10
Peripheral ulcerative keratitis	7
Sclerokeratitis	1
Delayed limbal vasculitis	<1

*(Reproduced from Pavan-Langston D., Dunkel E. "Varicella-Zoster Diseases: Anterior Segment of the Eye" *Ocular Infection and Immunity*, St. Louis, Mosby, 1996)

Anterior stromal infiltrates commonly occur following epithelial keratitis and may be single or multiple focal areas of stromal oedema and opacification that develop beneath areas of resolved epithelial keratitis.[54] A larger single circumscribed area of disciform stromal keratitis may also occur. Endotheliitis may accompany stromal keratitis and results in keratic precipitates, corneal oedema, and anterior uveitis. Intraocular pressure is often elevated. Peripheral ulcerative keratitis similar to that seen in patients with collagen vascular disease may occur with circumferential areas of epithelial loss and corneal thinning associated with a variable uveitis. Keratitis represents an immune response to sequestered antigen within the stroma and ranges in severity from mild and transient oedema and opacification to necrosis and severe destruction of the cornea. HIV infection impairs such responses and modifies the frequency and severity of stromal keratitis. The effects of antiretroviral therapy will further modify the patient's immune responses. Therapy of keratitis needs to be individualised using topical aciclovir and topical corticosteroids. Oral aciclovir at viral suppressive doses of 600 – 800 mg per day is useful in the management of keratitis.

Neurotrophic keratopathy is seen in about 25% of patients with herpes zoster ophthalmicus and is the result of impaired corneal sensation from neural destruction within the cornea and trigeminal ganglion.[54] Epithelial irregularity and haziness, persistent corneal epithelial defects, and stromal thinning occur. Lid margin and tear film abnormalities may compound the damage to corneal integrity. Exposure keratopathy from upper eyelid scarring and destruction may further add to the anaesthetic cornea. Management involves careful clinical assessment of the role of factors such as tear film, eyelash and lid margin abnormalities, the degree of exposure, the presence of infective epithelial disease, the presence of stromal abnormalities (see Fig. 2.5) and severity of corneal sensory deficit. Copious ocular lubricants, removal of aberrant lashes, treatment of meibomian gland dysfunction, control of secondary infection, treatment of infectious zoster keratitis, and consideration of central or lateral tarsorraphy are major management considerations.

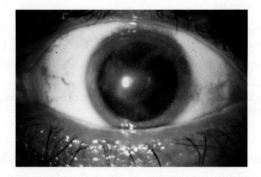

Fig. 2.5 Stromal opacities in herpes zoster ophthalmicus.

Uveitis occurs in about 50% of patients with herpes zoster ophthalmicus and is associated with characteristic iris stromal and pigment cell atrophy.[55] There can be localised sector-like areas of destruction or widespread involvement of the iris with loss of the posterior pigment layer, thinning of the iris stroma, and loss of iris sphincter function with a fixed pupil.[56] Widespread posterior synechiae may develop. Anterior uveitis is thought to result from direct iris invasion by varicella zoster and a resultant plasma cell-lymphocyte vasculitis. Iris angiography reveals widespread occlusive vasculitis that is thought to induce much of the iris damage seen clinically. HIV infection may result in impaired T-cell responses and allow more intense virus-mediated damage to occur. Uveitis develops early in the course of disease and is usually associated with keratitis but may occur in isolation. Elevated intraocular pressure is common. Initial therapy should include topical and systemic aciclovir. Uveitis is persistent and requires the use of topical corticosteroids for many months or years before the inflammation subsides. Cataract and glaucoma are very common complications.

Elevated intraocular pressure and glaucoma may occur from a number of mechanisms including direct zoster involvement inducing peripheral corneal endotheliitis and trabeculitis, trabecular obstruction from inflammatory cells, debris or pigment, angle closure from peripheral anterior synechiae, or secondary angle closure from pupil block.[47,54] Management is similar to that of other uveitic glaucomas and requires careful clinical assessment to determine the mechanisms responsible for elevated intraocular pressure, followed by treatment directed at the primary cause and topical ocular hypotensive medications to decrease the pressure. Refractory glaucoma requires surgery.

Optic neuritis is rare following HZO.[57] It presents three to 12 weeks following the onset of infection with severe visual loss, colour desaturation, and an afferent pupillary defect. There may be an optic papillitis or retrobulbar optic neuritis. Pathologically the optic nerve is involved by an inflammatory arteritis and leptomeningitis. The visual outcome is poor. Systemic corticosteroids may be beneficial in some patients, but their role is not defined in patients with HIV infection.

Cranial nerve palsies are uncommon and are seen in patients with more severe disease.[58] Third cranial nerve palsy is the most common and may or may not involve the pupil. Multiple nerves may be involved resulting in complete ophthalmoplegia. Cranial nerve palsies may be caused either by orbital involvement of nerves or retrograde spread of infection to involve the nerves within the subarachnoid space. Complete recovery normally occurs without specific treatment.

Zoster retinitis is common in patients with advanced HIV infection and may occur clinically as a spectrum of retinitis ranging from acute retinal necrosis to progressive outer retinal necrosis. Zoster retinitis is discussed in detail in chapter 5.

Management of HZO is complex and requires detailed clinical assessment to determine the clinical features and extent of involvement. Treatment involves the control of viral replication with systemic and topical aciclovir, control of destructive host cell inflammatory response with the use of topical and systemic corticosteroids, and specific treatment for complications such as raised intraocular pressure. Systemic corticosteroid therapy in HIV-infected patients is generally safe and well tolerated. As with most aspects of HIV management consultation between treating physicians is essential prior to introducing new systemic medication given the high potential for drug interactions in patients with HIV infection. Recently, famciclovir and valaciclovir have become available as oral therapy for HZO. These drugs have better bioavailability following oral administration than aciclovir and therefore need to be given less frequently. Their efficacy is very similar to that of aciclovir

In HIV infection, dysregulation and immune suppression alter the host response further complicating the management of HZO. Recent advances in antiretroviral therapy have further confounded the clinical manifestations and course of HZO in patients with HIV infection. Earlier in the HIV epidemic, HZO was typically severe and associated with persistant viral replication and a poor host response to infection. It was considered to be a marker of disease progression. There was often severe skin infection and ocular infection and little in the way of immune-mediated inflammatory manifestations. With the advent of combination antiretroviral therapy and its positive effects on immune function, severe HZO has become less frequent, but immune mediated inflammatory manifestations of infection more common.

Herpes Simplex Virus

Herpes simplex is a common ocular infection with a worldwide distribution. Both herpes simplex type-1 and-2 may infect the eye and establish latency in the trigeminal ganglion, although type-1 infection predominates in patients with ocular disease.[44] Type-1 virus has a predeliction for the eye and face and is spread by contact with infected secretions. The type-2 virus is spread predominantly by sexual transmission and results in genital herpes. There may be spread to the eye. Primary infection with herpes simplex is usually a childhood illness of the first five to ten years of life characterised by an upper respiratory illness accompanied by gingivostomatitis, pharnyngitis, rhinitis, and a variable vesicular skin eruption that clears in seven to ten days. There may be a follicular conjunctivitis and superfical ulcerative keratitis. Many infections are subclinical.[59]

Recurrent disease has many triggers and clinical forms.[60] Immunosuppression is a recognised trigger for both reactivation of previously acquired herpes simplex infection and for acqusition of herpes virus infection. HIV infection *per se* has not been shown to increase the risk of reactivation of herpetic eye disease, however, reactivations of eye disease in HIV-infected patients are more frequent.[61] Recurrences are more common in patients with a history of recurrent ocular disease. Patients may develop recurrent eyelid vesicular lesions without eye involvement. Epithelial infection is usually in the form of arborising curvilinear ulcers with terminal end bulbs. Such dendritic ulcers stain vividly with rose bengal and relatively less well with fluorescein. Large ulcers tend to lose the characteristic dendritic pattern and form large geographic areas of ulceration which retain the characteristic ulcer edge staining pattern of dendritic ulcers (see Fig. 2.6).

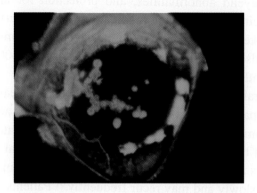

Fig. 2.6 Large peripheral dendriform ulcers from herpes simplex infection stained with fluorescein.

Stromal keratitis has several clinical forms.[62] Disciform keratitis is characterised by a solitary central circular area of stromal oedema with underlying Descemets folds and keratitic precipitates. There may be low-grade anterior uveitis. Interstitial keratitis comprises stromal opacification and infiltration by inflammatory cells and may result in stromal necrosis. Healing may be associated with stromal scarring, thinning, neovascularisation, and lipid deposition. Severe inflammation may result in descemetocoele formation and corneal perforation. Secondary bacterial or fungal infection may complicate ulcerative keratitis. Uveitis and elevated intraocular pressure is common. Patchy iris stromal loss, pigment layer loss, and synechiae are common.

Severe epithelial disease, the toxic effects of topical medications, corneal sensory impairment, tissue loss, and stromal disorganisation may result in the development of a large, indolent non-healing corneal ulcer with a characteristic smooth rolled-up edge termed a metaherpetic ulcer. Such ulcers are treated after careful clinical assessment to detect reversible factors such as medication toxicity and exposure. Tarsorraphy may be necessary.

Herpes simplex may infect the retina producing acute retinal necrosis or less fulminant forms of viral retinitis. This aspect of herpes simplex ocular infection is covered in detail in chapter 5.

The treatment of herpes simplex eye disease is complex and must be individualised to the clinical features of each patient.[26] Topical antiviral drugs are essential for active epithelial disease. Aciclovir eye ointment and trifluorothymidine drops are the most potent and best-tolerated topical medications currently available. These may be combined with epithelial debridement in selected patients. Treatment of stromal disease requires combination therapy with topical antivirals and topical corticosteroids. Treatment of secondary infection, correction of tear film and eyelid abnormalities, and protection for anaesthetic corneas are critical. Toxicity from topical medications and preservatives should be minimised. Severe keratitis and keratouveitis may require systemic aciclovir therapy. Oral aciclovir is also useful in viral suppressive doses of 600–800 mg per day to control frequently recurrent ocular disease.[63]

There are several important differences in the ocular disease of HIV-infected patients and other patients.[41] Epithelial disease predominates and stromal keratitis is distinctly less common. The epithelial lesions tend to be located in the perilimbal cornea rather than the central and paracentral cornea typical of herpes simplex disease. The ulcers are usually larger and more geographic in nature. The ulcers tend to heal more slowly and may recur frequently.[61] Patients with HIV infection who develop ocular herpes simplex disease should be treated with topical aciclovir or trifluorothymidine. Such patients require treatment for a longer time than the average patient. Topical corticosteroids should be used as needed for stromal disease, once epithelial lesions have healed. All HIV-infected patients developing herpes simplex eye disease should be maintained on long-term suppressive doses of oral aciclovir in order to minimise recurrences.[63]

Tuberculous Uveitis

Tuberculosis is common in HIV-infected patients and has resulted in a large increase in the number of patients with tuberculosis in areas where HIV infection is common. Tuberculosis progresses rapidly in HIV-infected patients, who may develop widespread infection and severe open lung disease within a few months of infection. Extrapulmonary tuberculosis is common. In the developing world, tuberculosis is endemic and is extremely common in HIV-infected patients (see chapter 9) and it is a common cause of death.

Almost any structure in the eye may be involved by tuberculosis and recognised clinical manifestations include conjunctival phlyctenulosis, interstitial keratitis, scleritis, anterior uveitis, posterior uveitis, and retinal vasculitis. Tuberculous uveitis is rare in the developed world and is only seen in patients with miliary tuberculosis and meningitis. Such patients are critically ill and develop single or multiple deep retinal and choroidal whitish-yellow masses. There is associated panuveitis and retinal vasculitis. Retinal vasculitis may also develop as a hypersensitivity response to tuberculosis in the absence of other signs of ocular infection by tuberculosis. The vasculitis is venous in nature and characterised by vascular sheathing, capillary closure, and frequent neovascularisation. Accurate data on the frequency of ocular involvement in HIV-infected patients is lacking, but clinical experience would indicate that ocular manifestations remain rare in patients with HIV infection and tuberculosis, at least in the developed world.

Cancer Associated Retinopathy and HIV Infection

There are anecdotal reports of a syndrome similar to cancer associated retinopathy (CAR) occurring in patients with HIV infection. The author has managed two patients with HIV infection who have developed CAR syndrome. Cancer associated retinopathy is characterised by progressive visual loss, photopsias, and the development of ring-like scotomas in the presence of normal fundi except for the late development of pigmentary changes.

First described in association with bronchogenic lung cancer, it has been seen in a range of tumours including large and small cell lung cancer, cervical and endometrial carcinoma, breast carcinoma, lymphoma and melanoma.[64–66] CAR has also rarely been seen in patients with vasculitis rather than cancer.[67] Although not completely documented, it appears that CAR can occur in patients with HIV infection. CAR is the result of an autoimmune response directed towards the outer retina, and patients with CAR have detectable autoantibodies directed against the retinal protein recoverin and almost certainly other retinal proteins.[68,69] Treatment with corticosteroids may delay the onset of blindness.

Actinic Neoplasms and HIV Infection

In areas such as Australia where severe actinic damage to the skin is common, sun-related neoplasms such as basal cell and squamous cell carcinomas are frequent. Although clearly difficult to document, there is a clinical impression that actinic-related carcinomas begin earlier and behave more aggressively in patients with HIV infection. Clinically, this means that formal excisional biopsy of suspicious eyelid lesions should be performed with histopathological examination of all specimens. Careful follow-up of positive skin lesions should be performed.

Lymphoma

Non-Hodgkin's lymphoma is common in HIV infection.[70] The lymphomas are derived from B-cells and the majority have evidence of Epstein-Barr viral infection suggesting a role for this infection in the generation of these lymphomas in patients with HIV infection.[71] The lymphomas are usually high-grade immunoblastic, Burkitt's type (small non cleaved) or large cell lyphomas. Lymphoma in HIV infection commonly presents as primary cerebral lymphoma with ocular manifestations, rarely with primary intraocular lymphoma and rarely with ocular involvement from systemic extranodal lymphoma. Cerebral lymphoma presents clinically and radiologically like cerebral toxoplasmosis, with signs and symptoms of raised intracranial pressure and focal neurological signs according to the site of involvement.

The eye and visual system may be involved in a number of ways by cerebral lymphoma (see also chapter 7). Acute raised intracranial pressure leads to the development of papilloedema and sixth cranial nerve palsies. Focal neurological syndromes typical of lymphoma may result in homonymous visual field defects from involvement of the posterior visual pathways. Brainstem involvement produces cranial nerve palsies or gaze disorders such as one and half syndromes and internuclear ophthalmoplegia. Neuroimaging demonstrates single or multiple ring-enhancing mass lesions within the brain. Diagnosis may be confirmed by stereotactic biopsy in selected patients, malignant cells on cerebrospinal fluid examination or failure of response to a trial of adequate toxoplasmosis therapy. Cerebral lymphoma has a poor prognosis. It is unresponsive to systemic chemotherapy and makes a variable short-lived response to systemic corticosteroids and radiation therapy. Lymphoma leads to death from involvement of vital structures.

The eye may rarely be the site of origin of primary lymphoma or may be involved by spread of systemic lymphoma. Primary lymphoma tends to involve initially the retina and vitreous, whereas systemic lymphoma usually spreads to the choroid prior to retinal involvement. Primary intraocular lymphoma may present with signs similar to that of viral retinitis, with vascular occlusions and a frosted angiitis or with isolated vitreous cellular infiltration.[32] The clinical signs are non-specific and may mimic opportunistic infections such as CMV retinitis or toxoplasmosis very closely. A failure of response to appropriate antimicrobial therapy or clinical signs which seem unusual or out-of-keeping with the presumed clinical diagnosis should alert the clinician to the possibility of lymphoma. Vitreous and endoretinal biopsy are required to make the diagnosis. Ocular lymphoma usually responds well to radiation therapy.

Primary intraocular lymphoma is virtually always associated with cerebral lymphoma which may be clinically silent at the time of ocular presentation. Neuroimaging and cerebrospinal fluid studies are essential for looking for central nervous system lymphoma. It may be necessary to look for evidence of systemic lymphoma in other patients.

Orbital Aspergillosis

Chronic sinus infection with aspergillus is common and most patients develop chronic mucosal non-invasive infection or allergic disease.[72] A small number of patients develop tissue invasive or fulminant aspergillus infection.[73] HIV infection is recognised as one of the predisposing factors for such tissue invasive infection and is usually lethal.

The clinical presentation depends upon the rapidity of spread and may range from slowly developing proptosis with a mass lesion and bony sinus destruction to rapidly progressive orbital cellulitis and ischaemic optic neuropathy.[72,74] Fulminant infection spreads rapidly to involve the meninges and brain. Aspergillus organisms invade blood vessels readily and produce an occlusive vasculitis that leads to widespread infarction and necrosis of involved orbital and central nervous system tissue.[75] Involvement of the brain is almost always fatal despite aggressive treatment.

A wide range of unusual fungi and bacteria may cause a similar clinical picture, as may tumors and orbital pseudotumours. Management involves obtaining good-quality imaging studies of the orbits and sinuses, ENT consultation, biopsy of involved tissue, if possible, and other medical consultation as indicated. Surgical drainage and orbital biopsy may be necessary for diagnostic and therapeutic purposes. Aggressive antimicrobial therapy is needed.

Optic Neuropathy

There are clinical reports of subtle visual field abnormalities in HIV-infected patients without signs of other ocular disease and pathological reports of optic nerve axon loss without obvious cause.[76] These field defects are clinically asymptomatic. There is no evidence to suggest that these diseases are directly the result of HIV infection, and at this time the cause is unknown.

The clinical syndrome of optic neuritis may occur from involvement by a number of different disease processes including CMV neuroretinitis, cryptococcal optic neuropathy, syphilitic perineuritis, hepatitis B-or C-induced optic neuropathy, and optic neuritis associated with herpetic retinitis. There is also a form of optic neuritis that presents as demyelinating optic neuritis with visual loss, abnormal colour vision, pain on eye movement, and a normal fundus. Both optic nerves are affected. The presentation, clinical course and neuropathology are similar to that of the optic neuritis of multiple sclerosis. The benefit of systemic corticosteroid therapy for this form of optic neuritis remains uncertain at this time. Treatment with antiretroviral therapy may be of benefit to patients with demyelinating optic neuropathy.

References

1. Stewart G.J., Irvine S.S., Scott M. *et al.* "Strategies of care in managing HIV," in: Stewart G.J. (Ed.), *Managing HIV.*, Australasian Medical Publishing Company, Sydney (1997).

2. Cooper D.A., Gold J., Maclean P. *et al.* "Acute AIDS retrovirus infection. Definition of a clinical illness associated with seroconversion," *Lancet* **1** (1985), 537–540

3. Ulirsch R.C., Jaffe E.S. "Sjogren's syndrome like illness associated with the acquired immunodeficiency syndrome-related complex," *Hum. Pathol.* **18** (1987), 1063–1068.

4. Kaye B.R. "Rheumatologic manifestations of infection with human immunodeficiency virus (HIV)," *Ann. Intern. Med.* **111** (1989), 158–163.

5. McCluskey P.J. "Intermediate uveitis," in: Lightman S., Towler H.M.A. (Eds.), *Uveitis.*, London, BMA Books (1998).

6. McCluskey P.J., Hall A.J., Lightman S. "HIV related eye disease," *Med. J Aust.* **164** (1996), 484–486.

7. Newman N.J., Lessell S. "Bilateral optic neuropathies with remission in two HIV positive men," *J. Clin. Neuroophthalmol.* **12** (1992), 1–5.

8. Dwyer D.E., Adelstein S., Cunningham A.L. *et al.* "The laboratory in monitoring HIV infection," in: Stewart G. (Ed.). *Managing HIV*, Australasian Medical Publishing Company, Sydney (1997).

9. Kestylen P., de Perre P.V., Sprecher-Goldberger S. "Isolation of the human T cell leukaemia/lymphotropic virus III from aqueous humour in two patients with perivasculitis of the retinal vessels," *Int. Ophthalmol.* **9** (1986), 247–251.

10. Srinivasan A., Kalyanaraman S., Dutt K. *et al.* "Isolation of HIV 1 from vitreous humour," *Am. J. Ophthalmol.* **108** (1989), 197–198.

11. Fujikawa L.S., Salahuddin S.Z., Palestine A.G. *et al.* "Isolation of T lymphotropic virus type III from the tears of a patient with the acquired immunodeficiency syndrome," *Lancet* **2** (1985), 529–530.

12. Laycock K.A., Pepose J.S. "HIV infection and AIDS: Background and recent developments," in: Stenson S.M., Friedberg D.N. (Eds.), *AIDS and the Eye*, Contact Lens Association of America, New orleans (1995).

13. Whitcup S.M., Butler K.M., Caruso R. *et al.* "Retinal toxicity in human immunodeficiency virus infected children treated with 2,2-dideoxyyinosine," *Am. J. Ophthalmol.* **113** (1992), 1–7.

14. Jacobs D.S., Piliero P.J., Kuperwaser M.G. "Acute uveitis associated with rifabutin use in patients with human immunodeficiency virus infection," *Am. J. Ophthalmol.* **118** (1994), 716–722.

15. Davis J.L., Taskintuna I., Freeman W.R. *et al.* "Iritis and hypotony after treatment with intravenous cidofovir for cytomegalovirus retinitis," *Arch. Ophthamol.* **115** (1997), 733–737.

16. Ng P., McCluskey P.J., McCaughan G. *et al.* "Ocular complications of heart, lung and liver transplantation," *Br. J. Ophthalmol.* **82** (1998), 423–428.

17. Carr A., Penny R. "Human immunodeficiency virus infection and acquired immunodeficiency syndrome," in: Bradley J., McCluskey J. (Eds.), *Clinical Immunology*, Oxford University Press (1997).

18. Chan H.L., Stern R.S., Arndt K.A. *et al.* "The incidence of erythema multiforme, Stevens-Johnson syndrome and toxic epidermal necrolysis: A population based study with particular reference to reactions caused by drugs among outpatients," *Arch. Dermatol.* **126** (1990), 43–47.

19. Bianchine J.R., Macaraeg P.V.G., Lasagna L. *et al.* "Drugs as aetiology factors in Stevens-Johnson Syndrome," *Am. J. Med.* **44** (1968), 390–405.

20. Asby D.W., Lazar T., "Erythema multiforme major (Stevens-Johnson syndrome)," *Lancet* i (1951),1091–195.

21. Coster D.J. "Stevens-Johnson syndrome," in: *Cicatrising Conjunctivitis* Bernauer W., Dart J.K.G., Elder M.J. (Eds), Basel, Karger (1997).

22. Wright P. Collin J.R. "The ocular complications of erythema multiforme (Stevens-Johnson syndrome) and their management," *Trans. Ophthalmol. Soc. UK* **103** (1983), 338–341.

23. Coster D.J., Williams K.A. "The surgical management of ocular surface disorders using conjunctival and stem cell allografts," *Br. J. Ophthalmol.* **79** (1995), 977–982.

24. McCluskey P.J. "HIV related eye disease," *Med. J. Aust.* **153** (1993), 111–113.

25. Itescu S., Brancato L.J., Buxbaum J. *et al.* "A diffuse infiltrative CD8 lymphocytosis in human immunodeficiency virus infection: A host immune response associated with HLA DR 5," *Ann. Intern. Med.* **112** (1990), 3–10.

26. Berger T.G., Veronique H., King C. *et al.* Itraconazole therapy for HIV associated eosinophilic folliculitis," *J. Am. Acad. Dermatol.* (1997).

27. Keat A. "Reiter's syndrome and reactive arthritis in perspective," *N. Engl. J. Med.* **39** (1983), 1606–1615.

28. Winchester R., Bernstein D.H., Fischer H.D. "The co-occurrence of Reiter's syndrome in acquired immunodeficiency," *Ann. Intern. Med.* **106** (1987), 19–26.

29. Lee D.A., Barker S.M., Su W.P.D. *et al.* "The clinical diagnosis of Reiter's syndrome," *Ophthalmol.* **93** (1986), 350–356.

30. Wakefield D., Montanaro A., McCluskey P.J. "Acute anterior uveitis and HLA B27," *Surv. Ophthalmol.* **36** (1991), 223–232.

31. Rosenbaum J.T. "HLA B27 Associated diseases," in: Pepose J.S., Holland G.N., Wilhelmus K.R. (Eds.), Ocular Infection and Immunity, St Louis, Mosby (1996).

32. McCluskey P.J., Wakefield D. "Posterior uveitis in the acquired immunodeficiency syndrome," *Int. Ophthalmol. Clin.* **35** (1995), 1–14.

33. Woods S.L., Wakefield D., McCluskey P.J. "The acquired immune deficiency syndrome: Ocular findings and infection control guidelines," *Aust. NZ J. Ophthalmol.* **14** (1986), 287–291.

34. Kupperman B.D., Petty J.G., Richman D.D. *et al.* "Correlation between CD4+ counts and the prevalence of cytomegalovirus retinitis and human immunodeficiency virus related non infectious vasculopathy in patients with acquired immunodeficiency syndrome," *Am. J. Ophthalmol.* **115** (1993), 575–582.

35. Pepose J.S., Holland G.N., Nestor M.S. *et al.* "Acquired immune deficiency syndome: Pathogenic mechanisms of ocular disease," **92** (1985), 472–484.

36. Jabs D.A., Quinn T.C. *Acquired Immunodeficiency Syndrome in Ocular Infection and Immunity*, Pepose J.S., Holland G.N., Wilhelmus K.R. (Eds.), St Louis, Mosby (1996).

37. Nussenblatt R.B., Lane H.C. "Human immunodeficiency virus disease: changing patterns of intraocular inflammation," **125** (1998), 374–382.

38. Teich S.A. "Conjunctival vascular changes in AIDS and AIDS related complex," *Am. J. Ophthalmol.* **103** (1987), 332–333.

39. Aristimuno B., Nirankari V.S., Hemady R.K. *et al.* "Spontaneous ulcerative keratitis in immunocompromised patients," *Am. J. Ophthalmol.* **115** (1993), 202–208.

40. Hersh P.S., Zagelbaum B., Sachs R. *et al.* "Corneal ulcers associated with the use of crack cocaine," *Ophthalmology.* **98** (1991), p. 104.

41. Stenson S.M. "Anterior segment manifestations of AIDS," in: Stenson S.M., Friedberg D.N. (Eds.), *AIDS and the Eye*. Contact Lens Association of New Orleans, Los Angeles, America, (1995).

42. Shuler J.D., Engstrom R.E., Holland G.N. "External ocular disease and anterior segment disorders associated with AIDS," *Int. Ophthalmol. Clin.* **29** (1989), 98–104.

43. Charles N.C., Friedberg D.N. "Epibulbar molluscum contagiosum in acquired immune deficiency syndrome," *Ophthalmology* **99** (1992), 1123–1126.

44. Liesegang T. "The biology and molecular aspects of herpes simplex and varicella zoster virus infections," *Ophthalmology* **98** (1992), 1216–1229

45. Kestelyn P., Stevens A.M., Bakkers E. *et al.* "Severe herpes zoster ophthalmicus in young african males: A marker for HTLV III seropositivity," *Br. J. Ophthalmol.* **71** (1987), 806–809.

46. Holland G.N. "Acquired immunodeficiency syndrome and ophthalmology: The first decade," *Am. J. Ophthalmol.* **114** (1992), 86–95.

47. Leisegang T.J. "Varicella zoster virus: Systemic and ocular features," *J. Am. Acad. Dermatol.* **11** (1984), 165–173.

48. Leisegang T.J. "Herpes zoster ophthalmicus," *Int. Ophthalmol. Clin.* **25** (1985), 77–96.

49. Cobo L.M., Foulks G.N., Leisgang T. *et al.* "Oral acyclovir in the treatment of acute herpes zoster ophthalmicus," *Ophthalmology* **93** (1986), 763–768.

50. Keczkes K., Basheer A. "Do corticosteroids prevent post herpetic neuralgia?" *Br. J. Ophthalmol.* **101** (1980), 551–557.

51. Esmann V., Geil J.P., Kroon S. *et al.* "Prednisolone does not prevent post herpetic neuralgia," *Lancet* **2** (1987), 126–130.

52. Threlkeld A.B., Eliot D., O'Brien T.P. "Scleritis associated with varicella zoster disciform stromal keratitis," *Am. J. Ophthalmol.* **113** (1992), 721–722.

53. Tuft S.J., Watson P.G. "Progression of scleral disease," *Ophthalmology.* **98** (1991), 467–471.

54. Leisegang T.J. "Corneal complications from herpes zoster ophthalmicus," *Ophthalmology.* **92** (1985), 316–321.

55. Womack L., Leisegang T.J. "Complications of herpes zoster ophthalmicus," *Arch. Ophthalmol.* **101** (1983), 42–49.

56. Marsh R.J., Easty D., Jones B. "Iritis and iris atrophy in herpes zoster ophthalmicus," *Am. J. Ophthalmol.* **78** (1974), 255–259.

57. Culbertson W.W., Atherton S.S. "Acute retinal necrosis and similar retinitis syndromes," *Ophthalmology.* **33** (1993), 129–143.

58. Marsh R.J., Dudley B., Kelly V. "External ocular motor palsies in ophthalmic zoster: A review," *Br. J. Ophthalmol.* **61** (1977), 677–682.

59. Osler B. "Herpes simplex: The primary infection," *Surv. Ophthalmol.* **21** (1976), 91–99.

60. Leisegang T.J. "Epidemiology of ocular herpes simplex: Natural history in Rochester Minn 1950 through 1982," *Arch. Ophthalmol.* **107** (1989), 1160–1165.

61. Hodge W.G., Margolis T.P. "Herpes simplex virus keratitis among patients who are positive or negative for human immunodeficiency virus: An epidemiologic study," *Ophthalmology.* **104** (1997), 120–124.

62. Pepose J.S., Leib D.A., Stuart M., Easty D. "Herpes simplex virus diseases: Anterior segment of the eye," in: *Ocular Infection and Immunity*, St Louis, Mosby (1996).

63. The herpetic eye disease study group, "Acyclovir for the prevention of recurrent herpes simplex eye disease," *N. Engl. J. Med.* (1998), 300–306.

64. Kornguth S.E., Klien R., Appen R. *et al.* "Occurrence of antiretinal ganglion cell antibodies in patients with small cell carcinma of the lung," *Cancer* **50** (1982), 1289–1292.

65. Keltner J.L., Roth A.M., Chang R.S. "Photoreceptor degeneration: Possible autoimmune disorder," *Arch. Ophthalmol.* **101** (1983), 564–569.

66. Berson E.L. Lessel S. "Paraneoplastic night blindness with malignant melanoma," *Am. J. Ophthalmol.* **106** (1988), 307–310.

67. Keltner J.L., Thirkill C.E., Roth A.M. "Autoimmune related retinopathy and optic neuropathy (Aaron syndrome)," *Invest. Ophthalmol. Vis. Sci.* 29 (1988), 178–181.

68. Thirkill C.E., Tait R.C., Tyler N.K. *et al.* "The cancer associated retinopathy antigen is a recoverin like protein," *Invest. Ophthalmol. Vis. Sci.* 33 (1992), 2768–2772.

69. Adamus G., Aptsiauri N., Guy J. *et al.* "Antienolase antibodies in cancer associated retinopathy," *Invest. Ophthalmol. Vis. Sci.* 34 (1993), 1485–1489.

70. National AIDS registry. *Australian HIV Surveillance Report* 11 (1995), P.22.

71. Levine A. "Acquired immunodeficiency syndrome related lymphoma," *Blood* 80 (1992), 8–20.

72. Sarti E.J., Lucente F.E. "Aspergillosis of the paranasal sinuses," *J. Ear Nose Throat* 67 (1988), 824–831.

73. Stein D.K., Sugar A.M. "Fungal infections in the immunocompromised host," *Diagn. Microbiol. Infect. Dis.* 12 (1989), 221S–228S.

74. Hedges T.R., Leung L.E. "Parasellar and orbital apex syndrome caused by aspergillosis," *Neurology* 26 (1976), 117–120.

75. Weinstein J.M., Morris G.L., ZuRhein G.M. *et al.* "Posterior ischaemic optic neuropathy due to aspergillus fumigatus," *J. Clin. Neuro-ophthalmol.* 9 (1989), 7–13.

76. Quiceno J.I., Capparelli E., Sadun A.A. *et al.* "Visual dysfunction without retinitis in patients with acquired immunodeficiency syndrome," *Am. J. Ophthalmol.* 113 (1992), 8–13.

CHAPTER 3

OVERVIEW OF HIV/AIDS OCULAR MANIFESTATIONS

Douglas A Jabs

Introduction

Ocular findings are common in patients with AIDS, and the majority will develop some type of ocular involvement. The most frequently encountered ocular finding is microangiopathy, which is most often detected in the retina. This microangiopathy has been referred to as "AIDS retinopathy", "HIV retinopathy", or "non-infectious HIV retinopathy". Opportunistic ocular infections, particularly cytomegalovirus (CMV) retinitis, are the primary causes of visual morbidity. Ocular and orbital structures may also be affected by neoplasms such as Kaposi's sarcoma and lymphoma, neurophthalmic lesions, and drug-related side effects from the drugs used for treating patients with HIV infection (see Table 3.1).

Ocular Microangiopathy

Ocular microangiopathy is the most frequently encountered ocular finding in patients with AIDS.[1-8] It is most often recognised in the retina and consists of cotton wool spots (see Fig. 3.1) and, less frequently, intraretinal haemorrhages.[1-5] Retinal microangiopathy is detected clinically in approximately one-half of patients with AIDS, but in less than 1% of patients with asymptomatic HIV infection.[1,5] HIV retinopathy is associated with low CD4 T-cell counts, particularly <100 cells/μl.[6,7] A higher frequency of microangiopathy (as high as 90% of patients) has been suggested by fluorescein angiographic studies and autopsy studies, but these studies are subject to selection bias.[3,4] Although less often recognised, conjunctival microangiopathy is also present and may occur as frequently as retinal microangiopathy.[8]

61

Table 3.1. Ocular manifestations of AIDS.

Lesion	Estimated Frequency (%)
Microangiopathy	
Conjunctival	75
Retinal	50–67
Opportunistic ocular infections	30
Cytomegalovirus retinitis	
Varicella-zoster virus	3–4
Herpes zoster ophthalmicus	<1
VZV retinitis	1–3
Toxoplasmic retinitis	<1
Pneumocystis choroidopathy	<1
Microsporidial keratitis	<1
Ocular syphilis	
Ocular neoplasms	1–4
Kaposi's sarcoma (lids, conjunctiva)	<1
Lymphoma (orbital, intraocular)	5–10
Neurophthalmic lesions	

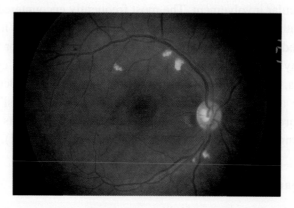

Fig. 3.1 Non-infectious retinal microangiopathy ("HIV retinopathy") in a patient with AIDS, manifested by cotton wool spots. (Taken from Jabs D.A.[1] with permission.)

Although the pathogenesis of the ocular microangiopathy is unknown, there have been three hypotheses: (1) circulating immune complex disease;[2-4] (2) infection of the retinal vasculature by HIV;[9] and (3) haemorheologic abnormalities.[10] Immune complex deposition disease such as pathogenesis of the retinal microangiopathy has been suggested by the presence of polyclonal B-cell activation in patients with AIDS, circulating immune complexes in patients with AIDS, and the finding of immunoglobulin deposition in the retinal vessels.[2,4,11,12] Although HIV infection of the retinal vascular endothelial cells has been demonstrated, some authors have argued that the amount of HIV infection is inadequate to account for the retinal vasculopathy.[3,13] Haemorheologic abnormalities have been associated with HIV microangiopathy, but their origin remains unclear.[10]

Clinically, HIV retinopathy is asymptomatic and does not appear to have a clinically evident effect on visual function.[1] However, subtle abnormalities of visual function, such as colour vision, contrast sensitivity, and automated perimetry, have been reported in patients with AIDS.[14,15] Autopsy studies have reported a loss of optic nerve fibers, and it has been speculated that this loss of optic nerve fibers and subtle abnormalities of visual function may be due to a cumulative insult from the microangiopathy.[16] Alternatively, these findings may be due to a direct HIV-related toxic effect on the optic nerve.

Occasionally, patients will have larger vessel retinal disease, such a branch vein occlusion or a central retinal vein occlusion.[1] Whether or not the frequency of this finding is increased in patients with AIDS as compared to the general population is uncertain.

Opportunistic Ocular Infections

Cytomegalovirus Retinitis

Epidemiology

CMV retinitis is the most common opportunistic ocular infection in patients with AIDS.[17] Prior to the advent of HAART, it was estimated that approximately 30% of patients would develop CMV retinitis sometime between the diagnosis of AIDS and death.[18–20] Although other organs may be affected by CMV, including the brain, lungs, and gastrointestinal tract, CMV retinitis accounts for 75% to 85% of all CMV disease in patients with AIDS.[19,20]

CMV retinitis is a late-stage manifestation of AIDS, typically associated with CD4 T-cell counts <50 cells/µl.[19–21] Prior to the use of HAART, the incidence of CMV retinitis among patients with CD4 T-cell counts <100 cells/µl was estimated at 10% per year and among patients with CD4 T-cell counts <50 cells/µl at 20% per year.[19,21] By 1996 combination antiretroviral therapy including the use of protease inhibitors, also known as HAART, had resulted in at least a 50% decrease in the incidence of CMV retinitis in major urban medical centres throughout the US.[22] HAART therapy results in improved immune function and substantial rises in CD4 T-cell counts in many patients, and this improved immune function has decreased the proportion of patients with very low CD4 T-cell counts, thereby decreasing the cohort of patients at risk for CMV retinitis. A similar but much more modest and more short-lived drop in the incidence of

CMV retinitis was seen when zidovudine was first introduced — an observation consistent with this hypothesis and the more modest effect of zidovudine monotherapy on HIV disease.[22]

CMV is a focal necrotising retinitis, which may or may not contain haemorrhages (see Fig. 3.2). Untreated CMV retinitis spreads throughout the retina over a period of several months resulting in total retinal destruction and blindness.[23] Although CMV retinitis may be associated with symptoms such as floaters, flashing lights, loss of visual field, or a vague sense of visual impairment, CMV retinitis may also be asymptomatic. Two studies have estimated the prevalence of asymptomatic and undiagnosed CMV retinitis at 13% to 15% of patients with CD4 T-cell counts <50 cells/μl.[7,24] Therefore, some experts have recommended routine evaluation of patients at high risk for CMV retinitis by an ophthalmologist in order to detect early asymptomatic disease. However, this approach is not universally accepted, and no long-term outcome studies have been performed to validate it. For those experts who recommend screening, patients with CD4 T-cell counts <50 cells/μl are typically seen every three to four months, patients with CD4 T-cell counts between 50 and 100 cells/μl twice annually, and those with CD4 T-cell counts >100 cells/μl (who are low risk for the development of CMV retinitis) only once annually.

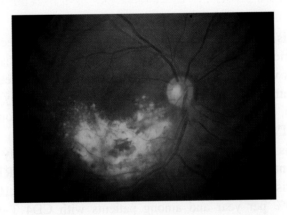

Fig. 3.2 Cytomegalovirus retinitis in a patient with AIDS. (Taken from Jabs D.A.[1] with permission.)

Treatment

The goal of treatment of CMV retinitis is to arrest the progression of the disease, minimise the amount of retinal damage, and preserve vision. Treatment with anti-CMV agents suppresses viral replication but does not eliminate the virus.[25] Therefore, discontinuation of therapy (at least in those patients who have not had immune reconstitution) results in prompt relapse of the retinitis.[26] Hence, long-term suppressive therapy has been required. However, there have been case reports of patients with CMV retinitis who have been treated with HAART, resulting in an improved immune function and have been able to discontinue anti-CMV agents and maintain successful control of the retinitis.[27,28] These case reports suggest that in some patients, immune reconstitution may result in adequate control of the retinitis and obviate the need for anti-CMV agents, at least until the immune system begins to fail once again. Conversely, there have been case reports of patients started on HAART, who have had large increases in CD4 T-cell counts, and then subsequently developed CMV retinitis.[29] These case reports suggest that selective immunity to CMV is not restored in all patients who have increased CD4 T-cell counts as a consequence of HAART and that not all patients can have medication discontinued. What proportion of patients responding to HAART can have anti-CMV drugs discontinued remains to be determined. For detailed description of treatment see chapter 6.

Ocular Toxoplasmosis

Epidemiology

In the US infection of the eye by *Toxoplasma gondii* occurs in approximately 1% of patients with AIDS, whereas in other countries where the baseline of seroprevalence of antibodies to *Toxoplasma gondii* is higher, a higher frequency of ocular toxoplasmosis has been reported.[1,30] For example, in France the frequency was reported at 3%.[30] Although ocular toxoplasmosis may occur at any stage of HIV infection, it is most often seen in patients with CD4 T-cell counts <100 cells/μl.[1,30-34] Concurrent toxoplasmic ocular encephalitis has been reported to occur in 29% to 56% of patients with AIDS and toxoplasmosis.[1,30] Patients with AIDS may develop ocular toxoplasmosis as either a primary infection or a metastatic focus of another source.[31] Patients with cerebral toxoplasmosis have been reported to have detectable Toxoplasma organisms in the blood, suggesting a mechanism for dissemination to other parts of the body.[35] In one large series of patients with ocular toxoplasmosis, only 4% of HIV-infected patients with toxoplasmic retinitis had retinal scars to suggest a local reactivation, and 12% had positive IgM antibodies suggesting a primary infection with *Toxoplasma gondii*.[30]

Clinical features

The clinical appearance of ocular toxoplasmosis in patients with AIDS (see Fig. 3.3) is variable, although the typical picture of a focal, white, full-thickness necrotising retinitis may be seen.[1] Patients may also have a diffuse necrotising retinitis, which can be mistaken for CMV disease,[32] or rarely a multifocal "miliary" appearance.[34] Vitritis and anterior uveitis are common but are not required for the diagnosis.

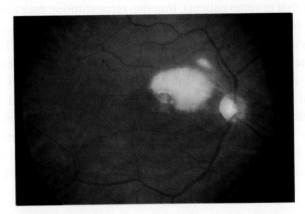

Fig. 3.3 Ocular toxoplasmosis in a patient with AIDS. (Taken from Jabs D.A.[1] with permission.)

Treatment

Most cases of toxoplasmosis retinitis in patients with AIDS respond to standard anti-toxoplasma treatment within four to six weeks. Regimens typically include pyrimethamine, sulfadiazine and/or clindamycin.[1] In the past, long-term maintenance therapy was typically required to prevent relapse of the disease. What effect HAART will have on the need for maintenance therapy in patients with ocular toxoplasmosis remains to be determined. Oral corticosteroid therapy, often given to immunocompetent hosts with ocular toxoplasmosis to reduce the "innocent bystander" damage to the retina is not needed in patients with AIDS. The infection responds well to antibiotics alone. The widespread use of oral cotrimoxazole as primary prophylaxis for *Pneumocystis carinii* pneumonia appears to have decreased the frequency of ocular toxoplasmosis in patients with AIDS.[22]

Varicella-Zoster Virus Retinitis

Epidemiology, clinical features and treatment

Varicella-zoster virus may affect the retina (see Fig. 3. 4), and the frequency of varicella-zoster virus retinitis is estimated at 0.6% of HIV-infected patients.[1,36–42] In HIV-infected patients, varicella-zoster virus retinitis may occur as one of two clinical syndromes. The first is the acute retinal necrosis, similar to that seen in immunologically normal hosts, which can occur at any stage of HIV infection.[1,38–42] This variant of varicella zoster virus retinitis can be successfully managed with intravenous aciclovir at a dosage of 500 mg/m^2 every eight hours for ten to 14 days, followed by long-term suppression with oral aciclovir.[36]

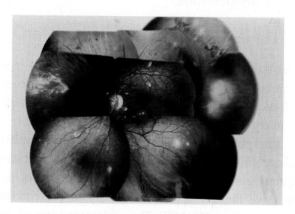

Fig. 3.4 Varicella-zoster retinitis in a patient with AIDS. The patient also had a small area of cytomegalovirus retinitis nasally. (Taken from Jabs D.A.[1] with permission.)

The second clinical syndrome of varicella-zoster virus retinitis is seen only in HIV-infected patients and occurs in patients with CD4 T-cell counts typically <50 cells/µl. It is sometimes known as the progressive outer retinal necrosis syndrome (PORN).[38–42] This variant is characterised by multifocal retinal lesions, which progress very rapidly, and is associated with little or no intraocular inflammation. Approximately two-thirds of these patients have bilateral disease, and the disease often begins in the posterior pole and involves the optic nerve. This variant of varicella-zoster virus retinitis does not appear to respond to intravenous aciclovir or other single-agent treatments.[1] Anecdotal reports have suggested that combination foscarnet and intravenous aciclovir may be effective in controlling the retinitis.[1,42] However, retinal detachments occur in approximately 70% of patients with this syndrome and often result in a poor visual outcome.[1]

Pneumocystis Choroidopathy

Epidemiology

Pneumocystis choroidopathy was first described in 1989.[43] It is an uncommon infection, clinically occurring in less than 1% of patients with AIDS, but it accounted for 22% of infectious choroidopathies identified in one autopsy series.[44] Most patients with *Pneumocystis carinii* choroidopathy have a history of *Pneumocystis carinii* pneumonia,[44] and in one aggregate series from several centres, 86% of patients with *Pneumocystis carinii* choroidopathy received aerosolised pentamidine as their Pneumocystis prophylaxis.[46] Pneumocystis choroidopathy typically is associated with other extra-pulmonary lesions and may be the initial and/or only sign of dissemination.[44]

Clinical features and treatment

The Pneumocystis lesions are one-third to two disc diameters in size, are creamy yellow to white in colour, round or oval, and located at the level of the choroid (see Fig. 3.5).[46] Typically they are multifocal, bilateral, and present in the posterior pole and midperiphery of the retina. There is no overlying vitritis. Pathologically, an eosinophilic, amorphic, acellular foamy infiltrate is identified in the inner choroid and choriocapillaris.[43,44] *Pneumocystis carinii* choroidopathy responds to systemic cotrimoxazole, pentamidine, or dapsone alone, or in combination.[46] Life-long maintenance therapy appears necessary to prevent recurrence unless the patient responds well to HAART. The widespread use of cotrimoxazole as the preferred prophylaxis for *Pneumocystis carinii* pneumonia has resulted in an apparent decrease in the frequency of Pneumocystis choroidopathy.[22]

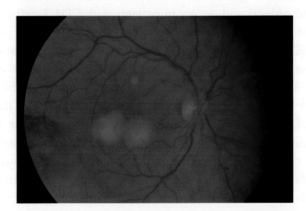

Fig. 3.5 Pneumocystis choroidopathy in a patient with AIDS. (Taken from Jabs D.A.[1] with permission.)

Microsporidial keratoconjunctivitis

Microsporidial keratoconjunctivitis is caused by the eukaryotic obligate intracellular protozoa of the Encephalitozoon species, usually *E. hellum* or *E. cuniculi*. It is an uncommon manifestation occurring in substantially less than 1% of patients with AIDS.[1,47-50] Clinically, it is characterised by a fine to coarse corneal punctate epitheliopathy associated with conjunctival hyperemia.[47-50] Agents of activity against these parasites include fumagillin, itraconazole, propamidine isethionate, and the benzimidazoles.[47-50] Topical fumagillin (Fumadil B) at a concentration of 3 mg/ml, installed hourly for one week and then tapered over several weeks, appears to be very effective. Although the required duration of therapy remains undefined, the persistence of spores with therapy suggests that indefinite suppressive therapy is needed.

Other Ocular Infections

Bacterial Infections

Ocular syphilis

The most common bacterial eye infection in HIV-infected patients is ocular syphilis, which may occur at any stage of HIV infection.[1,51-55] The ocular manifestations include iridocyclitis, retinitis, neuroretinitis, panuveitis, papillitis, perineuritis, and retrobulbar optic neuropathy.[51-55] However, 90% of HIV-infected patients present with uveitis as their primary ocular manifestations.[55] Although many patients with ocular syphilis are staged clinically as secondary syphilis, approximately two-thirds of the patients will have a positive CSF-VDRL and/or neurologic disease.[51-55] All patients with syphilitic uveitis should undergo a lumbar puncture and be treated with an antibiotic regimen for neurosyphilis.[55] In HIV-infected patients, this regimen is typically 24 million units of penicillin per day intravenously for ten to 14 days, with or without three subsequent doses of intramuscular penicillin.

Mycobacterial Infections

Mycobacterial infection of the choroid with *Mycobacterium tuberculosis* or *Mycobacterium avium* complex has been demonstrated on autopsy studies.[1,45,56,57] Clinically, these lesions are uncommon.[1] There are case reports of choroidal granulomata due to *Mycobacterium tuberculosis* producing disease.[56,57] One study estimated that only 5% of patients with active tuberculosis and HIV infection had clinical evident ocular lesions.[1] In those countries where tuberculosis is common among HIV-infected patients, the number of cases of ocular tuberculosis may be substantially greater.

Fungal Infections

Candida endophthalmitis

Candida retinitis and/or endophthalmitis is uncommon and has been reported to occur in less than 1% of patients with AIDS. Most HIV-infected patients with Candida endophthalmitis appear to be intravenous drug users, and the Candida infection related to intravenous drug use rather than to AIDS itself.[1]

Cryptococcal choroiditis

Infection of the eye with *Cryptococcus neoformans* is uncommon, occurring in less than 1% of patients with AIDS.[1] However, it has been reported to occur in 2.5% of patients with systemic cryptococcosis and as much as 6% of patients with cryptococcal meningitis.[58–60] Clinically, cryptococcal lesions of the choroid are deep, hypopigmented or yellow-white, often multifocal, and range in size from one-fifth to one disc diameter (see Fig. 3.6).[1,44,58-60] Pathologically, these lesions involve the choriocapillaris and inner choroidal vessels.[44] Treatment of cryptococcal infection with amphotericin or fluconazole results in clearing of the choroidal lesions, as well as the systemic disease. With treatment these lesions decrease in size and fade in colouration.[1,44,58]

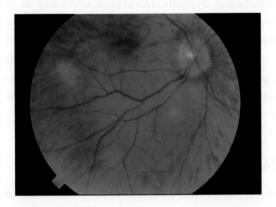

Fig. 3.6 Cryptococcal choroiditis in a patient with AIDS.

Other fungal infections

There have been isolated case reports both clinically and at autopsy of choroidal infection with *Histoplasma capsulatum* and *Aspergillus fumigatus*.[45,61,62] The clinical appearance of the Histoplasma lesions have been described as creamy-white, small (one-quarter disc diameter or less) lesions with distinct borders and occasional halos or haemorrhage.[61,62] The relative infrequency of case reports of these disorders suggests that these infections are quite uncommon.[1]

Viral Infections

Herpes zoster ophthalmicus

HZO has been reported to occur in 3% to 4% of patients with HIV infection at any stage of HIV disease.[1,62-64] Ocular complications have been reported in 49% of patients with HZO managed with antiviral agents, such as aciclovir. The most common complications are keratitis (26%), uveitis (23%), and scleritis (6%). The frequency of ocular complications does not appear to be substantially greater than that reported in non-HIV-infected patients with HZO.[1] However, in HIV-infected patients, HZO may cause a widespread necrotising and destructive cutaneous problem, resulting in damage to the eyelids and long-term problems with corneal exposure (see also chapters 2 and 4). In HIV-infected patients, HZO responds to standard treatments, including aciclovir and famciclovir. Some immune compromised HIV-infected patients may require intravenous aciclovir as opposed to oral aciclovir for severe ocular involvement, and chronic viral suppressive therapy may be required.

Herpes simplex keratitis

HSK does not appear to be more common in HIV-infected patients than in the general population.[1] However, when it does occur, it may be atypical, more severe, and take a longer time to heal. Therefore, a longer treatment course may be required.

Ocular Neoplasms

Kaposi's Sarcoma

Prior to the AIDS epidemic, KS was a rare conditions occurring in specific populations, particularly in elderly men of Mediterranean origin, African children, and renal transplant recipients. With the advent of the AIDS epidemic, a dramatic increase in KS was seen among men having sex with other men and was identified as one of the manifestations of AIDS. The disease had an aggressive course and a high frequency of visceral involvement. Although men who have sex with other men still represents the vast majority of patients with AIDS and

KS, cases have been described in other risk groups as well. Ocular involvement by KS has been reported in 15% to 22% of patients with AIDS and KS elsewhere, resulting in an overall frequency of 2% of patients with AIDS.[1,65-68] KS generally presents with multiple red to violet macules, papules, and/or nodules, and either the eyelids or conjunctiva may be involved. The characteristic pathologic findings on biopsy include bands of spindle cells and vascular structures embedded in collagen and reticular fibers.

Conjunctival KS may not require treatment. The lesions are slow growing, do not invade the eye, and often do not affect the vision. Conversely, eyelid involvement by KS often requires therapy as it causes functional problems with the eyelid and impairs vision. A variety of techniques have been successfully employed, including local excision, cryotherapy, radiation therapy, and local or systemic chemotherapy.[65-68]

Lymphoma

In patients with HIV infection, high-grade lymphoma is an AIDS-defining disorder. Orbital and intraocular involvement by lymphoma in patient with AIDS have been reported, but they appear to be uncommon and occur in less than 1% of patients with AIDS.[1,69-72] The clinical appearance of intraocular lymphoma is multifocal, yellow-white, multiple chorioretinal lesions associated with vitritis. Intraocular lymphoma may be associated with primary central nervous system lymphoma.[69,71]

Neurophthalmic Lesions

Neurophthalmic lesions have been reported in 5% to 10% of patients with AIDS.[1,5] The reported lesions include cranial nerve palsies, papilledema, optic neuropathy, hemianopsias, and cortical blindness[1,73-83] (see chapter 7). The most common aetiology for these neurophthalmic lesions in patients with AIDS is cryptococcal meningitis, which accounts for up to 54% of neurophthalmic lesions.[1] Of patients with AIDS and cryptococcal meningitis, approximately 25% will have a neurophthalmic lesion, most commonly papilledema.[1,58] Visual loss from cryptococcal meningitis occurs in 1% to 9% of patients, either due to direct invasion of the optic nerve by cryptococcus, elevated intracranial pressure, or adhesive arachnoiditis.[1,58,76-78] Other common causes of neurophthalmic lesions include herpes zoster ophthalmicus, syphilis, viral encephalitis, and central nervous system lymphoma.

Subtle ocular motility defects, including slowed saccades, fixational instability, and abnormal pursuit, also can be seen in patients with AIDS.[79-81] These lesions typically are detected by eye movement recordings using infrared oculography. They appear to be related to the HIV infection itself and not to opportunistic infections. It has been suggested that these subtle ocular motor defects may correlate with the severity of the AIDS dementia complex.[81] Although lacking definitive proof, case reports of optic neuropathies in HIV-infected patients have been described, which are without another obvious cause. These have been described as HIV optic neuropathy.[1,82,83]

Drug-Related Ocular Side Effects

Rifabutin Uveitis

Rifabutin is an antimycobacterial agent used largely as primary prophylaxis for *M. avium* complex infections. Its use has been associated with the development of uveitis.[84-89]

The uveitis has a variable severity but may mimic infectious endophthalmitis and present with a hypopyon. Rifabutin-associated uveitis may be seen in association with a rifabutin-associated polyarthralgia/polyarthritis syndrome,[84] but may also develop on its own. Fluconazole and clarithromycin, which raise the serum levels of rifabutin, have been described as cofactors for rifabutin-associated uveitis. 39% of 59 patients receiving rifabutin at 600 mg/day, clarithromycin, and ethambutol for the treatment of *M. avium* complex infections in the MAC Study Group of the Canadian HIV Trials Network developed iridocyclitis.[84] The incidence appears to be substantially lower with the more typical 300 mg/day dose. Rifabutin uveitis responds well to topical corticosteroids and discontinuing rifabutin or reducing the dose.

Cidofovir Uveitis

Intravitreous cidofovir has been given as an investigational treatment for CMV retinitis. The typical dose is 20 μg given every five to six weeks.[90,91] However, the 100 μg dose has been associated with uveitis, severe hypotony, and loss of vision. Even with the 20 μg dose, 14% of patients given intravitreous cidofovir injections developed iritis, which generally can be managed by topical corticosteroid therapy.[90-92]

Uveitis also has been associated with intravenous cidofovir therapy.[92] In one study, as many as 26% of patients treated with intravenous cidofovir developed uveitis and 9% developed hypotony.[92] In these patients, loss of vision was associated with the hypotony as well. Most patients were successfully managed with topical corticosteroids and cycloplegics, although intravenous cidofovir had to be discontinued in some patients. Although the reported frequency in this study may suffer from selection bias, patients receiving intravenous cidofovir should be monitored regularly for the occurrence of cidofovir-associated uveitis.

Other Reported Ocular Toxicity

Drugs associated with ocular toxicity in non-immunosuppressed patients, such as ethambutol, also may have similar toxicity profiles in patients with HIV infection. Clofazamine, which has been used to treat *M. avium* complex disease, has been associated with a bull's eye maculopathy in a single case report.[93] Didanosine (ddI), a nucleoside reverse transcriptase inhibitor, used to treat HIV, has been reported to cause retinal pigment epithelialopathy in children treated with high-dose ddI therapy.[94] In this report, 7% of children developed well-circumscribed areas of retinal pigment epithelial atrophy in the midperiphery.[94] However, no such toxicity has been reported in adults treated with didanosine. There is a single case report of zidovudine-associated cystoid macular oedema.[95]

References

1. Jabs D.A. "Ocular manifestations of HIV infection," *Trans. Am. Ophthalmol. Soc.* **93** (1995), 623–683.

2. Holland G.N., Pepose J.S., Petit T.H. *et al.* "Acquired immune deficiency syndrome. Ocular manifestations," *Ophthalmology* **90** (1983), 859–873.

3. Newsome D.A., Green W.R., Miller E.D. *et al.* "Microvascular aspects of acquired immune deficiency syndrome retinopathy," *Am. J. Ophthalmol.* **98** (1984), 590–601.

4. Pepose J.S., Holland G.N., Nestor M.S. *et al.* "Acquired immune deficiency syndrome. Pathogenic mechanisms of ocular disease," *Ophthalmology* **92** (1985), 472–484.

5. Jabs D.A., Green W.R., Fox R. *et al.* "Ocular manifestations of acquired immune deficiency syndrome," *Ophthalmology* **96** (1989), 1092–1099.

6. Freeman W.R., Chen A., Henderly D.E. *et al.* "Prevalence and significance of acquired immunodeficiency syndrome-related retinal microvasculopathy," *Am. J. Ophthalmol.* **107** (1989), 229–335.

7. Kuppermann B.D., Petty J.G., Richman D.D. *et al.* "Correlation between CD4 counts and prevalence of cytomegalovirus retinitis and human immunodeficiency

virus-related noninfectious retinal vasculopathy in patients with acquired immunodeficiency syndrome," *Am. J. Ophthalmol.* **115** (1993), 575–582.

8. Teich S.A. "Conjunctival vascular changes in AIDS and AIDS-related complex," *Am. J. Ophthalmol.* **103** (1987), 332–333.

9. Pomerantz R.J., Kuritzkes D.R., de-la-Monte S.M. *et al.* "Infection of the retina by human immunodeficiency virus type I," *N. Engl. J. Med.* **317** (1987), 1643–1647.

10. Engstrom R.E., Holland G.N., Hardy W.D. *et al.* "Haemorheologic abnormalities in patients with human immunodeficiency virus infection and ophthalmic microvasculopathy," *Am. J. Ophthalmol.* **109** (1990), 153–161.

11. Lane H.C., Masur H., Edgar L.C. *et al.* "Abnormalities of B-cell activation and immunoregulation in patients with the acquired immunodeficiency syndrome," *N. Engl. J. Med.* **309** (1983), 453–458.

12. Gupta S., Licorish K. "Circulating immune complexes in AIDS," *N. Engl. J. Med.* **310** (1984), 1530–1531.

13. Faber D.W., Wiley C.A., Lynn G.B. *et al.* "Role of HIV and CMV in the pathogenesis of retinitis and retinal vasculopathy in AIDS patients," *Invest. Ophthalmol. Vis. Sci.* **33** (1992), 2345–2353.

14. Quiceno J.I., Capparelli E., Sadun A.A. *et al.* "Visual dysfunction without retinitis in patients with acquired immunodeficiency syndrome," *Am. J. Ophthalmol.* **113** (1992), 8–13.

15. Geier S.A., Hammel G., Bogner J.R. "HIV-related ocular microangiopathic syndrome and color contrast sensitivity," *Invest. Ophthalmol. Vis. Sci.* **35** (1994), 3011–3021.

16. Tenhula W.N., Xu S., Madigan M.C. *et al.* "Morphometric comparisons of optic nerve loss in aquired immunodeficiency syndrome," *Am. J. Ophthalmol.* **113** (1992), 14–20.

17. Moore R.D., Chaisson R.E. "Natural history of opportunistic disease in an HIV-infected urban clinical cohort" *Ann. Intern. Med.* **124** (1996), 633–642.

18. Hoover D.R., Saah A.J., Bacellar H. *et al.* "Clinical manifestations of AIDS in the era of Pneumocystis prophylaxis," *N. Engl. J. Med.* **329** (1993), 1922–1926.

19. Gallant J.E., Moore R.D., Richman D.D. *et al.* "Incidence and natural history of cytomegalovirus disease in patients with advanced human immunodeficiency virus disease treated with zidovudine. The Zidovudine Epidemiology Group," *J. Infect. Dis.* **166** (1992), 1223–1227.

20. Hoover D.R., Peng Y., Saah A. *et al.* "Occurrence of cytomegalovirus retinitis after human immunodeficiency virus immunosuppression," *Arch. Ophthalmol.* **114** (1996), 821–827.

21. Pertel P., Hirschtick R., Phair J. *et al.* "Risk of developing cytomegalovirus retinitis in persons infected with the human immunodeficiency virus," *J. Acquir. Immune Defic. Syndr.* **5** (1992), 1069–1074.

22. Jabs D.A., Bartlett J.G. "AIDS and ophthalmology: A period of transition," *Am. J. Ophthalmol.* **124** (1997), 227–233.

23. Jabs D.A., Enger C., Bartlett J.G. "Cytomegalovirus retinitis and acquired immunodeficiency syndrome," *Arch. Ophthalmol.* **107** (1989), 75–80

24. Baldassano V., Dunn J.P., Feinberg J. *et al.* "Cytomegalovirus retinitis and low CD4 T-lymphocyte counts," *N. Engl. J. Med.* **333** (1995), 670.

25. Pepose J.S., Newman C., Bach M.C. *et al.* "Pathologic features of cytomegalovirus retinopathy after treatment with the antiviral agent ganciclovir," *Ophthalmology* **94** (1987), 414–424.

26. Jacobson M.A., O'Donnell J.J., Brodie H.R. *et al.* "Randomized prospective trial of ganciclovir maintenance therapy for cytomegalovirus retinitis," *J. Med. Virology.* **25** (1988), 339–349.

27. Whitcup S.M., Fortin E., Mussenblatt R.B. *et al.* "Therapeutic effect of combination antiretroviral therapy on cytomegalovirus retinitis [letter]," *JAMA* **277** (1997), 1519–1520.

28. Reed J.B., Schwab I.R., Gordon J. *et al.* "Regression of cytomegalovirus retinitis associated with protease-inhibitor treatment in patients with AIDS," *Am. J. Ophthalmol.* **124** (1997), 199–205.

29. Jacobson M.A., Mitchell S.M., Youle M.S. *et al.* "Cytomegalovirus retinitis after initiation of highly active antiretroviral therapy," *Lancet* **349** (1997), 1443–1445.

30. Cochereau-Massin I, LeHoang P., Lautier-Frau M. *et al.* "Ocular toxoplasmosis in human immunodeficiency virus- infected patients," *Am. J. Ophthalmol.* **114** (1992), 130–135.

31. Holland G.N., Engstrom R.E. Jr., Glasgow B.J. *et al.* "Ocular toxoplasmosis in patients with the acquired immunodeficiency syndrome," *Am. J. Ophthalmol.* **106** (1988), 653–667.

32. Parke D.W., Font R.L. "Diffuse toxoplasmic retinochoroiditis in a patient with AIDS," *Arch. Ophthalmol.* **104** (1986), 571–575.

33. Weiss A., Margo C.E., Ledford D.K. *et al.* "Toxoplasmic retinochoroiditis as an initial manifestation of the acquired immune deficiency syndrome," *Am. J. Ophthalmol.* **101** (1987), 248–249.

34. Berger B.B., Egwuagu C.E., Freeman W.R. *et al.* "Miliary toxoplasmic retinitis in acquired immunodeficiency syndrome," *Arch. Ophthalmol.* **111** (1993), 373–376.

35. Lamoril J., Molina J.M., De-Gouvello A. *et al.* "Detection by PCR of *Toxoplasma gondii* in blood in the diagnosis of cerebral toxoplasmosis in patients with AIDS," *J. Clin. Pathol.* **49** (1996), 89–92.

36. Jabs D.A., Schachat A.P., Liss R. *et al.* "Presumed varicella zoster retinitis in immunocompromised patients," *Retina* **7** (1987), 9–13.

37. Sellitti T.P., Huang A.J.W., Schiffman J. *et al.* "Association of herpes zoster ophthalmicus with acquired immunodeficiency syndrome and acute retinal necrosis," *Am. J. Ophthalmol.* **116** (1993), 297–301.

38. Forster D.J., Dugel P.U., Frangieh G.T. *et al.* "Rapidly progressive outer retinal necrosis in the acquired immunodeficiency syndrome," *Am. J. Ophthalmol.* **110** (1990), 341–348.

39. Johnston W.H., Holland G.N., Engstrom R.E. *et al.* "Recurrence of presumed varicella-zoster virus retinopathy in patients with acquired immunodeficiency syndrome," *Am. J. Ophthalmol.* **116** (1993), 42–50.

40. Margolis T.P., Lowder C.Y., Holland G.N. *et al.* "Varicella-zoster virus retinitis in patients with the acquired immunodeficiency syndrome," *Am. J. Ophthalmol.* **112** (1991), 119–131.

41. Engstrom R.E., Jr., Holland G.N., Margolis T.P. *et al.* "The progressive outer retinal necrosis syndrome. A variant of necrotizing herpetic retinopathy in patients with AIDS," *Ophthalmology* **101** (1994), 1488–1502.

42. Morley M.G., Duker J.S., Zacks S. "Successful treatment of rapidly progressive outer retinal necrosis in the acquired immunodeficiency syndrome," *Am. J. Ophthalmol.* **117** (1994), 264–265.

43. Rao N.A., Zimmerman P.L., Boyer D. *et al.* "A clinical, histopathologic, and electron microscopic study of *Pneumocystis carinii* choroiditis," *Am. J. Ophthalmol.* **107** (1989), 218–228.

44. Morinelli E.N., Dugel P.U., Riffenburgh R. *et al.* "Infectious multifocal choroiditis in patients with acquired immune deficiency syndrome" *Ophthalmology* **100** (1993), 1014–1021.

45. Dugel P.U., Rao N.A., Forster D.J. *et al.* "*Pneumocystis carinii* choroiditis after long-term aerosolized pentamidine therapy," *Am. J. Ophthalmol.* **110** (1990), 113–117.

46. Shami M.J., Freeman W., Friedberg D. *et al.* "A multicenter study of Pneumocystis choroidopathy," *Am. J. Ophthalmol.* **112** (1991), 15–22.

47. Friedberg D.N., Stenson S.M., Ornstein J.M. *et al.* "Microsporidial keratoconjunctivitis in acquired immunodeficiency syndrome," *Arch. Ophthalmol.* **108** (1990), 504–508.

48. Lowder C.Y., Meisler D.M., McMahon J.T. *et al.* "Microsporidia infection of the cornea in a man seropositive for human immunodeficiency virus," *Am. J. Ophthalmol.* **109** (1990), 242–244.

49. Metcalfe T.W., Doran R.M.L., Rowlands P.L. *et al.* "Microsporidial keratoconjunctivitis in a patient with AIDS," *Brit. J. Ophthalmol.* **76** (1992), 177–178.

50. Rastrelli P.D., Didier .E, Yee R.W. "Microsporidial keratitis," *Ophthalmol. Clin. N. Am.* **7** (1994), 617–633.

51. Passo M.S., Rosenbaum J.T. "Ocular syphilis in patients with human immunodeficiency virus infection," *Am. J. Ophthalmol.* **106** (1988), 1–6.

52. Carter J.B., Hamill R.J., Matoba A.Y. "Bilateral syphilitic optic neuritis in a patient with a positive test for HIV," *Arch. Ophthalmol.* **105** (1987), 1485–1486.

53. Becerra L.I., Ksiasek S.M., Savino P.J. *et al.* "Syphilitic uveitis in human immunodeficiency virus-infected and noninfected patients," *Ophthalmology* **96** (1989), 1727–1730.

54. McLeish W.M., Pulido J.S., Holland S. *et al.* "The ocular manifestations of syphilis in the human immunodeficiency virus type 1-infected host," *Ophthalmology* **97** (1990), 196–203.

55. Shalaby I.A., Dunn J.P., Semba R.D. *et al.* "Syphilitic uveitis in human immunodeficiency virus-infected patients," *Arch. Ophthalmol.* **115** (1997), 469–473.

56. Croxatto J.O., Mestre C., Puente S. *et al.* "Nonreactive tuberculosis in a patient with acquired immune deficiency syndrome," *Am. J. Ophthalmol.* **105** (1986), 659–660.

57. Blodi B.A., Johnson M.W., McLeish W.M. *et al.* "Presumed choroidal tuberculosis in a human immunodeficiency virus infected host," *Am. J. Ophthalmol.* **108** (1989), 605–607.

58. Kestelyn P., Taelman H., Bogaerts J. *et al.* "Ophthalmic manifestations of infections with *Cryptococcus neoformans* in patients with the acquired immunodeficiency syndrome," *Am. J. Ophthalmol.* **116** (1993), 721–727.

59. Carney M.D., Coombs J.L. "Cryptococcal choroiditis," *Retina* **10** (1990), 27–32.

60. Charles N.C., Boxrud C.A., Small E.A. "Cryptococcosis of the anterior segment in acquired immune deficiency syndrome," *Ophthalmology* **99** (1992), 813–816.

61. Specht C.S., Mitchell K.T., Bauman A.E. *et al.* "Ocular histoplasmosis with retinitis in a patient with acquired immune deficiency syndrome," *Ophthalmology* **98** (1991), 1356–1359.

62. Macher A., Rodrigues M.M., Kaplan W. *et al.* "Disseminated bilateral chorioretinitis due to *histoplasma capsulatum* in a patient with the acquired immunodeficiency syndrome," *Ophthalmology* **92** (1985), 1159–1164.

63. Cole E.L., Meisler D.M., Calabrese L.H. *et al.* "Herpes zoster ophthalmicus and acquired immune deficiency syndrome," *Arch. Ophthalmol.* **102** (1984), 1027–1029.

64. Sandor E.V., Millman A., Croxson S. *et al.* "Herpes zoster ophthalmicus in patients at risk for the acquired immune deficiency syndrome (AIDS)." *Am. J. Ophthalmol.* **101** (1986), 153–155.

65. Schuler J.D., Holland G.N., Miles S.A. *et al,* "Kaposi sarcoma of the conjunctiva and eyelids associated with the acquired immunodeficiency syndrome," *Arch. Ophthalmol.* **107** (1989), 858–862.

66. Dugel P.U., Gill P.S., Frangieh G.T. *et al.* "Ocular adnexal Kaposi's sarcoma in acquired immunodeficiency syndrome," *Am. J. Ophthalmol.* **119** (1990), 500–503.

67. Dugel P.U., Gill P.S., Frangieh G.T. *et al.* "Treatment of ocular adnexal Kaposi's sarcoma in acquired immunodeficiency syndrome," *Ophthalmology* **99** (1992), 1127–1132.

68. Ghabrial R., Quivey J.M., Dunn J.P., Jr, *et al.* "Radiation therapy of acquired immunodeficiency syndrome-related Kaposi's sarcoma of the eyelids and conjunctiva," *Arch. Ophthalmol.* **110** (1992), 1423–1426.

69. Schanzer M.C., Font R.L., O'Malley R.E. "Primary ocular malignant lymphoma associated with the acquired immune deficiency syndrome," *Ophthalmology* **98** (1991), 88–91.

70. Antle C.M., White V.A., Horsman D.E. *et al.* "Large cell orbital lymphoma in a patient with acquired immune deficiency syndrome. Case report and review," *Ophthalmology* **97** (1990), 1494–1498.

71. Stanton C.A., Sloan III D.B., Slusher M.M. *et al.* "Acquired immunodeficiency syndrome-related primary intraocular lymphoma," *Arch. Ophthalmol.* **110** (1992), 1614–1617.

72. Matzkin D.C., Slamovits T.L., Rosenbaum P.S. "Simultaneous intraocular and orbital non-Hodgkin lymphoma in the acquired immune deficiency syndrome," *Ophthalmology* **101** (1994), 850–855.

73. Keane J.R. "Neuro-ophthalmologic signs of AIDS: 50 patients," *Neurology* **41** (1991), 841–845.

74. Mansour A.M. "Neuro-ophthalmic findings in acquired immunodeficiency syndrome," *J. Clin. Neuro-ophthalmol.* **10** (1990), 167–174.

75. Winward K.E., Hamed L.M., Glaser J.S. "The spectrum of optic nerve disease in human immunodeficiency virus infection," *Am. J. Ophthalmol.* **107** (1989), 373–380.

76. Lipson B.K., Freeman W.R., Beniz J. *et al.* "Optic neuropathy associated with cryptococcal arachnoiditis in AIDS patients," *Am. J. Med.* **107** (1989), 523–527.

77. Rex J.H., Larsen R.A., Dismukes W.E. *et al.* "Catastrophic visual loss due to *Cryptococcus neoformans* meningitis," *Medicine* **72** (1993), 207–224.

78. Cohen D.B., Glasgow B.J. "Bilateral optic nerve cryptococcosis in sudden blindness in patients with acquired immune deficiency syndrome," *Ophthalmology* **100** (1993), 1689–1694.

79. Hamed L.M., Schatz N.J., Galetta S.L. "Brainstem ocular motility defects in AIDS," *Am. J. Ophthalmol.* **106** (1988), 437–442.

80. Nguyen N., Rimmer S., Katz B. "Slowed saccades in the acquired immunodeficiency syndrome," *Am. J. Ophthalmol.* **107** (1989), 356–360.

81. Currie J., Benson E., Ramsden B. *et al.* "Eye movement abnormalities as a predictor of the acquired immunodeficiency syndrome dementia complex," *Arch. Neurology.* **45** (1988), 949–953.

82. Sweeney B.J., Manji H., Gilson R.J.C. *et al.* "Optic neuritis and HIV-1 infection," *J. Neurol. Neurosurg. Psych.* **56** (1993), 705–707.

83. Newman N., Lessell S. "Bilateral optic neuropathies with remission in two HIV-1 positive men," *J. Clin. Neuro-ophthalmol.* **12** (1992), 1–5.

84. Shafran S.D., Deschenes J., Miller M.E. *et al.* "The MAC Study Group of the Canadian HIV Trials Network: Uveitis and pseudojaundice during a regimen of clarithromycin, rifabutin and ethambutol," *N. Engl. J. Med.* **330** (1994), 438–439.

85. Jacobs D.S., Piliero P.J., Kupperwaser M.G. *et al.* "Acute uveitis associated with rifabutin use in patients with human immunodeficiency virus infection," *Am. J. Ophthalmol.* **118** (1994), 716–722.

86. Rifai A., Peyman G.A., Daun M. *et al.* "Rifabutin-associated uveitis during prophylaxis for *Mycobacterium avium* complex infection," *Arch. Ophthalmol.* **113** (1995), P. 707.

87. Karbassi M., Nikou S. "Acute uveitis in patients with acquired immunodeficiency syndrome receiving prophylactic rifabutin," *Arch. Ophthalmol.* **113** (1995), 699–701.

88. Saran B.R., Maguire A.M., Nichols C. *et al.* "Hypopyon uveitis in patients with acquired immunodeficiency syndrome treated for systemic *Mycobacterium avium* complex infection with rifabutin," *Arch. Ophthalmol.* **112** (1994), 1159–1165.

89. Siegal F.P., Eilbott D., Burger H. *et al.* "Dose-limiting toxicity of rifabutin in AIDS-related comples: Syndrome of arthralgia/arthritis," *AIDS* **4** (1990), 433–441.

90. Kirsch L.S., Arevalo J.F., De-Clercq E. *et al.* "Phase I/II study of intravitreal cidofovir for the treatment of cytomegalovirus retinitis in patients with the acquired immunodeficiency syndrome," *Am. J. Ophthalmol.* **119** (1995), 466–476.

91. Davis J.L., Taskintuna I., Freeman W.R. *et al.* "Iritis and hypotony after treatment with intravenous cidofovir for cytomegalovirus retinitis," *Arch. Ophthalmol.* **115** (1997), 733–737.

92. Rahhal F.M., Arevalo J.F., Chavez-De-La Paz E. *et al.* "Treatment of cytomegalovirus retinitis with intravitreous cidofovir in patients with AIDS. A preliminary report," *Ann. Intern. Med.* **125** (1996), 98–103.

93. Cunningham C.A., Friedberg D.N., Carr R.E. "Clofazimine-induced generalized retinal degeneration," *Retina* **10** (1990), 131–134.

94. Whitcup S.M., Butler K.M., Caruso R. *et al.* "Retinal toxicity in human immunodeficiency virus-infected children treated with 2,3-dideoxyinosine," *Am. J. Ophthalmol.* **113** (1992), 1–7.

95. Lalonde R.G., Deschenes J.G., Seamone C. "Zidovudine-induced macular edema," *Ann. Intern. Med.* **114** (1991), 297–298.

CHAPTER 4

OCULAR SURFACE, ANTERIOR SEGMENT, ADNEXAL AND ORBITAL DISORDERS IN AIDS

Andrew B Tullo

Introduction

When the nature and consequence of infection with HIV was first recognised, it might have been predicted that the ocular surface would be a likely site of opportunistic infection, as there are many organisms which cause disease in the cornea and conjunctiva of the immunocompetent individual. The fact that this is not often the case is of considerable interest. It supports the understanding that protective mechanisms other than those dependent on cell-mediated immunity are likely to play a dominant role in protecting the ocular surface. These mechanisms include blinking, tear irrigation as well as factors found in the tears such as lactoferrin, lysozyme and immunoglobulins.[1,2]

A number of studies have looked for alterations in the ocular surface physiology of patients with AIDS.[3] Whilst tear secretion may alter, no differences were observed in the ocular flora between HIV-negative patients and patients with AIDS, even including those with diminished tear production.[4]

Recent work has begun to reveal the special mechanisms which confer immunological privilege on the eye. For example, the ability of receptors in corneal cells to cause potentially damaging T-cells to undergo apoptosis[5] in the immunocompetent individual may explain why the severe depletion of CD4 cells seen in AIDS does not profoundly alter the response to infection in the anterior segment. The increasing sophistication of laboratory tests, including the use of PCR, and the accessibility of the eye for biopsy, has led to problematic interpretation of results particularly when dealing with agents which cannot be easily grown in the laboratory.[6] Indeed, difficulty has already been faced in the interpretation of the presence of HSV DNA in the cornea[7] in immunocompetent individuals using PCR. Nevertheless, it is these recent developments that were responsible for the realisation that AIDS-related Kaposi's sarcoma was likely to be caused by a transmissible agent other than HIV, before the likely causative agent was subsequently identified.[8]

Infection with HIV may present the unexpected opportunity to test a hypothesis. The involvement of EBV has been suspected in the pathogenesis of keratoconjunctivitis sicca[9] However, when this agent was sought in the tears of patients with AIDS with and without symptoms of dry eye, it was not found, though HIV itself was usually present.[10]

Reviews on the anterior eye in AIDS,[11–14] including this one, are of necessity based on little more that collections of case studies. The advent of HAART (see chapter 1) may diminish the task at least in the intermediate term or perhaps modify further the clinical features. This chapter will also include manifestations in the anterior segment, adnexae and orbits in HIV infection, which are also sites of infrequent involvement and where the clinical signs may be unusual.

Ocular Surface Disorders

Conjunctival Microangiopathy

Microvascular changes in the bulbar conjunctiva may be present in 75% of patients with AIDS[15] and are similar to those seen in sickle-cell disease. They include irregular calibre and course, microaneurysms, telangiectasiae and poor flow (see Fig. 4.1). Comparisons have been drawn between these changes and those seen in the retina.[16–18] The suggestion that changes are due to infection of vascular endothelial cells by HIV has yet to be proven, as has the clinical significance of these changes. It will be of interest to see if the recent improved management of HIV infection with HAART, which can result in significant reduction of the blood viral load, has any influence on the time of onset and degree of conjunctival vascular changes.

Dry Eye

The prevalence of dry eye in AIDS patients is said to be as high as 40%. The conventional criteria of tear break-up time, corneal and conjunctival staining, and the Schirmer's test, are often abnormal in AIDS patients who, if symptomatic, usually respond to tear replacement therapy. Signs and symptoms do not appear to be related to CD4 counts.[19–211] Punctal occlusion with silicone plugs may not be suitable as infection with these has already been reported in patients who are immunocompetent.[22] For the obviously symptomatic patient who is a contact lens wearer, it would seem sensible to reduce lens wearing time or cease their use altogether.

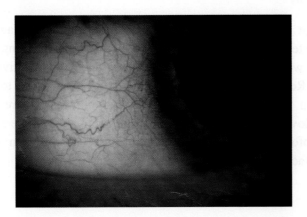

Fig. 4.1 Conjunctival vessels showing tortuosity, irregular calibre, telangiectasiae and poor flow.

Infection

Herpes simplex keratitis

The incidence, pathogenesis and clinical features of HSK have been extensively discussed in the ophthalmic literature. Experience of HSK in immunosuppressed kidney transplant patients suggested that the condition may indeed be more common and more severe.[23] An initial report[24] suggested that HSK may be similarly influenced in patients with AIDS, i.e. with larger and more peripheral corneal lesions occuring. However, the number of cases was limited and no control group was used. More recently, however, in a larger study it was concluded that HSK in patients with AIDS and AIDS-related complex was no different in both terms of incidence and response to treatment when compared to a non-immunocompromised control group of hospital-based patients,[25] but the overall recurrence rates were significantly higher amongst the HIV-positive group. If it is assumed that after a first episode of HSK, a site of chronic or latent infection is established, the higher rate of recurrence suggests that immunosuppression by HIV infection may impair those mechanisms which are normally responsible for controlling such an infection.[25]

An investigation of possible or probable HSK should ideally be by culture. Topical acycloguanosine (aciclovir) is the treatment of choice, but interferon has also been suggested[26] following its successful use in a 15-year-old patient with bilateral disease who failed to respond to antiviral agents despite the isolate showing *in vitro* drug sensitivity.

Cytomegalovirus

CMV has not been described as a cause of ocular surface disease in immunocompetent individuals, and only rarely in AIDS.[27] Single cases have been reported which include infection of the caruncle, conjunctiva and bilateral keratitis.[28-29] Recognition of this type of infection may prove to be important as it is known from experience with CMV retinitis that the response of this agent to aciclovir is poor. The newer purines and pyrimidine derivatives, in particular cidofovir, may find a useful role as a broad-spectrum antiviral agent in ocular surface disease in AIDS (see chapter 6).

Adenovirus

Adenoviral infection is not normally associated by ophthalmologists with sexually transmitted diseases. However, in a large prospective study of patients attending a sexually transmitted disease clinic, several patients were found to have both genital and conjunctival infection with adenovirus type 37.[30] This serotype belongs to the same subgenus D which also includes the ocular epidemic types 8, 10 and 19.[31] In addition, type 8 itself has been recovered from the urine of one HIV-positive patient and from multiple sites including the eye of another.[32] It, therefore, seems prudent to remain alert to the possibility of adenovirus as a cause of oculogenital disease in both HIV-positive and HIV-negative patients, not least because it is from AIDS patients that the new serotypes also classified as belonging to subgenus D, have been identified.[33]

Bacterial Infection

The list of bacteria that can cause corneal infection in immunocompetent patients is extensive. Those that have been reported as a cause of microbial conjunctivitis and keratitis in AIDS[34-35] are, as yet, limited (see Table 4.1) and to date no organism has emerged which is characteristic in AIDS. Infection with *Pseudomonas aeruginosa* may be especially fulminant with and without contact lens wear[36-37] and when the patient is neutropenic, the severity of disease may be enhanced.[38] In the largest series to date, unusual features of bilaterality, recurrence, and polymicrobial infection were identified in a group of 13 patients all but one of whom were intravenous drug abusers.[39]

Table 4.1 Causes of bacterial keratitis reported in HIV-infected or AIDS patients. [13]

- *Pseudomonas aeruginosa*
- *Staphylococcus aureus*
- *Staphylococcus epidermidis*
- α-Streptococcus
- *Neisseria gonorrhoea*
- α-Hemolytic streptococcus
- Capnocytophagia
- Bacillus
- Micrococcus

Fungal Infection

The initial report of a spontaneous fungal corneal ulcer suggested that this relatively rare condition in the West might occur without anticedent ocular surface disease or a dirty injury.[40] In a series of four HIV-positive patients (all were young female intravenous drug abusers) with microbial keratitis, three eyes were infected with *Candida albicans*.[41] Cryptococcal keratitis has been described in a 30-year-old man with AIDS who also had cryptococcal meningitis and disseminated cutaneous lesions,[42] whilst conjunctival granuloma due to cryptococcus was reported in a prostitute before she subsequently became seropositive to HIV.[43]

Any microbial keratitis in patients with HIV and AIDS should be vigorously investigated by culture, as response to appropriate treatment is often good.

Protozoal Infection

Chronic diarrhoea and weight loss commonly complicate the late stages of HIV infection. The most common causative agents are coccidia, which includes microsporidia. Although microsporidia has been recognised as an animal pathogen, it was virtually unknown as a human agent until the HIV epidemic.[44] It is of interest that coccidia which are obligate intracellular protozoal parasites and include toxoplasma and cryptosporidia, are commonly encountered in HIV infection. However, microsporidia have been reported to cause ocular surface disease particularly in patients with low CD4 counts, but in addition have also been reported as a cause of keratoconjunctivitis in patients not infected with HIV.[45-46] Ocular features range from mild conjunctivitis to punctate corneal epithelial keratopathy.[47-49] This is characteristically a bilateral coarse epithelialopathy with white infiltrates and may affect vision. Culture is difficult but identification of Gram-positive intracytoplasmic organisms and PAS-positive granules together with help from immunofluorescence and electron microscopy are all useful.[50-51]

The presence of microsporidia in the conjunctiva and/or cornea is likely to be associated with infection of the urinary and respiratory tracts and in particular, the nasal sinuses. Consequently, systemic rather than local treatment may well be required, e.g with Albendazole.[52] Successful topical treatments described include Propamidine and Fumagillin,[49,53,54] which need to be given intensively.

Pneumocystis carinii, which is common in patients with AIDS, may spread to the choroid and also the orbit. It has recently been reported as the cause of a placoid-like lesion of the tarsal conjunctiva in a 33-year-old homosexual man with total CD4 depletion.[55] The effect of treatment could not be evaluated before he died.

Neoplasia

Squamous cell neoplasia

The contribution of the papilloma virus in the causation of cervical cancer is widely recognised though its contribution to ocular surface neoplasia seem less certain.[56-57] When a viral aetiology is suspected it might have been expected that immunocompromise would have led to an increase in ocular surface neoplasia. Interestingly reports of such lesions in HIV patients have so far been limited almost exclusively to African patients (see chapter 9).[58-60] In one patient a necrotising scleritis was associated with the lesion.[61]

Others

Corneal transplantation

It has been appreciated for some time that HIV can be found in the corneas of HIV-infected patients.[62-63] Although there are no reported cases of seroconversion of the graft recipient despite inadvertent transmission from seropositive donors,[63] it is now standard practice to screen all donors for HIV as well as Hepatitis B and C (Eye Bank Association of America Medical Standards and European Eye Bank Association Directory, 1998). Surrogate markers such as syphilis and social history are deemed inadequate.[64]

Stevens-Johnson syndrome (SJS)

SJS has been reported as a result of treatment with dapsone and trimethoprim-sulphamethoxazole as well as others in HIV-infected patients. Despite profound immunosuppression and alteration in cell-mediated immunity, AIDS may paradoxically allow the development of particularly severe SJS and toxic epidermal necrolysis including the ocular features.[65-66]

Calcification

The eyes of three patients with AIDS were found at postmortem to have an unusual corneal and scleral calcarious degeneration. Calcium deposits were present in the corneal stroma but the Bowman's layer was spared, as is usually seen in primary and secondary corneal calcification. The calcified areas were positive to von Kossa, alizarin red, alcian blue, and colloidal iron stains. Electron probe analysis of the three cases showed the presence of calcium and phosphorus in a ratio characteristic for hydroxyapatite. No predisposing factors could be found. The possible role of associated alterations in the mucopolysaccharide content or composition in the calcified areas is unclear.[67]

Epitheliopathy

A form of corneal epithelial phospholipidosis confirmed by electron microscopy, has been described in two patients in which ganciclovir and aciclovir given systemically are implicated.[68]

Anterior Segment

Patients with AIDS can present with anterior segment abnormalities that may occur either as a consequence of their disease or its treatment.

Anterior Uveitis

Asymptomatic linear and stellate corneal endothelial deposits forming a reticular pattern (with or without an accompanying iritis) are found in over 80% of patients with CMV retinitis.[69-70] Although the corneal features are essentially pathognomonic for the presence of CMV retinitis, they are not adequately sensitive and do not resolve after effective treatment.

Cidofovir is a potent, long-acting, anti-CMV drug which is used in the treatment of CMV retinitis (see chapter 6). Anterior uveitis (see Fig. 4.2) and hypotony, the risks of which are dose dependant, have been described following both intravitreal[71] and intravenous[72] injection of cidofovir. These adverse events occur secondary to a toxic effect of cidofovir on the non-pigmented epithelium of the ciliary body. The concomitant use of oral probenecid (in patients not allergic to sulfa derivatives) competitively inhibits the uptake of cidofovir into the non-pigmented epithelium of the ciliary body and significantly decreases the incidence of iritis and hypotony.

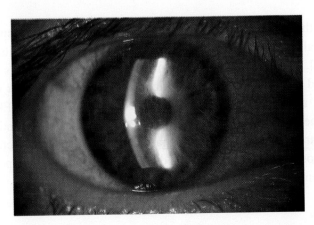

Fig. 4.2 Anterior uveitis caused by intravenous Cidofovir and characterised by plastic exudate and iris hyperaemia.

Rifabutin is used in the prophylaxis and treatment of MAI infection.[73] 15% of patients taking rifabutin will develop a reversible, dose-related, topical corticosteroid-responsive, anterior uveitis. The co-administration of macrolides and azoles increases the risk of uveitis developing. One patient who developed anterior uveitis was also found to have retinal vasculitis.[74]

Infection

Cryptococcus is a rare form of human ocular infection which usually occurs in immunocompromised individuals and which typically affects the posterior segment (see chapter 5). Intraocular cryptococcosis presented in one AIDS patient with an iris inflammatory mass and secondary glaucoma.[75]

Disseminated histoplasmosis in an HIV-positive patient is an AIDS-defining illness; fortunately, ocular involvement occurs rarely (see chapter 5). The treatment of ocular infection with cryptococcus and/or histoplasmosis includes the administration of systemic and intraocular amphoteracin-B possibly combined with vitrectomy when the patient has endophthalmitis.[76]

Tuberculosis (TB) is the most common opportunistic infection affecting HIV-positive patients in the developing world (see chapter 9). The anterior segment manifestations of tuberculous ocular disease are protean and include granulomatous keratic precipitates, anterior chamber inflammation, and iris nodules.[14] Ocular TB should be treated under the guidance of an infectious disease specialist, using a regimen appropriate for central nervous system involvement with TB.

There is a higher incidence and earlier presentation of ocular syphilis and neurosyphilis in HIV-positive patients (see also chapter 5).[77] Anterior segment manifestations of syphilis are similar in HIV-positive and immunocompetent patients and include interstitial keratitis and granulomatous or non-granulomatous iridocyclitis.[78] All patients with ocular syphilis should have a lumbar puncture performed to exclude concurrent neurosyphilis. The treatment for ocular syphilis is the same as that for neurosyphilis.

It should be borne in mind that the impairment of the immune response observed in HIV-positive patients may make the results of diagnostic tests (such as those which rely upon obtaining indirect evidence of underlying infection, e.g. Heaf test[79] and the serological tests for syphilis) more difficult to interpret.

Masquerade Uveitis

An AIDS patient presented with an anterior chamber hypopyon and uveitis which was found to be the presenting feature of a metastatic NHL.[80]

Cataract

Acute onset bilateral cataract in an infant with vertically transmitted HIV and CMV retinitis has been described in which it is speculated that CMV or HIV itself may be responsible.[81]

Adnexae and Orbit

Adnexal and orbital abnormalities will develop in approximately 6% of HIV-positive patients and will be the first manifestation of HIV infection or AIDS in 1%.[82] The progression to AIDS is associated with the development of opportunistic infections and neoplasms which occur at an earlier age and frequently follow an unusually aggressive course.[83] The decision to proceed with surgery must not be taken lightly as this group of patients are characterised by poor wound healing and are at greater risk of wound infection. Collaboration with specialists in pathology, microbiology, infectious diseases, otolaryngology, neurosurgery, radiology, and radiotherapy will help reduce the mortality and morbidity associated with the development of adnexal and orbital disease in patients with AIDS.

Adnexae

Infection

Molluscum contagiosum

Molluscum contagiosum is a cutaneous infection caused by a DNA virus of the poxvirus group which affects 10% to 20% of symptomatic HIV-infected individuals.[84] The appearance of mollusca are usually associated with very low CD4 cell counts[85] but have been reported as a presenting feature of HIV infection.[86] Whilst individual lesions retain their characteristic morphology, atypical presenting features in patients with AIDS include onset in adulthood, florid proliferation, unusual distribution including the bulbar conjunctiva,[87] abnormally large lesions (see Fig. 4.3), and resistance to treatment.[88-89]

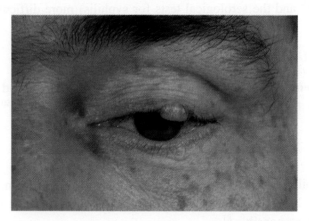

Fig. 4.3 Giant lid margin molluscum in patient with AIDS without keratoconjunctivitis.

Cutaneous infection with cryptococcus, histoplasmosis or coccidioidomyosis can masquerade as mollusca and biopsy is recommended in atypical cases, especially when accompanied by headache, confusion, or pulmonary infiltrates. Impairment of the normal T-cell mediated response to molluscum virus[90] may help explain why, in contrast to immunocompetent individuals, the association of periocular mollusca and keratoconjunctivitis is rarely observed in patients with AIDS. In contrast to the findings of other workers, excellent results using hyperfocal cryotherapy have been described for the treatment of multiple facial molluscum lesions in patients with AIDS.[91]

Herpes zoster ophthalmicus

Herpes zoster ophthalmicus (HZO) caused by the varicella-zoster virus (VZV) is recognised as a marker for HIV infection particularly in sub-Saharan Africa, where 92% of patients with HZO were found to be HIV positive[92] (see chapter 9). In addition to being more prevalent in the immunocompromised population, HZO often follows a more severe and protracted course.[93] A higher incidence of corneal involvement (89% versus 65%) and postherpetic neuralgia (43% versus 20%) has been reported in patients who were HIV positive (see chapter 2). Atypical features include age at onset < 50 years, bilaterality,[94] ocular involvement without cutaneous manifestations,[95] a higher incidence of disseminated VZV, and neurological sequelae including cranial nerve palsies and VZV encephalitis.[15] In addition, the final visual acuity may also be worse with 49% of HIV-positive Malawian patients achieving <6/60 following HZO. The severe anterior segment inflammation and poor visual outcome observed in this group of patients is thought to be due to the combination of the general unavailability of antiviral drugs and the relative integrity of the immune system. Treatment includes the prolonged systemic administration of antiherpetic agents such as aciclovir or famciclovir.[96] A 17% incidence of acute retinal necrosis following HZO in patients who were HIV positive has been reported[97]. It is therefore recommended that these patients undergo weekly dilated fundoscopy.

Neoplasia

Kaposi's sarcoma

KS is a multicentric vascular neoplasm which is almost exclusively seen in patients with AIDS, 95% of whom are homosexual.[98] It is the most frequently encountered AIDS-related malignancy occurring in up to one-third of patients and is most commonly observed at a non-ophthalmic site.[99] The pathogenesis of KS is linked to KS-associated herpes virus, also called the human herpes virus 8 (HHV-8). HHV-8 DNA sequences have been detected in over 95% of cases of AIDS-associated KS, classic KS and the KS that occurs in HIV-negative homosexual men.[100] Typically, KS involves only the skin, however, particularly when associated with reduced CD4 cell counts it can follow a rapidly progressive course with involvement of extracutaneous sites such as the gastrointestinal tract and the CNS.[101] Ocular involvement occurs in between 5% and 24% of patients with AIDS, the vast majority of lesions affect the conjunctiva and/or the eyelid (see Fig. 4.4).[102–103] Lacrimal sac[104] and orbital[105–106] involvement are rarely encountered. KS lesions are non-tender, can be single or multiple, nodular or plaque-like, and range from pink to dark purple in colour. Associated ocular complications include entropion, ectropion, trichiasis and exposure keratopathy.[102,104-106] Slowly growing eyelid and conjunctival lesions which are not associated with visual symptoms need only be observed.

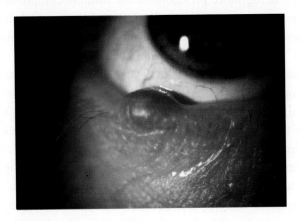

Fig. 4.4 Kaposi's sarcoma of lid which resolved after radiotherapy.

Local treatment options include cryotherapy, intralesional vinblastine and surgical excision all of which can be effective providing the tumour is completely treated.[107] The importance of ensuring complete excision has been emphasised and the use of preoperative fluorescein angiography recommended in the surgical planning of the excision of advanced (> 3 mm in height) bulbar conjunctival KS lesions.[107]

The mainstay of treatment for adnexal KS is radiotherapy. Complete success in 33% and partial success in 67% has been reported in patients treated with a single treatment of 800 cGy. 22% of these patients (usually in association with the development of more profound immunosuppression) developed recurrences at a mean of eight months post-treatment. Side effects of radiotherapy include radiation dermatitis and conjunctivitis, loss of cilia, and alteration in skin pigmentation.[103]

The efficacy of treatment of disseminated KS with chemotherapy and/or immunotherapy[109] is limited by adverse effects, in particular, the inevitable worsening of an already immunocompromised state. In patients receiving HAART, spontaneous regression of KS lesions has been reported and it therefore suggested that local treatment could be deferred for a period of one to two months after HAART is initiated.[110]

Lymphoma

Non-Hodgkin's lymphoma (NHL) is an uncommon manifestation of AIDS but remains significantly more prevalent in this group than in the general population.[15]

Adnexal and/or orbital NHL is rare with eyelid involvement usually occuring secondary to spread from an orbital NHL. The only case of primary eyelid NHL reported, presented with a rapidly progressive erythematous, tender thickening of the affected eyelid and responded to a course of radiotherapy with 4000 cGy.[111]

Carcinoma

A 31-year-old male patient presented with a basal cell carcinoma affecting the lower eyelid without any clinical evidence of the basal cell naevus syndrome.[105] Squamous cell carcinoma is the third most common neoplasm associated with HIV infection and has been reported to have occured on the eyelid in a patient with AIDS.[112]

Others

Other adnexal manifestations of HIV infection include trichomegaly,[113] neurogenic ptosis,[114] Bell's palsy, and long palpebral fissures (HIV dysmorphism).[115]

Orbit

Infection

Orbital cellulitis

HIV-related orbitopathy is most often encountered in a setting of profound immunosupression and a mean CD4 cell count of 18.4/μl has been reported in HIV patients with orbital infections.[116] When compared with the prevalence of ocular infections (30%), the relative risk of orbital infection in patients with AIDS is small. The visual morbidity and mortality associated with orbital infection in this group is, however, significantly worse than that in immunocompetent individuals. The risk of permanent visual loss after orbital infection in patients with AIDS is between 63% and 71% with the one-year mortality at 50%.[116]

Presenting features include periorbital pain, swelling, and localised tenderness which is accompanied by non-axial proptosis, diplopia, and visual impairment. CT and/or MR scanning are the investigations of choice. The majority of orbital infections result from spread from contiguous sinuses, however, panophthalmitis, endogenous endophthalmitis, conjunctival ulceration, and syphilis have all been reported to give rise to orbital cellulitis in patients with AIDS.[116] The causative organisms are much more likely to be opportunistic and include *Proprionibacterium* acnes, *Treponema pallidum, Aspergillus fumigatus, Rhizopus arrhizus, Toxoplasma gondii*, and *Pneumocystis carinii*.[116,117]

Aspergillosis is the most common cause of orbital infection in patients with AIDS. Typically, CT scanning demonstrates bony destructive disease which is associated with sino-orbital pathology. These appearances are however non-specific and may be mimicked by a malignant neoplasm, which underscores the importance of obtaining orbital/sinus biopsies for histological analysis and culture. Despite treatment with systemic antifungal agents such as amphoteracin B, the prognosis is poor with the majority of patients succumbing to the effects of CNS involvement. One patient with subacute orbital cellulitis presented with a slowly progressive granulomatous type of orbitopathy secondary to infection with *Pneumocystis carinii*, and was successfully treated with trimethoprim and sulfamethoxazole.[118]

Neoplasia

Lymphoma

NHL develops in 3% to 10% of HIV-positive patients and is the second most commonly encountered neoplasm.[119] It is a diagnostic feature of AIDS and is the most common orbital manifestation of AIDS.[120] In contrast to the NHL which develops in immunocompetent individuals, AIDS-related lymphomas typically occur at an earlier age, are much more likely to demonstrate extranodal involvement, and be high grade.[121] The presentation of orbital NHL in patients with AIDS can differ from that encountered in the immunocompetent individual with the acute onset of pain accompanied by the rapid development of proptosis, diplopia, and visual loss.[122,123] The typical radiographic appearances in the orbit are depicted in Fig. 4.5 and associated CNS lesion in Fig. 4.6. Radiotherapy is the treatment of choice with adjunctive chemotherapy being considered for disseminated or high-grade disease. Even with optimum treatment the prognosis is dismal, with a median survival of seven months, and only 10% still alive after two years.[105,124]

Although there is a report of a primary orbital Hodgkin's lymphoma (HL),[125] it is usually encountered as part of the terminal phase of systemic HL.[126]

Carcinoma

Other orbital malignancies reported include metastatic gastric adenocarcinoma,[127] squamous carcinoma, and adenoid cystic carcinoma of the lacrimal gland.[128]

Others

Orbital myositis,[129] and non-specific orbital inflammatory disease[130] (both of which were steroid-responsive) have been described in HIV-positive patients. An unusually aggressive parasellar eosinophilic granuloma which was partially responsive to radiotherapy has been reported in a HIV-infected intravenous drug abuser.[131]

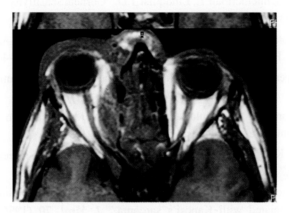

Fig. 4.5 MRI scan demonstrating a well-defined extraconal lesion occupying the posterior two-thirds of the medial aspect of the right orbit in with an extensive lesion which involves the ipsilateral ethmoid sinuses. Biopsy showed lymphoma.

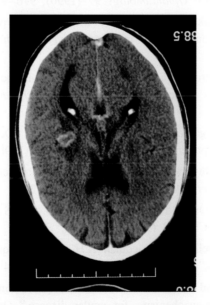

Fig. 4.6. CT head scan (from the same patient as Fig. 4.5) demonstrating a well-circumscribed ring-enhancing lesion located in the peri-thalamic region of the right cerebral hemisphere which involves the posterior limb of the internal capsule, suggestive of lymphoma.

References

1. McClellan K.A. "Mucosal defence of the outer eye," *Surv. Ophthalmol.* **42** (1997), 233–246.

2. Comerie-Smith S.E., Nunez J., Hosmer M. *et al.* "Tear lactoferrin levels and ocular bacterial flora in HIV positive patients," *Adv. Exp. Med. Biol.* **350** (1994), 339–344.

3. Thorneberg T., Schneiderman T., Lindquist T.D. "Corneal sensitivity in HIV positive patients," *Invest. Ophthalmol. Vis. Sci.* **34** (1993), S1026.

4. Gritz D.C., Scott T.J., Sedo S.F. *et al.* "Ocular flora of patients with AIDS compared with those of HIV negative patients," *Cornea* **16** (1997), 400–405.

5. Griffiths T.S., Ferguson T.A. "The role of FasL-induced apoptosis in immune privilege," *Immunol. Tdy.* **18** (1997), 240–244.

6. Gao S.-J., Moore P.S. "Molecular approaches to the identification of uncultuarable infectious agents," *Emerg. Infect. Dis.* **2** (1996), 159–167.

7. Cleator G.M., Klapper P.E., Dennett C. *et al.* "Corneal donor infection by herpes simplex virus," *Cornea* **13** (1994), 294–304.

8. Moore P.S., Gao S.J., Dominingues G. *et al.* "Primary Characterisation of a herpes like agent associated with Kaposi's sarcoma," *J. Virol.* **70** (1996), 549–558.

9. Pflugfelder S.C., Crouse C., Pereira I. *et al.* "Amplification of Epstein-Barr virus genomic sequences in blood cells, lacrimal glands, and tears from primary Sjogren's Syndrome patients," *Ophthalmology* **97** (1990), 976–998.

10. Willoughby C., Baker K., Kaye S.B. *et al.* "Human herpesviruses in the tear film in Sjogren's syndrome and HIV infection," *Invest. Ophthalmol. Vis. Sci.* **39** (1998), S(434).

11. Shuler J.D., Engstrom R.E., Holland G.N. "External ocular disease and anterior segment disorders associated with AIDS," *Int. Ophthalmol. Clin.* **29** (1989), 98–104.

12. Gabrieli C.B., Angarano G., Moramarch A. *et al.* "Ocular manifestations in HIV-seropositive patients," *Ann. Ophthalmol.* **22** (1990), 173–176.

13. Chronister C.L. "Review of external ocular disease associated with AIDS and HIV infection," *Optometry Vis. Sci.* **73** (1996), 225–230.

14. Ryan-Graham M., Durrand M., Pavan-Langston D. "AIDS and the anterior segment," *Int. Ophthalmol. Clin.* **38** (1998), 241–263.

15. Schuman J.S., Orellana J., Friedman A.H. *et al.* "Acquired immunodeficiency syndrome (AIDS)," *Surv. Ophthalmol.* **31** (1987), 384–410.

16. Pepose J.S., Holland G.N., Nestor M.S. *et al.* "Acquired immune deficiency syndrome AIDS. Pathogenic mechanisms for ocular disease," *Ophthalmology* **92** (1985), 472–484.

17. Teich S.A. "Conjunctival vascular changes in AIDS and AIDS related complex," *Am. J. Ophthalmol.* **103** (1987), 332–333.

18. Engstrom R.E., Holland G.N., Nestor M.S. *et al.* "Hemorheologic abnormalities in patient with human immunodeficiency virus infection and ophthalmic microvasculopathy," *Am. J. Ophthalmol.* **109** (1990), 153–161.

19. Couderc L.J., D'Agay M.F., Danon F. *et al.* "Sicca complex and infection with human immunodeficiency virus," *Arch. Intern. Med.* **147** (1987), 898–901.

20. Lucca J.A., Farris R.L., Bielory L. *et al.* "Keratoconjunctivitis sicca in male patients infected with human immunodeficiency virus type 1," *Ophthalmology* **97** (1990), 1008–1010.

21. Geier S.A., Libera S., Klauss V. *et al.* "Sicca syndrome in patients with human immunodeficiency virus," *Ophthalmology* **102** (1995), 1319–1324.

22. Soparkar C.N., Patrinely J.R., Hunts J. *et al.* "The perils of permanent punctal plugs," *Am.Ophthalmol.* **123** (1997), 120–121.

23. Howcroft M.R., Breslin C.W. "Herpes simplex keratitis in renal transplant recipients," *Can. Med. Assoc. J.* **124** (1981), 292–294.

24. Young T.K., Robin J.B., Holland G.N. *et al.* "Herpes simplex keratitis in patients with acquired immunodeficiency syndrome," *Ophthalmology* **96** (1989), 1476–1479.

25. Hodge W.G., Margolis T.P. "Herpes simplex virus keratitis among patients who are positive or negative for human immunodeficiency virus," *Ophthalmology* **104** (1997), 120–124.

26. McLeish W., Pflugfelder S.C., Crouse C. *et al.* "Interferon treatment of herpetic keratitis in a patient with acquired immunodeficiency syndrome," *Am. J. Ophthalmol.* **109** (1990), 93–95.

27. Wilhelmus K.R., Ront R.L., Lehmann R.P. *et al.* "Cytomegalovirus keratitis in acquired immunodeficiency syndrome," *Arch. Ophthalmol.* **114** (1996), 869–872.

28. Espana-Gregori E., Vera-Sempere F., Cano-Parra J. *et al.* "Cytomegalovirus infection of the caruncle in the acquired immunodeficiency syndrome," *Am. J. Ophthalmol.* **117** (1994), 406–407.

29. Brown H., Glasgow B., Holland G. *et al.* "Cytomegalovirus infection of the conjunctiva in AIDS," *Am. J. Ophthalmol.* **117** (1994), 406–407.

30. Swenson P.D., Lownes M.S., Celum C.L. *et al.* "Adenovirus types 2, 8 and 38 associated with genital infections in patients attending a sexually transmitted disease clinic," *Clin. Microbiol. Rev.* **33** (1995), 2728–2731.

31. Kemp M.C., Hierholzer J.C., Cabradilla C.P. *et al.* "The changing aetiology of epidemic keratoconjunctivitis: Antigenic and restriction enzyme analyses of adenovirus types 19 and 37 isolated over a 10 year period," *J. Infect. Dis.* **148** (1983), 24–33.

32. Hierholzer J.C. "Adenovirus in the immunocompromised host," *Clin. Microbiol. Rev.* **5** (1992), 262–274.

33. Hierholzer J.C., Wigand R., Anderson L.J. *et al.* "Adenovirus from patients with AIDS: A plethora of serotypes and a description of 5 new serotypes of subgenus D types 43–47," *J. Infect. Dis.* **158** (1988), 804–813.

34. Hemady R.K., Griffin N., Aristimuno B. "Recurrent corneal infections in patients with the acquired immunodeficiency syndrome," *Cornea* **12** (1993), 266–269.

35. Lau R.K.W., Goh B.T., Estreich S. *et al.* "Adult gonococcal keratoconjunctivitis with AIDS," *Br. J. Ophthalmol.* **74** (1990), p. 52.

36. Nanda M., Pflugfelder S.C., Holland S. "Fulminant pseudomonal keratitis and scleritis in human immunodeficiency virus-infected patients," *Arch. Ophthalmol.* **109** (1991), 504–505.

37. Maguen E., Salz J.J., Nesburn A.B. "Pseudomonas corneal ulcer associated with rigid gas permeable, daily wear lenses in a patient infected with human immunodeficiency virus," *Am. J. Ophthalmol.* **113** (1992), 336–337.

38. Cano-Parra J., Espana E., Esteban M. *et al.* "Pseudomonas conjunctival ulcer and secondary orbital cellulitis in a patient with AIDS," *Br. J. Ophthalmol.* **78** (1994), 72–73.

39. Hemady R.K. "Microbial keratitis in patients infected with the human immunodeficiency virus," *Ophthalmology* **102** (1995), 1026–1030.

40. Parrish C., O'Day D., Hoyle T. "Spontaneous fungal corneal ulcer as an ocular manifestation of AIDS," *Am. J. Ophthalmol.* **104** (1987), p. 302.

41. Aristimuno B., Nirankari V.S., Hemady R.J. *et al.* "Spontaneous ulcerative keratitis in immunocompromised patients," *Am. J. Ophthalmol.* **115** (1995), 202–208.

42. Muccioli C., Belfort R.M., Neves R. *et al.* "Limbal and choroidal cryptococcus infection in the acquired immunodeficiency syndrome," *Am. J. Ophthalmol.* **120** (1995), 539–540.

43. Balmes R., Bialasiewicz A.A., Busse H. "Conjunctival cryptococcus preceding human immunodeficiency virus seroconversion," *Am. J.Ophthalmol.* **113** (1992), 719–721.

44. Hamour A.A., Mandal B.K. "Coccidian parasites in patient with AIDS: Cryptosporidiosis, microsporidiosis, isosporiasis and cycloporiasis," *BIPR Clin. Infect. Dis.* **3** (1996), 137–153.

45. Weber R., Kuster H., Visvesvara G.S. *et al.* "Disseminated microsporidiosis due to encephalitozoom hellem: Pulmonary colonization, microhematuria and mild conjunctivitis in patients with AIDS," *Clin. Infect. Dis.* **17** (1993), 415–419.

46. Silverstein B.E., Emmett T., Cunningham C.A. Jr, *et al.* "Microsporidial keratoconjunctivitis in a patient without human immunodeficiency virus infection," *Am. J. Ophthalmol.* **124** (1997), 395–397.

47. Canning E.U., Curry A., Lacey C.JN. *et al.* "Ultrastructive *Encephalitozoon sp.* infecting the conjunctiva, corneal and nasal epithelia of a patient with AIDS," *Europ. J. Protistol.* **28** (1992), 226–237.

48. McCluskey P.J., Goonan P.V., Marriott D.J.E. *et al.* "Microsporidial keratoconjunctivitis in AIDS," *Eye* **7** (1993), 80–83.

49. Diesenhouse M., Wilson L., Corrent G. *et al.* Treatment of microsporidial keratoconjunctivitis with topical fumagillin," *Am. J. Ophthalmol.* **115** (1993), 293–298.

50. Scwartz D.,Visvesvara G., Diesenhouse M. *et al.* "Pathologic features and immunofluorescent antibody demonstration of ocular microsporidiosis (encephalitozoon hellem) in seven patients with acquired immunodeficiency syndrome," *Am. J. Ophthalmol.* **115** (1993), 285–292.

51. Shah G., Pfister D., Probst L. *et al.* "Diagnosis of ocular microsporidiosis by confocal microscopy and the chromatrope stain," *Am. J. Ophthalmol.* **121** (1996), 89–91.

52. Gritz D.C., Holsclaw D.S., Neger R.E. *et al.* "Ocular and sinus microsporidial infection cured with systemic albendazole," *Am. J. Ophthalmol.* **124** (1997), 241–243.

53. Metcalfe T.W., Doran R.M.L., Rowland P.L. *et al.* "Microsporidial keratoconjunctivitis in a patient with AIDS," *Br. J. Ophthalmol.* **76** (1992), 177–178.

54. Rosberger D., Serdarevic O., Erlandson R. "Successful treatment of microsporidial keratoconjunctivitis with topical fumagillin in a patient with AIDS," *Cornea* **12** (1993), 261–265.

55. Ruggli G.M., Weber R., Messmer E.P. *et al.* "*Pneumocystis carinii* infection of the conjunctiva in a patient with acquired immunodeficiency syndrome," *Ophthalmology* **104** (1997), 1853–1856.

56. Lee G.A., Hirst L.W. "Ocular surface squamous neoplasia," *Surv. Ophthalmol.* **39** (1995), 429–450.

57. McDonnell J.M., McDonnell P.J., Sun Y.Y. "Human papilloma DNA in tissues in ocular surface swabs of patients with conjunctival epithelial neoplasia," *Invest. Ophthalmol. Vis. Sci.* **33** (1992), 184–189.

58. Winward K.E., Curtin V.T. "Conjunctival squamous cell carcinoma in a patient with human immunodeficiency virus infection," *Am. J. Ophthalmol.* **107** (1989), 554–555.

59. Kestelyn P., Stevens A.M., Ndayambaje A. *et al.* "HIV and conjunctival malignancies," *Lancet* **336** (1990), 51–52.

60. Waddell K.M., Lewallen S., Lucas S.B. *et al.* "Carcinoma of the conjunctiva and HIV infection in Uganda and Malawi," *Br. J. Ophthalmol.* **80** (1996), 496–497.

61. Kim R.Y., Seiff S.R., Howes E.L. *et al.* "Necrotising scleritis secondary to conjunctival squamous cell carcinoma in acquired immunodeficiency syndrome," *Am. J.Ophthalmol.* **109** (1990), 231–232.

62. Cantrill H.I., Henry K., Jackson B. *et al.* "Recovery of human immunodeficiency virus from ocular tissues in patients with acquired immunodeficiency syndrome," *Ophthalmology* **95** (1988), 1458–1462.

63. Simons R.J. "HIV transmission by organ and tissue transplantation," AIDS **7** (1993), S35–8.

64. Mannis M.J., Sugar J. "Syphilis, serologic testing and the setting of standards for eye banks," *Am. J. Ophthalmol.* **199** (1995), 93–95.

65. Rzany B., Mockenhaupt M., Stocker U. *et al.* "Incidence of Stevens-Johnson Syndrome and toxic epidermal necrolysis in patients with the acquired immunodeficiency syndrome in Germany (letter)," *Arch. Dermatol.* **129** (1993), p. 1059.

66. Belfort R., de Smet M., Whitcup S. *et al.* "Ocular complications of Stevens-Johnson syndrome and Toxic Epidermal Necrolysis in patients with AIDS," *Cornea* **10** (1991), 536–538.

67. Percorella I., McCartney A.C.E., Lucas S. *et al.* "Acquired Immunodeficiency Syndrome and ocular calcification," *Cornea* **15** (1996), 305–311.

68. Wilhelmus K., Keener M., Jones D. *et al.* "Corneal lipidosis in patients with acquired immunodeficiency syndrome.,"*Am. J. Ophthalmol.* **119** (1995), 14–19.

69. Walter K., Coutler V., Palay D. *et al.* "Corneal endothelial deposits in patients with cytomegalovirus retinitis," *Am. J. Ophthalmol.* **121** (1996), 391–396.

70. Mitchell S., Barton K., Lightman S. "Corneal endothelial changes in cytomegalovirus retinitis," *Eye* **8** (1994), 41–43.

71. Davis J.L., Taskintuna I., Freeman W.R. *et al.* "Iritis and hypotony after treatment with intravenous cidofovir for cytomegalovirus retinitis," *Arch. Ophthalmol.* **115** (1997), 785–786.

72. Chavez de la Paz E., Arevalo J.F., Kirsch L.S. *et al.* "Anterior nongranulomatous uveitis following intravitreal HPMPC (cidofovir) for the treatment of cytomegalovirus retinitis: Analysis and prevention," *Ophthalmology* **104** (1997), 539–544.

73. Kelleher P., Helbert M., Sweeney J. *et al.* "Uveitis associated with rifabutin and macrolide therapy for mycobacterium avium intracellulare infection in AIDS patients," *Genitourin. Med.* **72** (1996), 419–421.

74. Arevalo J.F., Russack V., Freeman W.R. "New ophthalmic manifestations of presumed rifabutin-related uveitis," *Ophthalmic Surg. Lasers* **28** (1997), 321–324.

75. Charles N.C., Boxrud C.A., Small E.A. "Cryptococcus of the anterior segment in acquired immune deficiency syndrome," *Ophthalmology* **99** (1992), 813–816.

76. Specht C., Mitchell K., Bauman A. *et al.* "Ocular histoplasmosis with retinitis in a patient with acquired immune deficiency syndrome.," *Ophthalmology* **98** (1991), 1356–1359.

77. Shalaby I., Dunn J., Semba R. *et al.* "Syphilitic uveitis in human immuno-deficiency virus-infected patients," *Arch. Ophthalmol.* **115** (1997), 469–473.

78. McLeish W., Pulido J., Holland S. *et al.* "The ocular manifestations of syphilis in the human immunodeficiency virus type-1 infected host," *Ophthalmology* **97** (1990), 196–203.

79. Graham N.M., Nelson K., Solomon L. *et al.* "Prevalence of tuberculin positivity and skin test anergy in HIV-1-seropositive and seronegative intravenous drug users," *JAMA* **267** (1992) 369–373.

80. Espana-Gregori E., Hernandez M., Menezo-Rozalen J.L. *et al.* "Metastatic anterior chamber non-Hodgkin's lymphoma in a patient with acquired immunodeficiency syndrome," *Am. J. Ophthalmol.* **124** (1997), 243–245.

81. Tong L., Hodkins P., Taylor D. "Acute onset bilateral cataracts in an infant with vertically transmitted HIV with CMV retinitis despite treatment," *Eye* **12** (1998), p. 150.

82. Mansour A.M. "Adnexal findings in AIDS," *Ophthal. Plast. Reconstr. Surg.* **9** (1993), 273–279.

83. Jabs D.A., Bartlett J.G. "AIDS and ophthalmology: a period of transition," *Am. J. Ophthalmol.* **124** (1997), 227–233.

84. Philips T.J., Dover J.S. "Recent advances in dermatology," *N. Engl. J. Med.* **326** (1992), 167–178.

85. Smith K.J., Skelton H.G., Yeager J. *et al.* "Molluscum contagiosum: Ultrastructural evidence for its presence in skin adjacent to clinical lesions in patients infected with human immunodeficiency virus type 1," *Arch. Dermatol.* **128** (1992), 223–227.

86. Leahey A.B., Shane J.J., Listhaus A. *et al.* "Molluscum contagiosum eyelid lesions as the initial manifestation of acquired immunodeficiency syndrome," *Am. J. Ophthalmol.* **124** (1997), 240–241.

87. Charles N.C., Freidberg D.N. "Epibulbar molluscum contagiosum in acquired immune deficiency syndrome, case report and review of the literature," *Ophthalmology* **99** (1992), 1123–1126.

88. Kohn S.R. "Molluscum contagiosum in patients with acquired immunodeficiency syndrome," *Arch. Ophthalmol.* **105** (1987), p. 458.

89. Robinson M.R., Udell I.J., Garber P.F. *et al.* "Molluscum contagiosum of the eyelids in patients with acquired immunodeficiency syndrome," *Ophthalmology* **99** (1992), 1745–1747.

90. Charteris D.C., Bonshek R.E., Tullo A.B. "Ophthalmic molluscum contagiosum: Clinical and immunopathological features," *Br. J. Ophthalmol.* **79** (1995), 476–481.

91. Bardenstein D.S., Elmets C. "Hyperfocal cryotherapy of multiple molluscum contagiosum lesions in patients with the acquired immune deficiency syndrome," *Ophthalmology* **102** (1995), 1031–1034.

92. Van de Perre P., Bakkers E., Batungwanao J. *et al.* "Herpes zoster in African patients: An early manifestation of HIV infection," *Scand. J. Infect. Dis.* **20** (1988), 277–282.

93. Cole E.L., Meisler D.M., Calabrese L.H. *et al.* "Herpes zoster ophthalmicus and acquired immune deficiency syndrome," *Arch. Ophthalmol.* **102** (1984), p.1027.

94. Yau T.H., Butrus S.I. "Presumed bilateral herpes zoster ophthalmicus," *Cornea* **15**(6) (1996), 633–634.

95. Silverstein B.E., Chandler D., Neger R. *et al.* "Disciform keratitis: A case of herpes zoster sine herpete," *Am. J. Ophthalmol.* **123** (1997), 254–255.

96. Pavan-Langston D. "Viral disease of the cornea and the external eye," in: Albert, Philadelphia, D.M., Jakobiek F.A. (Eds), *Principles and Practice of Ophthalmology, Vol 1.* Saunders (1994), 117–161.

97. Sellitti T., Huang A., Schiffman M. *et al.* "Association of herpes zoster ophthalmicus with acquired immune deficiency syndrome and acute retinal necrosis," *Am. J. Ophthalmol.* **116** (1993), 297–301.

98. Friedman-Kien A.E., Saltzman B.R. "Clinical manifestations of classical, endemic African and epidemic AIDS-related Kaposi's sarcoma," *J. Am. Acad. Dermatol.* **22** (1990), 1237–1250.

99. "Centres for disease control update: Acquired immunodeficiency syndrome and human immunodeficiency virus infection in the United States," *MMWR* **38** (1989), 1–4.

100. Moore P.S., Chang Y. "Detection of herpesvirus-like DNA sequences in Kaposi's sarcoma in patients with and without HIV infection," *N. Engl. J. Med.* **332** (1995), 1181–1185.

101. So Y.T., Choncair A., Davis R.L. *et al.* "Neoplasms of the central nervous system in AIDS," in: Rosenblum M.L., Levy R.M., Bresden D.E. (Eds), *AIDS and the Nervous System*, Raven Press, New York (1988), 285–301.

102. Dugel P.U., Gill P.S., Frangieh G.T. *et al.* "Ocular adnexal Kaposi's sarcoma in acquired immunodeficiency syndrome," *Am. J. Ophthalmol.* **110** (1990), 500–503.

103. Ghabriel R., Quivey J.M., Dunn J.P. Jr. *et al.* "Radiation therapy of acquired immunodeficiency syndrome-related Kaposi's sarcoma of the eyelids and conjunctiva," *Arch. Ophthalmol.* **110** (1992), 1423–1426.

104. Herman D.C., Palestine A.G. "Ocular manifestations of Kaposi's sarcoma," *Ophthalmol. Clin.* **1** (1989), 73–80.

105. Mansour A.M. "Orbital findings in acquired immunodeficiency syndrome," *Am. J. Ophthalmol.* **110** (1990), 706–707.

106. Freeman W.R., Lerner C.W., Mines J.A. *et al.* "A prospective study of the ophthalmological findings in the acquired immunodeficiency syndrome," *Am. J. Ophthalmol.* **97** (1984), 133–142.

107. Dugel P.U., Gill P.S., Frangieh G.T. *et al.* "Treatment of ocular adnexal Kaposi's sarcoma in the acquired immunodeficiency syndrome," *Ophthalmology* **99** (1992), 1127–1132.

108. Macher A.M., Palestine A., Masur H. *et al.* "Multicentric Kaposi's sarcoma of the conjunctiva in a male homosexual with the acquired immunodeficiency syndrome," *Ophthalmology* **90** (1983), 879–880.

109. Krown S.E, Real F.X., Vadhan-Raj S. *et al.* "Kaposi's sarcoma and the acquired immunodeficiency syndrome: Treatment with recombinant interferon alpha and analysis of prognostic factors," *Cancer* **57** (1986), 1662–1665.

110. Corey L., Holmes K. "Therapy for human acquired immunodeficiency virus — What have we learned?" *N. Engl. J. Med.* **335** (1996), 1142–1143.

111. Goldberg S.H., Fieo A.G., Wolz D.E. "Primary eyelid non-Hodgkin's lymphoma in a patient with acquired immunodeficiency syndrome," *Am. J. Ophthalmol.* **113** (1992), 216–217.

112. MacLean H., Dhillon B., Ironside J. "Squamous cell carcinoma of the eyelid and the acquired immunodeficiency syndrome," *Am. J. Ophthalmol.* **121** (1996), 219–221.

113. Casanava J.M., Puig T., Rubio M. "Hypertrichosis of the eyelashes in acquired immunodeficiency syndrome," *Arch. Dermatol.* **123** (1987), 1599–1601.

114. Antworth M.V., Beck R.W. "Third nerve palsy as a presenting sign of acquired immunodeficiency syndrome," *J. Clin. Neuro. Ophthalmol.* **7** (1987), 125–128.

115. Marion M.W., Wiznia A.A., Hutcheon R.G. *et al.* "Human T-cell lymphotrophic virus type III (HTLV-III) embryopathy," *Am. J. Dis. Child.* **10** (1986), 638–640.

116. Kronish J.W., Johnson T.E., Gilberg S.M. *et al.* "Orbital infections in patients with human immunodeficiency virus infection," *Ophthalmology* **103** (1996), 1483–1492.

117. Freiberg D.N., Warren F.A., Lee M.H. *et al.* "*Pneumocystis carinii* of the orbit," *Am. J. Ophthalmol.* **113** (1992), 595–596.

118. Levin L.A., Avery R., Shore J. *et al.* "The spectrum of orbital aspergillosis: A clinicopathological review," *Surv. Ophthalmol.* **41** (1996), 142–154.

119. Levine A.M. "Non-Hodgkin's lymphomas and other malignancies in the acquired immunodeficiency syndrome," *Semin. Oncol.* **14** (1987), 34–39.

120. Kronish J.W. "Eyelid and orbital considerations in AIDS," in: Bosniak S. (ed.), *Principles and Practice of Ophthalmic Plastic Reconstructive Surgery*, WB Saunders, Philadelphia; (1996), 525–534.

121. Khojasteh A., Reynolds R.D., Khojasteh C.A. "Malignant lymphoreticular lesions in patients with immune disorders resembling acquired immunodeficiency syndrome (AIDS), a review of 80 cases," *South. Med. J.* **79** (1986), 1070–1075.

122. Turok D.I., Meye D.R. "Orbital lymphoma associated with acquired immunodeficiency syndrome," *Arch. Ophthalmol.* **110** (1992), p. 611.

123. Font R.L., Laucirica R., Patrinely. "Immunoblastic B-cell malignant lymphoma involving the orbit and maxillary sinus in a patient with acquired immunodeficiency syndrome," *Ophthalmology* **100** (1993), 966–970.

124. Tien D.R. "Large cell lymphoma in AIDS," *Ophthalmology* **98** (1991), p. 412.

125. Park K.L., Goins K.M. "Hodgkin's Lymphoma of the orbit associated with acquired immunodeficiency syndrome," *Am. J. Ophthalmol.* **116** (1993), 111–112.

126. Patel S., Rootman J. "Nodular sclerosing Hodgkin's disease of the orbit," *Ophthalmology* **90** (1983), p. 1433.

127. Singer M.A., Warren F., Accardi F. *et al.* "Adenocarcinoma of the stomach confirmed by orbital biopsy in a patient seropositive for human immunodeficiency virus," *Am. J. Ophthalmol.* **110** (1990), 707–709.

128. Gilberg S.M., Kronish J.W., Tse D.T. *et al.* "Orbital manifestations in acquired immunodeficiency syndrome," Scientific poster, American Academy of Ophthalmology annual meeting, Dallas, October 1992.

129. Benson W.H., Linberg J.V., Weinstein G.W. "Orbital pseudotumour in a patient with AIDS," *Am. J. Ophthalmol.* **105** (1988), 697–698.

130. Fabricus E.M., Hoegel I., Pfaeffl W. "Ocular myositis as first presenting symptom of human immunodeficiency virus (HIV-I) infection and its response to high-dose cortisone treatment," *Br. J. Ophthalmol.* **75** (1991), 696–697.

131. Gross F.J., Waxman J.S., Rosenblatt M.A. *et al.* "Eosinophilic granuloma of the cavernous sinus and orbital apex in an HIV positive patient," *Ophthalmology* **96** (1989), 462–467.

CHAPTER 5

DIFFERENTIAL DIAGNOSIS AND MANAGEMENT OF INFLAMMATION AFFECTING THE RETINA AND/OR CHOROID

Anthony J Hall

Introduction

The most common form of retinitis in AIDS patients is that caused by CMV (see chapter 6). Retinitis or choroiditis can also be caused by other viral, protozoal, bacterial, and fungal infections, or by neoplastic infiltration. The diagnosis of these infections is based on a number of features, including ophthalmoscopic appearance, accompanying systemic disease, clinical history, and the degree of underlying immunodeficiency (see Table 5.1). Rapid and accurate diagnosis may be clinically difficult. It is nonetheless essential in preserving functional vision, as some forms of retinitis are rapidly progressive (especially acute retinal necrosis (ARN) and progressive outer retinal necrosis (PORN)) and since appropriate treatment varies by diagnosis.[1,2]

Accurate ocular diagnosis may also offer a clue to what may be an undiagnosed co-existing systemic infection. In one series of 235 consecutive autopsies of patients with AIDS, 18 of the 235 (7.7%) had histological evidence of infectious choroiditis.[2] Only four of these 18 (22%) cases of infectious choroiditis were diagnosed premortem and in the vast majority (15 of the 18, or 83%) of cases the cause of the infectious choroiditis was also the cause of death.

Classic microbiological confirmation of the cause of retinitis may be possible during life by retinal or vitreous biopsy or vitreous aspiration. Newer molecular diagnostic techniques (polymerase chain reaction-based assays of vitreous and anterior chamber samples) are becoming available and although their routine

Table 5.1 Differential diagnosis of retinitis and/or choroiditis in AIDS patients.

Disease	Fundal features	Vitritis	Progression	Systemic association	CD4 /μl	Treatment
• CMV	Diffuse/unifocal/ multifocal retinitis with haem + granular border	minimal	Slow		<100	See chapter 6
• Toxoplasmosis	Focal dense retinitis	Yes	Slow	Cerebral toxoplasmosis	<200	As for cerebral toxoplasmosis
• HIV micro-vasculopathy	Multiple, well-defined cotton wool spots with small haemorrhages	No	Regresses	Nil	<250	Nil
• ARN	Widespread dense peripheral retinitis	Yes	Rapid early detachment	Nil, rarely cutaneous zoster HSV encephalitis		High-dose aciclovir
• PORN	Multifocal outer retinitis	No	Rapid early detachment	Zoster VZV encephalitis	<50	Combination antivirals
• Syphilis	Papillitis, retinitis choroiditis, or uveitis	Yes		2ʳʸ syphilis or neurosyphilis	Any	As for neurosyphilis
• Fungal retinitis (candida)	Focal or multifocal vitritis, papillitis, or retinitis	Yes		Usually fungaemic	Any	Systemic and local antifungals
• Intraocular lymphoma	Diffuse or multifocal choroiditis	Yes	Slow	Cerebral lymphoma	<50	Radiotherapy plus chemotherapy
• Cryptococcal choroiditis	Multifocal discrete pale choroidal lesions	No	Slow	Cryptococcal meningitis	<200	As for cryptococcal meningitis
• Pneumocystis choroiditis	Multifocal discrete pale flat choroidal lesions	No	Slow	Inhaled PCP prophylaxis	<250	Systemic PCP therapy
• Histoplasmosis	Multifocal choroiditis	No	Slow	Systemic histoplasmosis		Systemic antifungals
• Atypical mycobacterial choroiditis	Single or multiple pale flat or raised choroidal lesions	No	Slow	Systemic MAC	<200	Systemic multi-drug therapy
• Tuberculous choroiditis	Mulitfocal yellow/white choroiditis	Yes		Milliary TB		As for TB

place is still to be ascertained it is clear that they will offer a powerful diagnostic tool in difficult cases.[3]

The clinical features of CMV retinitis are described in detail in chapter 6. This chapter summarises the other intraocular manifestations of AIDS and their clinical features.

Retinitis

HIV Microvasculopathy

CMV retinitis is the most significant ocular manifestation of AIDS but cotton wool spots (the hallmark of HIV related microvasculopathy) are also very common (see Fig. 5.1). The presence of cotton wool spots in patients with AIDS was recognised right at the beginning of the AIDS epidemic. The prognostic significance of cotton wool spots in HIV-infected subjects has been assessed by longitudinal studies. A close correlation exists between cotton wool spots and decrease in CD4 lymphocytes and an increasing morbidity and mortality. Cotton wool spots are uncommon in patients with AIDS without marked cellular immunodeficency[4] and appear to be much less common in patients whose HIV viral load is decreased on HAART. The half-life of cotton wool spots in AIDS has been studied in a prospective study, and the average time to disappearance is 6.9 weeks.[5] HIV retinopathy differs from diabetic retinopathy in having smaller sized cotton wool spots with much shorter half-life, suggesting a patchy involvement of the retinal capillaries in AIDS as compared to widespread capillary disease seen in diabetic retinopathy.

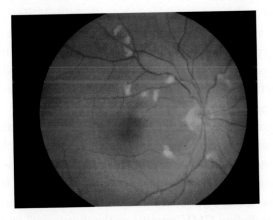

Fig. 5.1 HIV-related cotton wool spots.

Cotton wool spots have been associated with circulating vasoconstrictors[6] and rheological abnormalities and focal immune complex-mediated retinal vascular damage,[7] but their true aetiology is still unclear. There appears to be a higher incidence of CMV DNA in cotton wool spots than in the retina elsewhere in AIDS patients.[8] What is clear is that although they are common they rarely cause visual morbidity[9] and when they do it is usually of a chronic non-specific type. Cotton wool spots may be associated with conjunctival blood flow abnormalities and may be associated with or accompanied by cerebral blood flow abnormalities.[10,11]

Non-CMV Herpes Viral Retinitis

Non-CMV viral retinitis has become the second most common retinal infection in AIDS. There are two general forms of non-CMV herpes viral retinitis. The first is progressive outer retinal necrosis (PORN) and the second is similar to the acute retinal necrosis (ARN) recognised in immunocompetent patients.

Progressive outer retinal necrosis

This form of viral retinitis has a distinct clinical course characterised by fulminant progressive outer retinal necrosis without vitritis or retinal vasculitis (see Fig. 5.2). The initial lesions are characterised by areas of multifocal deep retinal opacification which rapidly coalesce.[12] Initially, peripheral lesions are more common than posterior pole lesions, but posterior spread is frequent and rapid. Progress in PORN may be by spread of existing lesions or by rapid multifocal development of new lesions. Bilaterality is common at presentation and occurs frequently and early in those patients who have unilateral disease at presentation. There is usually minimal anterior chamber activity and vitritis is also minimal or absent. Severe visual loss and retinal detachment usually occur within a matter of weeks.[13] Initial visual acuity may be good, but in the majority of patients the final visual outcome is very poor.[14] Macular lesions may appear quite white with a foveal cherry red spot. In the peripheral lesions there is often an appearance of perivascular sparing or clearing.

The patients usually have a low CD4 count (<40 cells/µl) and very frequently there is a co-existing or recent cutaneous, cerebral or visceral herpes-zoster viral infection. Occasionally, PORN may be preceded by herpes-zoster viral optic neuritis.[15] The diagnosis is usually made on clinical grounds, but if confirmation is required then the use of PCR-based assays on the vitreous may offer an accurate method of both excluding CMV retinitis as the diagnosis[16] and confirming VZV

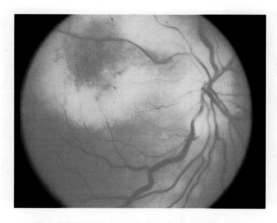

Fig. 5.2 Progressive outer retinal necrosis.

as the causative organism.[17] It is clear that the majority, if not all cases of PORN, are due to varicella-zoster virus.[17]

Treatment is very difficult and the prognosis poor, but there is strong suggestion that aggressive treatment with multiple anti-CMV antiviral agents helps to improve the prognosis, and unlike in acute retinal necrosis, there is little evidence that aciclovir alone is useful.[15] Successful treatment with intravitreal ganciclovir combined with oral sorivudine has been described as has the use of high-dose intravitreal ganciclovir alone. Resolution may leave a white plaque-like retinal change with an appearance of perivascular lucency — the so-called "cracked mud" appearance. It appears that using laser retinopexy is not useful in preventing retinal detachment, possibly because of the widespread and posterior position of the retinitis with its rapid and often multifocal progression. Successful management of the associated retinal detachment requires vitrectomy and silicone oil tamponade.[18] While surgical management is usually anatomically successful, there is often only a marginal visual benefit.

Acute retinal necrosis

The presentation of acute retinal necrosis in AIDS patients is similar to that of ARN recognised in immunocompetent patients. It is characterised by confluent peripheral retinitis with vitritis, papillitis and retinal vasculitis (see Fig. 5.3). There is a rapid posterior progression with increasing vitritis and early retinal detachment. In the majority of cases there is a recent varicella-zoster viral cutaneous infection.[19] As many as 17% of AIDS patients with HZO go on to develop zoster retinitis. Careful screening of these patients for retinitis has been recommended.[20] It appears that like PORN, ARN in AIDS patients is usually

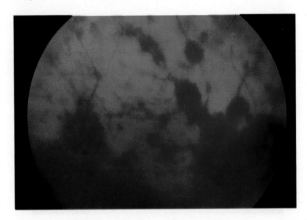

Fig. 5.3 Acute retinal necrosis.

due to varicella-zoster virus (VZV), but it may be due to herpes simplex virus (HSV). In these patients there is frequently a history of herpes simplex viral encephalitis,[21] or they may indeed develop subsequent HSV encephalitis.[3] Occasionally, ARN is preceded by herpes-zoster viral optic neuritis.[22] As in immunocompetent patients there is a high incidence of early secondary retinal detachment. The diagnosis is usually made on clinical grounds, but if confirmation is required then the use of PCR-based assays on vitreous samples may offer an accurate method of both excluding CMV retinitis as the diagnosis[16] and confirming VZV as the causative organism.[18]

Patients usually respond to high doses (5–10 mg/kg eight hourly) of intravenous aciclovir and, unlike in PORN, laser retinopexy can be effective in preventing retinal detachment.

Toxoplasmosis

Toxoplasmosis retinochoroiditis is an infrequent opportunistic infection of the eye in AIDS patients accounting for between 1% to 3% of retinal infections seen in AIDS patients.[23] The frequency of ocular toxoplasmosis appears to be higher in tropical areas. There may be an increasing incidence of ocular toxoplasmosis in AIDS patients over the years.

Ocular toxoplasmosis in AIDS patients is usually unilateral and often but not invariably, associated with significant anterior uveitis and vitritis.[24] The retinal lesions may be single, multifocal, or diffuse (even mimicking acute retinal necrosis) and are usually *not* associated with or adjacent to an old chorioretinal scar.[25] Retinal vascular sheathing may be present but haemorrhage is minimal or absent (see Fig. 5.4). Ocular toxoplasmosis may present with optic nerve head disease and precipitous visual loss.[26] Uncommonly ocular toxoplasmosis in AIDS patients

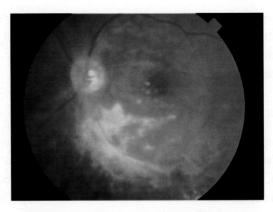

Fig. 5.4 AIDS-related ocular toxoplasmosis.

may cause a fulminant necrotising retinitis leading to panophthalmitis and an orbital cellulitis like clinical picture[27] or a miliary retinitis.[28] Rhegmatogenous detachment may occur but is much less frequent than in viral retinitis. Concurrent cerebral toxoplasmosis occurs in a significant number of patients with ocular toxoplasmosis (29% to 56 %) (see chapter 7). Ocular toxoplasmosis, however, occurs in a minority (10% to 20%) of patients with cerebral toxoplasmosis. It can also occur in combination with other retinal infection/(s) such as CMV.

Specific toxoplasmosis serology (IgG) is nearly always positive (but the anti-toxoplasma IgM may or may not be raised) and the most important element in the diagnosis is the clinical appearance. The origin of ocular toxoplasmosis in AIDS patients is uncertain but the lack of old pigmented scars, the development of bilateral or multifocal disease, and the frequent association with cerebral toxoplasmosis suggest that the lesions may occur as part of haematogenous dissemination of either primary acquired toxoplasmosis or reactivated non-ocular toxoplasmosis.

Ocular toxoplasmosis can be effectively treated with pyrimethamine, clindamycin, a sulfonamide, or spiramycin. Stable scar formation can be expected after two to three weeks of therapy. Subsequent long-term maintenance therapy with pyrimethamine and sulfadiazine is needed to prevent relapse. There is a high incidence of allergy to sulphonamide drugs in AIDS patients that often limits their long-term use. Although there is often a significant uveitis, steroids are generally not required.

Histoplasmosis

Disseminated histoplasmosis is one of the uncommon life-threatening opportunistic infections associated with AIDS. *Histoplasma capsulatum* may cause retinitis, optic neuritis, uveitis, or diffuse iridocyclitis. The retinitis appears as distinct creamy, white intraretinal and subretinal infiltrates.[29] It nearly always occurs in association with disseminated histoplasmosis. Pathologically, there is massive involvement of the choroidal vasculature.[30]

Syphilitic retinitis

There is a strong epidemiological association between syphilis and HIV infection. The natural course of syphilitic infection is more aggressive in HIV-infected patients.[31] The ocular manifestations of syphilis in HIV-infected patients are many and retinitis is not an uncommon manifestation. Syphilitic retinitis may occur at a wide range of CD4 cell counts. It may manifest as a necrotising peripheral retinitis with dense overlying vitritis, a unifocal or multifocal placoid-like retinitis at the posterior pole, a retinal vasculitis, serous retinal detachment, or a neuroretinitis.[32] The retinitis commonly occurs as part of secondary syphilis or neurosyphilis and there may or may not be a history of apparently treated syphilis in the past. Ocular involvement other than retinitis is also common and occurs in up to 40% of AIDS patients with neurosyphilis.[33] Other typical ocular involvement includes cranial nerve palsies, papilloedema, iridocyclitis without retinitis, optic neuritis and, conjunctivitis.[34]

The diagnosis can usually be successfully made by positive syphilis serology (RPR, VDRL or FTA-ABS) although seronegative cases have been described. Ocular syphilis may be frequently accompanied by neurosyphilis in AIDS patients[32] (see chapter 7). It has been recommended that all patients with AIDS and ocular syphilis be tested for neurosyphilis and that more aggressive treatment regimens be given for syphilis in AIDS patients than in other immunocompetent patients.[34] This treatment generally involves high dose (12–24 million units daily) intravenous penicillin for ten to 14 days. As with other patients with syphilis, treatment may be accompanied by a Jarisch-Herxheimer reaction. Response to therapy is monitored both clinically and by demonstrating a serological response with a two-dilution decrease in the rapid plasma reagin (RPR) test.

Multifocal Choroiditis

Multifocal choroiditis is not a common clinical picture in AIDS patients, being recognised in most series between 1% and 2% of patients.[2,35] It is seen much more often in postmortem studies (7.7% of postmortems in one study[2] and it would appear that it is probably under recognised premortem because it is relatively asymptomatic. In the same postmortem study the causative organisms were found to be *Cryptococcus neoformans, Pneumocystis carinii, Mycobacterium tuberculosis, Histoplasma capsulatum, Candida albicans, Aspergillus fumigatus, Toxoplasma gondii,* and MAI. In 15 of these 18 patients, the cause of death was considered to be due to systemic dissemination of the organism causing the choroiditis. In five of these 18 patients there was also simultaneous CMV retinitis. In life, the most common recognised causative organisms are *Pneumocystis carinii* and *Cryptococcus neoformans*.

Pneumocystis Carinii Choroiditis

Pneumocystis carinii pneumonia (PCP) was historically the most important and commonest of all AIDS-related opportunistic infections. Until the advent of effective antiretroviral regimens the most important therapeutic measure for AIDS patients was the use of effective anti-PCP prophylaxis. Most patients have systemic (usually oral) prophylaxis. Some patients were treated with inhaled pentamidine as their PCP prophylaxis. These patients were at risk of non-pulmonary pneumocystis infection.

Multifocal choroiditis occurred as part of this disseminated non-pulmonary pneumocystis infection. The characteristic fundus changes in this infection consisted of numerous slightly elevated, plaque-like, yellow-white lesions located in the choroid and are unassociated with signs of intraocular inflammation (Fig. 5.5). The lesions varied in size from 300–3000 microns. The vision is rarely affected unless there is subfoveal involvement.[36] There may be an associated febrile illness with multifocal nodules in the spleen and liver. The diagnosis is made by the clinical features in the setting of the use of inhaled PCP prophylaxis and the

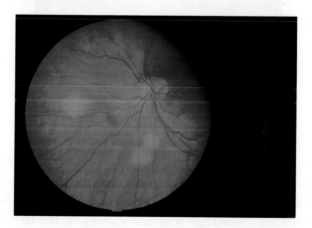

Fig. 5.5 *Pneumocystis carinii* choroiditis.

characteristically slow but total response to systemic PCP therapy. Fluorescein angiography of the lesions shows early hypofluorescence with late staining of the lesions, which appear deep to the retinal circulation.

Histopathologically, the affected eyes have many choroidal infiltrates that are eosinophilic, acellular, vacuolated, and frothy. Such infiltrates may be noted within the choroidal vessels and choriocapillaries. Electron microscopy shows thick-walled cystic organisms and large numbers of trophozoites.[37]

Cryptococcal Choroiditis

Cryptococcal meningitis is frequently associated with ocular signs, but these are usually related to papilloedema or other neurophthalmic manifestations. Some patients with cryptococcal meningitis develop multifocal choroiditis. These patients may present with visual loss, but that is usually due to the accompanying optic nerve involvement rather than the choroiditis. The choroiditis is clinically similar to pneumocystis choroiditis and appears as multiple yellow-white choroidal infiltrates 500–1500 microns in size (see Fig. 5.6). There is no associated anterior chamber or vitreous infiltrate and no haemorrhage.[38] Cryptococcal choroiditis rarely progresses to frank endophthalmitis.

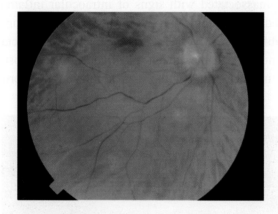

Fig. 5.6 Cryptococcal choroiditis.

Systemic investigation reveals features of cryptococcal meningitis with yeasts and cryptococcal antigen found in the CSF and often in the blood. Fluorescein angiogram reveals early blockage with late staining of the lesions and usually of the disc as well.

The lesions respond slowly (over one to five months) to systemic treatment of the cryptococcal meningitis, usually with intravenous amphotericin B, or intravenous or oral fluconazole depending on the degree of systemic illness. The long-term visual outcome depends on the optic nerve involvement.

Candida

Mucosal infection with *Candida albicans* is extraordinarily common in AIDS patients, but despite that, intraocular candida infection is rare. Affected patients generally have a history of intravenous drug abuse or candida sepsis from an indwelling central line. The clinical features are similar to those seen in immunocompetent patients running a spectrum from severe endophthalmitis with a dense focus of white retinitis (see Fig. 5.7) through a milder vitritis with a "string of pearls" to a small subretinal or pre-retinal inflammatory focus.

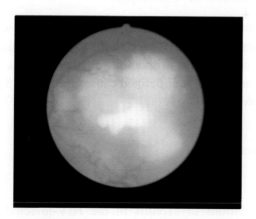

Fig. 5.7 *Candida albicans* endophthalmitis in an HIV-infected patient using intravenous drugs.

The diagnosis can be made non-invasively if candida can be isolated from the blood or intravenous catheter tip. If not, then the candida can be isolated from the vitreous at vitrectomy. The treatment depends on the severity of the ocular involvement and the systemic disease. The source of the candida infection should be removed. The treatment of severe disease is with vitrectomy and intravitreal amphotericin B, while milder disease can be treated with intravitreal amphotericin B without vitrectomy. Accompanying systemic disease can be treated with intravenous amphotericin B, or oral or intravenous fluconazole, again depending on severity.

Mycobacterial Choroiditis

Widespread infection with atypical mycobacteria is common in AIDS patients and in some areas tuberculosis remains a common problem in these patients. In spite of the high incidence of atypical mycobacterial sepsis in AIDS patients clinical descriptions of mycobacterial choroiditis are rare. Atypical mycobacterial choroiditis is characterised by small, usually asymptomatic, elevated white choroidal granulomas. The diagnosis is made by the exclusion of pneumocystis or cryptococcus as the cause and the finding of atypical mycobacteria on blood cultures. The treatment is with the usual multi-drug regimens for atypical mycobacterial infection.

Choroidal tuberculosis seems to have a more virulent presentation with an intense anterior chamber reaction and vitritis accompanying multifocal choroiditis.[39] This occurs as part of miliary tuberculosis and the treatment is aimed at the systemic tuberculosis. Topical steroids may be required.

Uveitis without Retinitis or Choroiditis

Intraocular inflammation is common in patients infected with HIV, but it is usually accompanied by an obvious retinitis or choroiditis. Less commonly intraocular inflammation occurs without an obvious retinitis. When this occurs it may be due to a number of well-defined causes (see Table 5.2) or the aetiology may remain obscure.

Opportunistic Infections

Syphilis

The ocular manifestations of syphilis in the HIV-infected host are protean; iridocyclitis, intermediate uveitis, panuveitis, retinitis, retinal vasculitis, serous retinal detachment, chorioretinitis, optic neuritis, and retinal vascular occlusions have all been described. Syphilis may cause uveitis without retinitis or choroiditis in patients with HIV infection usually as part of secondary syphilis. The uveitis is usually posterior, often with disc involvement or occlusive retinal vasculitis. Despite the immunodeficiency associated with AIDS the syphilis serology is usually still positive although one case of RPR negative secondary syphilis in an AIDS patient has been reported.[40] There is usually concomitant laboratory evidence of CNS syphilis even in the absence of clinical features suggestive of neurosyphilis.[41] Treatment with regimens for neurosyphilis are required for syphilitic uveitis in HIV-infected patients whether or not there is evidence of CNS involvement.[42]

Table 5.2 Summary of causes of uveitis without retinitis or choroiditis in HIV-infected patients.

Major Category	Diagnoses	Features	Treatment
• Opportunistic infections	1. Syphilis	1. Suggestive serology +/− neurosyphilis	1. Neurosyphilis treatment
	2. Herpes Zoster Ophthalmicus	2. Rash +/− keratitis	2. ACV
	3. Toxoplasmosis without chorioretinitis	3. CNS toxoplasmosis	3. Conventional toxoplasmosis treatment
• Directly HIV related	Uveitis alone or uveo-myelitis	CD4 100–400/µl No other diagnosis	antiretrovirals +/− steroids
• Drug related	1. Rifabutin	1. Acute anterior uveitis +/− arthritis	1. Topical steroids +/− cessation of rifabutin
	2. Cidofovir related	2. Seen in patients on systemic or ocular cidofovir.	2. Topical steroids
	3. Anti-sense drugs	3. Uveitis following intra-ocular injection	3. Nil
	4. HAART and CMV retinitis	4. CMVR and increased CD4	
• Non-HIV related	Reiters syndrome or idiopathic	Normal CD4 count B27 +ve Recent predisposing infection	Conventional iritis treatment
• Masquerade	1. Intra-ocular lymphoma	1. CNS lymphoma	1. CNS treatment + ocular radiation
	2. With/preceding chorioretinitis	2. Chorioretinal lesions	2. Appropriate treatment for retinitis
	3. Metastatic endophthalmitis	3. Systemic sepsis + positive vitreous cultures	3. Systemic antibiotics
	4. Postsurgical endophthalmitis	4. Unexplained post operative inflammation	4. Intraocular antibiotics

Herpes zoster ophthalmicus

HZO is a common early manifestation of declining immune function in HIV infection and more than half of patients with concomitant HIV infection and HZO will develop uveitis.[43] The uveitis is, however, usually associated with or preceded by a typical dermatomal rash. The uveitis may be chronic and require prolonged treatment.[44] Topical steroids are used if a reduction in the anterior segment inflammation is considered clinically useful and secondary glaucoma may occur and require treatment.[45] Long-term suppressive treatment with oral aciclovir may be used to prevent recurrence and patients should be made aware of the risk of serious retinitis.

Toxoplasmosis

Toxoplasmosis has been reported to cause intense anterior uveitis and secondary pressure rise without a definite choroidal focus in a patient with AIDS and cerebral toxoplasmosis. The patient failed to respond to topical treatment and died one month after developing uveitis.[46]

Drug Related

Rifabutin-related anterior uveitis

Acute anterior uveitis has been identified as a dose-related side effect of rifabutin in patients taking rifabutin for (or as prophylaxis against) atypical mycobacterial (MAC) infection.[47] Uveitis occurs at doses of >1800 mg/day if rifabutin is being given alone or at doses of 300–600 mg/day if the patient is being treated concurrently with clarithromycin (300–1000 mg/day) or fluconazole (50–200 mg/day). The disease is usually bilateral and may be associated with arthralgia.[48] It responds to topical steroids and mydriatics and in recalcitrant cases may require cessation of the rifabutin. The interaction with clarithromycin and fluconazole may be due to inhibition of hepatic cytochrome P-450 by these drugs causing an increase in serum levels of rifabutin. The exact cause of the uveitis is unknown, but there is evidence to suggest that it is due to the interaction between rifabutin and mycobacterium rather than due to direct toxicity of the drug.[49] If this is so, then rifabutin uveitis may be the human equivalent of endotoxin-induced uveitis seen in experimental animals.[50]

Cidofovir

Iritis and uveitis are relatively common side effects of both intravenous and intraocular cidofovir. The iritis may be quite severe and associated with marked posterior synechiae. It usually requires treatment with intensive topical steroids and if patients are to remain on cidofovir then topical steroids may be required in the long term. The iritis may be preceded by or accompanied by hypotony or at least lowered intraocular pressure (see also chapter 2).

Intraocular inflammation has been reported as a complication of intraocular therapy with fomivirsen (ISIS 2922), a CMV anti-sense drug. This appears to be dose related and settles with treatment with topical steroids.

An abnormally brisk anterior chamber or vitreous reaction may accompany CMV retinitis after concurrent treatment with HIV protease inhibitors has caused a degree of immune restoration. This abnormal vitritis accompanies an increase in the CD4 count (generally to above 100 cells/μl) and usually occurs when the retinitis is quiet. The increase in the uveitis in such patients generally heralds a period of quiescence of the CMV retinitis.[51] This increase in vitreous activity may be analogous to that seen in transplant patients with CMV retinitis when there is a decrease in their immunosuppressive medications.

Directly HIV Related

A small number of patients have been described in the literature with what is possibly a directly HIV-related uveitis.[52-55] This may present as an anterior uveitis or as an intermediate uveitis and usually occurs with CD4 counts in the range of 100–400 cells/μl. There appears to be a distinct group of patients with anterior uveitis, vitritis, and prominent peripheral pre-retinal infiltrates (see Fig. 5.8). These patients follow an indolent course and rarely have significant visual loss.[56] Some of them have had HIV isolated from the ocular tissues or other affected sites,[55] some have had a clinical response to antiretrovirals, and some an associated transverse myelitis.[57]

The ocular inflammation in these cases may be due to an unidentified opportunistic infection or to direct HIV infection of the eye or to an autoimmune uveitis caused at least in part by the immune dysregulation seen in early AIDS.

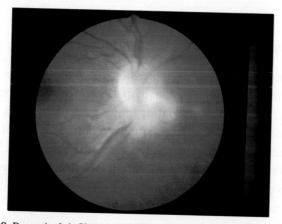

Fig. 5.8 Pre-retinal infiltrate in HIV-associated intermediate uveitis.

The latter theory is supported by the fact that the HIV-related uveitis is seen relatively early in the course of AIDS when immune dysregulation (rather than straightforward immune deficiency) is greatest and not later when the HIV viral load is greater and more direct HIV tissue invasion and a greater propensity to opportunistic infection could be expected. Treatment with antiretroviral drugs may be successful as may be treatment with topical steroids and cycloplegic agents.

Non HIV Related

Reiter's syndrome

There is an increased risk of Reiter's syndrome in AIDS patients which may well be due to increased risk of predisposing infections (e.g. chlamydia and yersinia) in sexually active homosexual men rather than due to a true immunological abnormality leading to an increased risk of disease.[58] There would appear to be no increased risk of Reiter's syndrome in intravenous drug users with AIDS[59] and our current knowledge of the immunopathology of Reiter's syndrome suggests that CD4 T-cell mechanisms (that are involved in AIDS-related immune dysregulation) are unlikely to play a role.

Other causes

HIV-positive patients are obviously also at risk of uveitis from the same spectrum of causes as non-HIV-infected patients, and these causes should be looked for and excluded.

Masquerade

Metastatic endophthalmitis

Unlike in patients with immunosuppression following chemotherapy, bacterial septicaemia is relatively uncommon in patients with immunodeficiency from AIDS. Similarly, metastatic bacterial or fungal endophthalmitis (as distinct from metastatic choroiditis) is surprisingly rarely reported. When it does occur it is usually in the setting of obvious and severe systemic sepsis.[60] A wide range of organisms have been reported including *M. Avium*,[61] Cryptococcus,[62] and Candida.[63] Such patients usually present with an acute onset unilateral panuveitis, which may be accompanied by focal choroidal lesions. The diagnosis can be made by culturing the causative organism from the involved systemic organ, the blood or the eye, as unlike postoperative endophthalmitis, treatment for metastatic endophthalmitis with systemic antibiotics appears to be as efficacious as with intravitreal antibiotics.[64]

Oculo-Cerebral lymphoma

Intraocular B-cell lymphoma may occur in AIDS patients, but it is uncommon and appears to be nearly always associated with cerebral involvement.[65] It may be associated with vitritis without retinal involvement or with small, focal, yellowish-white choroidal infiltrates and retinal vasculitis. The diagnosis is usually considered in the setting of eye disease occurring with already diagnosed cerebral lymphoma or undiagnosed uveitis or atypical retinitis not responding to the usual anti-CMV treatment (see chapter 7).

Cytological examination of the vitreous may be diagnostic showing neoplastic cells characteristic of large cell type malignant lymphoma.[65] Examination of the cerebrospinal fluid may also be helpful in revealing large cell malignant lymphoma. Cerebral imaging (especially magnetic resonance imaging) may reveal focal lesions suggestive of CNS lymphoma. The ocular disease responds well to whole eye radiotherapy. In many cases the lymphoma may be related to Epstein-Barr viral infection.[66]

Associated with retinitis

A degree of intraocular inflammation is often seen with CMV retinitis and this may be severe,[67] particularly in patients using protease inhibitors. Similarly, toxoplasmic, HSV and VZV viral retinitis are associated with intraocular inflammation and at times the focal chorioretinal pathology may be missed. In these cases treatment is obviously aimed at the underlying retinal infection.

Postoperative endophthalmitis

Patients having intraocular therapy for CMV retinitis (see chapter 6) are at increased risk of endophthalmitis because of the commonly associated neutropenia and it may occur after intraocular surgery[68] or intraocular injection alone.[69] The disease is characterised by a sustained increase in intraocular inflammation post procedure and responds to intraocular antibiotics if the causative organism is of low virulence (e.g. *Staph epidermitis*). Intravitreal ganciclovir injections alone without secondary infection do not cause inflammation.

This list of causes of uveitis in patients with HIV infection is short and in time more causes will develop or be found. Management depends on the proper evaluation for likely causes. Only if this is negative and only when the morbidity from the uveitis is significant should speculative topical or systemic immunosuppression be used.

References

1. de Smet M.D. "Differential diagnosis of retinitis and choroiditis in patients with acquired immunodeficiency syndrome," *Am. J. Med.* **92** (1992), 17S–21S.

2. Morinelli E.N., Dugel P.U., Riffenburgh R. *et al.* "Infectious multifocal choroiditis in patients with acquired immune deficiency syndrome," *Ophthalmology* **100** (1993), 1014–1021.

3. Knox C.M., Chandler D., Short G.A. *et al.* "Polymerase chain reaction based assays of vitreous samples for the diagnosis of viral retinitis — Use in diagnostic dilemmas," *Ophthalmol* **105** (1998), 37–45.

4. Pivetti-Pezzi P., Tamburi S., Accorinti M. *et al.* "Immunological and viral markers of HIV infection and retinal microangiopathy," *Euro. J. Ophthalmol.* **3** (1993), 138–142.

5. Mansour A.M., Rodenko G., Dutt R. "Half-life of cotton-wool spots in the acquired immunodeficiency syndrome," *Int. J. STD AIDS* **1** (1990), 132–133.

6. Geier S.A., Rolinski B., Sadri I. *et al.* "Ocular microangiopathy syndrome in patients with AIDS is associated with increased plasma levels of the vasoconstrictor endothelin-1," *Klin. Mon. Augen.* **207** (1995), 353–360.

7. Pepose J.S., Holland G.N., Nestor M.S. *et al.* "Acquired immune deficiency syndrome. Pathogenic mechanisms of ocular disease," *Ophthalmology* **92** (1985), 472–484.

8. Gonzalez C.R., Wiley C,A., Arevalo J.F. *et al.* "Polymerase chain reaction detection of cytomegalovirus and human immunodeficiency virus-1 in the retina of patients with acquired immune deficiency syndrome with and without cotton-wool spots," *Retina* **16** (1996), 305–311.

9. Freeman W.R., Chen A., Henderly D.E. *et al.* "Prevalence and significance of acquired immunodeficiency syndrome-related retinal microvasculopathy," *Am. J. Ophthalmol.* **107** (1989), 229–235.

10. Geier S.A., Schielke E., Tatsch K. *et al.* "Brain HMPAO-SPECT and ocular microangiopathic syndrome in HIV-1-infected patients AIDS," **7** (1993), 1589–1594.

11. Geier S.A., Klauss V., Goebel F.D. "Ocular microangiopathic syndrome in patients with acquired immunodeficiency syndrome and its relationship to alterations in cell adhesion and in blood flow," *Ger. J. Ophthalmol.* **3** (1994), 414–421.

12. Holland G.N. "The progressive outer retinal necrosis syndrome," *Int. Ophthalmol.* **18** (1994), 163–165.

13. Engstrom R.E., Holland G.N., Margolis T.P. *et al.* "The progressive outer retinal necrosis syndrome: a variant of necrotizing herpetic retinopathy in patients with AIDS," *Ophthalmol* **101** (1994), 1488–1502.

14. Moorthy R.S., Weinberg D.V., Teich S.A. *et al.* "Management of varicella zoster virus retinitis in AIDS," *B. J. Ophthalmol.* **81** (1997), 189–194.

15. Shayegani A., Odel J.G., Kazim M. *et al.* "Varicella-zoster virus retrobulbar optic neuritis in a patient with human immunodeficiency virus," *Am. J. Ophthalmol.* **122** (1996), 586–588.

16. McCann J.D., Margolis T.P., Wong M.G. *et al.* "A sensitive and specific polymerase chain reaction based assay for the diagnosis of cytomegalovirus retinitis," *Am. J. Ophthalmol.* **120** (1995), 219–226.

17. Short G.A., Margolis T.P., Kuppermann B.D. *et al.* "A polymerase chain reaction based assay for the diagnosis of varicella-zoster virus retinitis in patients with AIDS," *Am. J. Ophthalmol.* **123** (1997), 157–164.

18. Spaide R.F., Martin D.F., Teich S. *et al.* "Successful treatment of progressive outer retinal necrosis syndrome," *Retina* **16** (1996), 479–487.

19. Batisse D., Eliaszewicz M., Zazoun L. *et al.* "Acute retinal necrosis in the course of AIDS: Study of 26 cases," *AIDS.* **10** (1996), 55–60.

20. Sellitti T.P., Huang A.J., Schiffman J. *et al.* "Association of herpes zoster ophthalmicus with acquired immunodeficiency syndrome and acute retinal necrosis," *Am. J. Ophthalmol.* **116** (1993), 297–301.

21. Margolis T.P., Atherton S.S. "Herpes simplex diseases: Posterior segment of the eye," in: Pepose JS, Holland GN, Wilhelmus KR (Eds.), *Ocular Infection and Immunity*, Mosby Year Book Inc, Philadelphia, (1996), 1155–1168.

22. Friedlander S.M., Rahhal F.M., Ericson L. *et al.* "Optic neuropathy preceding acute retinal necrosis in acquired immunodeficiency syndrome," *Arch. Ophthalmol.* **114** (1996), 1481–1485.

23. Rodgers C.A., Harris J.R. "Ocular toxoplasmosis in HIV infection," *Int. J. STD AIDS* **7** (1996), 307–309.

24. Cochereau-Massin I., LeHoang P., Lautier-Frau M. *et al.* "Ocular toxoplasmosis in human immunodeficiency virus-infected patients," *Am. J. Ophthalmol.* **114** (1992), 130–135.

25. Gagliuso D.J., Teich S.A., Friedman A.H. *et al.* "Ocular toxoplasmosis in AIDS patients," *Trans. Am. Ophthalmol. Soc.* **88** (1990), 63–86.

26. Wei M.E., Campbell S.H., Taylor C. "Precipitous visual loss secondary to optic nerve toxoplasmosis as an unusual presentation of AIDS," *Aust. NZ J. Ophthalmol.* **24** (1996), 75–77.

27. Moorthy R.S., Smith R.E., Rao N.A. "Progressive ocular toxoplasmosis in patients with acquired immunodeficiency syndrome," *Am. J. Ophthalmol.* **115** (1993), 742–747.

28. Berger B.B., Egwuagu C.E., Freeman W.R. *et al.* "Miliary toxoplasmic retinitis in acquired immunodeficiency syndrome," *Arch. Ophthalmol.* **111** (1993), 373–376.

29. Specht C.S., Mitchell K.T., Bauman A.E. *et al.* "Ocular histoplasmosis with retinitis in a patient with acquired immune deficiency syndrome," *Ophthalmology* **98** (1991), P1356–1359.

30. Font R.L., Parsons M.A., Keener M.J. *et al.* "Involvement of anterior chamber angle structures in disseminated histoplasmosis: Report of three cases," *Ger. J. Ophthalmol.* **4** (1995), 107–115.

31. Johns D.R., Tierny M., Felsenstein D. "Alteration in the natural history of neurosyphilis by concurrent infection with the human immunodeficiency virus," *N. Eng. J. Med.* **316** (1987), 1569–1572.

32. Levy J.H., Liss R.A., Maguire A.M. "Neurosyphilis and ocular syphilis in patients with concurrent human immunodeficiency virus infection," *Retina* **9** (1989), 175–180.

33. Katz D.A., Berger J.R. "Neurosyphilis in acquired immunodeficiency syndrome," *Arch. Neurol.* **46** (1989), 895–898.

34. McLeish W.M., Pulido J.S., Holland S. *et al.* "The ocular manifestations of syphilis in the human immunodeficiency virus infected host," *Ophthalmology* **97** (1990), P196–203.

35. Muccioli C., Belfort Junior R., Lottenberg C. *et al.* "Ophthalmological manifestations in AIDS: Evaluation of 445 patients in one year," *Revista Da Associacao Medica Brasileira* **40** (1994), 155–158.

36. Shami M.J., Freeman W., Friedberg D. *et al.* "A multicenter study of Pneumocystis choroidopathy," *Am. J. Ophthalmol.* **112** (1991), 15–22.

37. Rao N.A., Zimmerman P.L., Boyer D. *et al.* "A clinical, histopathologic, and electron microscopic study of *Pneumocystis carinii* choroiditis," *Am. J. Ophthalmol.* **107** (1989), 218–228.

38. Carney M.D., Combs J.L., Waschler W. "Cryptococcal choroiditis," *Retina* **10** (1990), 27–32.

39. Blodi B.A., Johnson M.W., McLeish W.M. *et al.* "Presumed choroidal tuberculosis in a human immunodeficiency virus infected host," *Am. J. Ophthalmol.* **108** (1989), 605–607.

40. Hicks C.B., Benson P.M., Lupton G.P., *et al.* "Seronegative secondary syphilis in a patient infected with the human immunodeficiency virus (HIV) with Kaposis Sarcoma," *Ann. Int. Med.* **107** (1987), 492–494.

41. Beccera L.I., Ksiasek S.M., Savino P.J. *et al.* "Syphilitc uveitis in human immunodeficiency virus-infected and non infected patients," *Ophthalmol* **96** (1989), 1727–1730.

42. Richards B.W., Hessburg T.J., Nussbaum J.N. "Recurrent syphilitic uveitis," *NEJM* **320** (1989), p. 62

43. Kestelyn P., Stevens A.M., Bakkers E. *et al.* "Severe herpes zoster ophthalmicus in young african adults: A marker for HTLV-III seropositivity," *Br. J. Ophthalmol.* **71** (1987), 806–809.

44. Schuman J.S., Orellano J., Freidman A.H. *et al.* "Acquired Immunodeficiency Syndrome (AIDS)," *Surv. Ophthalmol.* **31** (1987), 384–410.

45. Bergaust B., Westby R.K. "Zoster ophthalmicus: local treatment with cortisone," *Acta. Ophthalmol.* **45** (1967), 787–793.

46. Rehder J.R., Burnier M., Pavesio C.E. *et al.* "Acute unilateral toxoplasmic iridocyclitis in an AIDS Patient," *Am. J. Ophthalmol.* **106** (1988), 740–741.

47. Saran B.R., Maguire A.M., Nichols C. *et al.* "Hypopyon uveitis in patients with acquired immunodeficiency syndrome treated for systemic Mycobacterium avium complex infection with rifabutin," *Arch. Ophthalmol.* **112** (1994), 1159–1165.

48. Kelleher P., Helbert M., Anderson J. *et al.* "Uveitis and rifabutin." AIDS, **8** (1994), S18.

49. Opremcak E.M., Cynamon M. "Uveitogenic activity of rifabutin and clarithromycin in the *Mycobacterium avium*-infected beige mice," *Invest. Ophthalmol. Vis. Sci.* **36** (1995), S317.

50. Rosenbaum J.T., McDevitt H.O., Guss R.B. *et al.* "Endotoxin induced uveitis in rats as a model for human disease," *Nature* **286** (1980), 611–613.

51. Zegans M.E., Walton R.C., Holland G.N. *et al.* "Transient vitreous inflammatory reactions associated with combined antiretroviral therapy in patients with AIDS and cytomegalovirus retinitis," *Am. J. Ophthalmol.* **125** (1998), 292–300.

52. Farrell P.L., Heinemann M.H., Roberts C.W. *et al.* "Response of Human Immunodeficiency Virus-Associated Uveitis to Zidovudine," *Am. J. Ophthal.* **106** (1988), 7–10.

53. Martenet A.C. "Unusual ocular lesions in AIDS," *Int. Ophthalmol.* **14**(5–6), (1990), 359–363.

54. O'Hara M.A., Raphael S.A., Nelson L.B. "Isolated anterior uveitis in a child with acquired immunodeficiency syndrome," *Ann. Ophthalmol.* **23** (1991), 71–73.

55. Rosberger D.F., Heineman M., Freidberg D.N. *et al.* "Uveitis associated with human immunodeficiency virus infection," *Am. J. Ophthalmol.* **125** (1998), 301–305.

56. Levinson R.D., Vann R., Davis J.L. *et al.* "Chronic multifocal retinal infiltrates in patients infected with human immunodeficiency virus," *Am. J. Ophthalmol.* **125** (1998), 312–324.

57. Hall A.J., Stawell R.J. "Human immunodeficiency virus-related uveomyelitis," *Arch. Ophthalmol.* **112**(9), (1994), 1144–1145.

58. Clark M.R., Solinger A.M., Hochberg M.C. "Human immunodeficiency virus infection is not associated with Reiter's syndrome," *Rheum. Dis. Clin. North Am.* **18** (1992), 267–275.

59. Monteagudo I., Rivera J., Lopez-Longo J. *et al.* "AIDS and rheumatic manifestations in patients addicted to drugs. An analysis of 106 cases," *J. Rheumatol.* **18** (1991), 1038–1041.

60. Shivaram U., Cash M. "Purpura fulminans, metastatic endophthalmitis, and thrombotic thrombocytopenic purpura in an HIV-infected patient," *NY. J. Med.* **92** (1992), 313–314.

61. Cohen J.I., Saragas S.J. "Endophthalmitis due to mycobacterium avium in a patient with AIDS," *Ann. Ophthalmol.* **22** (1990), 47–51.

62. Denning D.W., Armstrong R.W., Fishman M. *et al.* "Endophthalmitis in a patient with disseminated cryptococcosis and AIDS who was treated with itraconozole," *Rev. Infect. Dis.* **13** (1991), 1126–1130.

63. Heinemann M.H., Bloom A.F., Horowitz J. "Candida endophthalmitis in a patient with AIDS," *Arch. Ophthalmol.* **105** (1987), 1172–1173.

64. Greenwald M.J., Wohl L.G., Cell C.H. "Metastatic bacterial endophthalmitis; a contemporary reappraisal," *Surv. Opthalmol.* **31** (1986), 81–101.

65. Sechanzer M.C., Font R.L., O'Malley R.E. "Primary ocular malignant lymphoma associated with the acquired immune deficiency syndrome," *Ophthalmology* **98** (1991), 88–91.

66. Nadal D., Caduff R., Frey E. *et al.* "Non-Hodgkin's lymphoma in four children infected with the human immunodeficiency virus. Association with Epstein-Barr Virus and treatment," *Cancer* **73** (1994), 224–230.

67. Daicker B. "Cytomegalovirus panuveitis with infection of corneo-trabecular endothelium in AIDS," *Ophthalmologica* **197** (1988), 169–175.

68. Anand R., Nightingale S.D., Fish R.H. *et al.* "Control of cytomegalovirus retinitis using sustained release of intraocular ganciclovir," *Arch. Ophthalmol.* **111** (1993), 223–227.

69. Cantrill H.L., Henry K., Melroe H.N. *et al.* "Treatment of cytomegalovirus retinitis with intravitreal ganciclovir," *Ophthalmology* **96** (1989), 367–374.

CHAPTER 6

CYTOMEGALOVIRUS RETINITIS

Baljean Dhillon, Ahmed Kamal and Thomas Kuriakose

Introduction

The entire CMV genome has been sequenced,[1] however, it is still not clear why this particular herpes virus has emerged as the major ocular opportunistic infection associated with AIDS. CMV is a major cause of morbidity and mortality amongst patients with AIDS. The retina is the commonest site of infection[2] CMV is species-specific and several different strains may cause disease in humans. CMV infection is acquired through close contact and in the majority of immunocompetent individuals causes a relatively trivial illness before assuming a "latent" state. Shared DNA sequences homologous with sites on the human genome[3] may influence the property of latency. However, severe immunosuppression leads to viral reactivation and tissue-invasive human disease. Virostatic therapy is effective and suppresses viral replication, but does not eradicate existing virus, and in this sense CMV disease is controllable but not curable.

CMV retinitis (CMVR) may be the AIDS-defining diagnosis though, it more commonly occurs months after the diagnosis of AIDS. If left untreated, patients with unilateral CMVR are likely to develop disease in their second eye and ultimately become blind.[4] It has now become accepted practice to treat sight-threatening CMVR with ganciclovir, foscarnet or cidofovir which are effective in delaying the progress of this destructive infection. Systemic treatment for CMV disease also reduces extraretinal CMV-related morbidity and mortality and subjectively improves quality of life.[5] The goal of CMVR management is to maintain infection control and preserve vision without subjecting the individual to unacceptable toxicity or complications related to therapy. In the majority of patients it is possible to retain functional vision until the terminal phase of illness.[6] Although side effects of therapy are common, the vast majority of patients with CMVR and AIDS co-operate and comply with therapy.

Since the early descriptions of CMVR in AIDS, the concept of this disease has shifted from a blinding pre-terminal event to a manageable chronic condition associated with a life survival measurable in months or even years — nor is a central line always necessary in the management of CMVR in an era of ever-increasing treatment options.

Virology and Pathogenesis

CMV is an enveloped double-stranded DNA virus, classified as human herpes virus type 5, and has the largest genome in this family.[7,8] The control of protein synthesis from the genome involves a complex cascade system.[9] The immediate-early proteins synthesised first may be the only sign of CMV infection in the absence of replication.[10] DNA polymerase and structural proteins are synthesised further down the cascade. Glycoproteins on the surface of the enveloped nucleocapsids contain immunogenic antigens.[11] Alterations to the terminal sequences of the CMV genome differentiate between different humans strains.[12] The role of complement in neutralising CMV and the modulating effect of specific anti-CMV antibody has led to a better understanding of CMV neutralisation[13] and specific cytotoxic T-lymphocytes are important in preventing CMV disease in AIDS.[14]

In the majority of individuals with AIDS-related CMV infection, it is assumed that reactivation of CMV from an extraocular site, leads to viraemia and seeding to a number of potential target sites in the retina, gastrointestinal, respiratory, nervous system and endocrine tissues. Blood-borne spread to the eye may be facilitated by impaired haemorheology[15] / microvacular disease[16] indicating breakdown of the inner blood-retinal barrier, which increases both the access and contact time between CMV-infected macrophages[17] and neuroretina. Co-infection of retinal cells with other herpes viruses[18] and HIV[19] may influence disease severity.

The histopathological features of CMVR are characterised by full-thickness retinal necrosis with cytomegaly. Neuroretinal spread is thought to be paravascular[20] rather than adjacent infection of retinal vascular endothelial cells directly.[21] Low-grade lymphocytic and neutrophilic infiltrates may be present in the retina.[17,22] Sites of perivascular sheathing associated with CMVR are composed of neutrophils but lack CMV antigen.[21,22]

Epidemiology

The use of antiretroviral agents together with the early recognition and treatment of opportunistic infection has led to increased survival of patients with AIDS.

The number of patients with newly diagnosed CMVR referred to a major US centre has dropped with the current practice of using combination antiretroviral therapy,[23] though at present it is not clear how this treatment will affect the incidence of CMVR over the longer term (see chapter 1). The median survival of patients with AIDS after the diagnosis of CMV disease is one year or longer[2,24] and as with other evolving statistics concerning CMVR, is likely to underestimate the current clinical experience.[25] Given the increasing number of patients with HIV infection, and their longer survival, it is likely that the incidence of CMVR will depend on many factors including antiretroviral prescribing practice and the use of anti-CMV prophylaxis. A previous communication reported an increasing CMVR attack rate with prolonged survival,[26] and supports the impression that the majority of patients with AIDS would develop CMVR if their survival was sufficiently long.

Reports from the US of CMVR prevalence among AIDS patients of up to 40%[4,5,17,27] vary widely due to differences in patient recruitment, detection methods, and populations studied. Geographical variations in survival which relate to the availability and use of drugs to treat opportunistic infections would also influence the prevalence of CMVR. Studies carried out prospectively or postmortem would yield the most accurate prevalence data. Regional series from London and Edinburgh estimated the minimum risk of developing sight-threatening CMVR amongst patients with AIDS as 17%[2,28] despite differences between the two populations in terms of HIV transmission group. In Edinburgh, 38% of AIDS in the region is associated with homosexual/bisexual behaviour, though constituted 75% of patients with CMVR in the region; this is probably a reflection of the higher prevalence of sexually acquired CMV infection. It could also represent greater immunosuppression in the homosexual/bisexual group because of the longer duration of infection.[26] In this region CMVR is the presenting diagnosis in approximately 3% of patients with AIDS and 17% of patients with CMVR and AIDS.

The epidemiology of AIDS-related CMV infection derived from Europe and the US is unlikely to reflect the pattern of disease in South East Asia, South America, and Africa (see chapter 9). Also, it is becoming clear that the incidence of CMVR is changing in the more affluent parts of the world with the wider use of combination antiretroviral therapy, and strategies for CMVR surveillance may need to be modified (see below).

Symptoms

In comparison to the more severe systemic symptoms associated with AIDS the onset of CMVR is associated with few visual symptoms; unless the patient is aware of their significance, relatively minor visual symptoms may be considered too trivial to disclose to their physician. In Edinburgh, from a cohort of 24 patients with CMVR and AIDS, 16 had unilateral retinitis at presentation and although 59% of this group had macula and/or optic nerve-threatening disease less than half the group showed visual symptoms.[28] Visual blurring, photopsia, floaters, and scotomata are usually only noticed on occlusion of the unaffected eye, or when CMVR affects both eyes. Larger studies have confirmed the relative preservation of vision and unilaterally at the time of CMVR presentation — patients with more retinal involvement could not be distinguished from those with less severe disease on the basis of systemic parameters other than chronic fever and weight loss.[29] Although untreated CMVR is relentlessly progressive, the spread is relatively slow, and may partly explain the absence of acute visual symptoms. The size and location of CMVR influence the rate of progression.[30] The insidious and silently progressive nature of CMVR may result in advanced disease before symptoms become apparent, resulting in delayed diagnosis and treatment.

Signs

Patients with established CMVR may show mild vitreous activity and anterior chamber activity with endothelial deposits.[29] though posterior synechiae formation is not observed. Although CMV produces a spectrum of fundal appearances, the clinical picture usually allows a diagnosis to be made without the need for viral isolation from the eye. However, uncertainty may arise — early lesions of CMVR in evolution may mimic the cotton wool spots of HIV retinopathy. Weekly follow-up will confirm the diagnosis of CMVR if the signs of enlargement, retinal oedema and necrosis and vasculitis are observed. In the early stages, the retina shows white granular patches with irregular margins and variable overlying haemorrhage. CMVR tends to spread along one or more of the vascular arcades (most commonly the temporal branches), resulting in wedge-shaped areas of necrosis with the apices pointing posteriorly (see Fig. 6.1 and 6.2). Vascular sheathing may be subtle, or florid enough to appear as frosted branch angiitis.[31]

CMVR may present as extensive, oedematous lesions which progress more rapidly than the indolent granular lesion.[30] Progression occurs by centrifugal or "brushfire" spread from the original focus. The advancing edge consists of oedematous, opaque retina and this border may show faint gray/white "satellite" retinal opacities (see Fig. 6.3). The resulting central atrophic scar shows variable pigment epithelial disturbance with areas of retinal gliosis, which appears densely white and may even show intraretinal calcific changes.[32] Retinal vasculature within the affected area show attenuation and eventually become "ghost" vessels (see Fig. 6.4). CMVR produces a full-thickness retinal necrosis and can lead to rhegmatogenous retinal detachment. This is more likely to occur with CMVR affecting a large peripheral area of retina and in these patients the cumulative probability of detachment is 50% one year after the diagnosis of CMVR.[33] Small centrally located CMVR does not carry such a high risk of retinal detachment.

Evaluation

Close observation and accurate documentation of the retinal signs are the key to effective management of CMVR. The patients may be sick and unable to tolerate prolonged examination and therefore the clinician must be able to carry out a swift but accurate assessment. Following assessment of the best corrected visual acuity, the pupils are dilated for fundus examination.

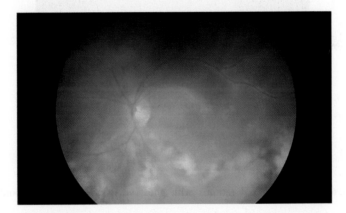

Fig. 6.1 Fulminant inferior CMV retinitis with superior retinal vascular sheathing.

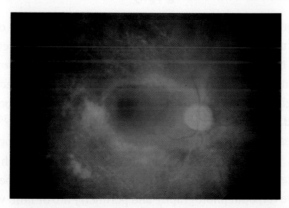

Fig. 6.2 Advanced circumferential CMV retinitis with macular sparing.

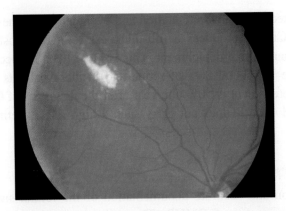

Fig. 6.3 CMV retinitis in evolution with satellite lesions and focal retinal vascular lesions.

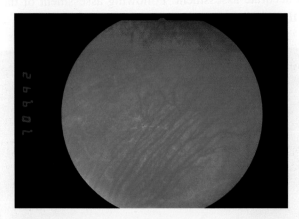

Fig. 6.4 Creeping CMV retinitis with ghost vessels and no active border.

Clinical Examination and Photography

The most important evaluation procedure is binocular indirect ophthalmoscopy. If a central focus of CMVR shows features of questionable activity and if the patient is able to sit at a slit-lamp, a hand-held 78-dioptre *or* 90-dioptre lens in used to examine the fundi, which may then be photographed. Perimetry can be of use though few patients are able to perform it well and perimetric defects may be elicited in HIV-infected individuals without retinitis.[34] Correlation of the retinal appearance with a corresponding field defect supports the diagnosis of CMVR; this invariably produces an absolute scotoma which enlarges as the infection progresses.[35] When photography is not possible, perimetry can be attempted. However, both photography and perimetry are of little value in mapping the progression of peripheral retinitis anterior to the equator, which is inaccessible to the fundus camera and may cause no scotoma. Also, it is not practical to perform photography or perimetry in patients with advanced AIDS who require bedside examination, and at this stage there is a high risk of recurrence. Therefore, it is always necessary to document not only the characteristics of the retinitis, as described above, but also precisely record the site and extent of the CMVR by clear and accurate drawing.

A classification for recording the site which divides the retina into three zones as been described — a posterior area which encompasses the disc and macular (zone 1), extending 3000 μ from the fovea and 1500 μ from the disc; midperipheral retina (zone 2) extending anterior to zone 1 up to the equator, and far peripheral retina (zone 3) extending anterior to the equator.[36] For peripheral CMVR the site is further defined by documenting the retinal site and clock hours involved; retinal vessels and vortex vein ampullae adjacent to the infection border served as landmarks to identify the demarcation line between affected and unaffected retina. The vascular landmarks adjacent to the CMVR border are noted, using the smallest visible arteriolar and venular branches to describe the boundary position, particularly the border closest to the macula and optic nerve.

Fundus Fluorescein Angiography

This investigation is not necessary in the majority of patients. It may be helpful in distinguishing between CMVR and toxoplasmosis retinochoroiditis if the clinical picture is uncertain. The fluorescein angiogram appearance of CMVR shows evidence of retinal vascular occlusion and permeability alterations in the area of retinitis.[37] Hyperfluorescence starts at the centre and extends to the borders, and the final hyperfluorescent area is smaller than the lesion observed on the red free photographs.[28] The underlying choroid is still present, and alterations in the retinal pigment epithelium produce this angiographic picture.

The fluorescein angiography of toxoplasmosis retinochoroiditis shows no permeability alterations or evidence of artery obstruction in the area of focal periarterial exudate or plaques,[37] and obscure the hyperfluorescence, which starts at the edge of the lesion and progresses towards the centre with marked fluorescein staining in the area of retinitis. The area of late hyperfluorescence is larger than the lesion seen on the control photographs.[28] The angiographic changes are produced by complete destruction of the retina and choroid, characteristic of a toxoplasmosis scar.

Laboratory Investigations

Serological testing or isolation of CMV from the throat or urine are not required for making the diagnosis of CMVR, which is a sign of systemic infection — of 24 patients with AIDS and CMVR studied in Edinburgh, 19 patients had raised CMV IgG levels indicating past infection and nine patients had detectable CMV IgM indicating newly acquired infection. 95% of homosexual men and 80% of HIV-positive injection drug users in Edinburgh show evidence of past CMV infection (Regional virus Laboratory, unpublished data).

The development of *in situ* nucleic acid hybridisation and nucleic acid amplification by PCR has allowed laboratory diagnosis on ocular fluids and tissue.[40,41] Standardised PCR-based assays are sufficiently sensitive and specific to be of more diagnostic value[42,43] than antibody-based assays in the form of the Goldmann-Witmer quotient.[44] Until these techniques are widely available, ophthalmologists must rely on their clinical skills to distinguish between CMVR and other infections affecting the retina and/or the choroid caused by toxoplasmosis, syphilis, candida, pneumocystis, varicella-zoster, and herpes simplex, which may cause concurrent infection (see chapter 5). Ocular lymphoma may also mimic CMVR.

Treatment

In most instances the treatment for CMVR is for the duration of the patient's life (unless they respond to HAART, see chapter 1) and decisions regarding therapy should actively involve the patient and their partner. Even if CMVR is peripheral and not immediately sight threatening, treatment should not be delayed; CMVR threatening the macula and disc should be treated immediately. A heavy commitment is required from the patient, ophthalmologist, and referring physician to monitor the therapeutic response and toxic effects of therapy for the duration of the patient's life. The problem of progressive CMVR during maintenance therapy remains a major management challenge.

Systemic Anti-CMV Therapy

At the time of diagnosis of retinitis extraocular CMV disease may also be manifest in the gut, central nervous system, or lung. Subclinical involvement of these organs is often difficult to prove, and occasionally local reactivation of CMV retinitis occurs in the absence of systemic infection. Currently, there are three intravenous treatment option for CMVR — ganciclovir, foscarnet and, more recently, cidofovir.

Ganciclovir and foscarnet

Ganciclovir is a nucleoside analogue which acts by competitive inhibition of CMV DNA polymerase. The UL97 gene produce protein kinase mediates monophosphorylation and drug activation. UL97 gene mutation appears to confer ganciclovir resistance. A controlled retrospective study of ganciclovir[36] confirmed previous uncontrolled reports of treatment benefit for CMVR. Foscarnet inhibits CMV DNA polymerase and does not require phosphorylation to become actively virostatic. Foscarnet is also effective in slowing the progression of CMVR.[45]

Intravenous ganciclovir and foscarnet suppress, but do not eradicate, CMV disease. Following high-dose induction therapy for two to three weeks — 10 mg/kg/day of ganciclovir, or 180 mg/kg/day of foscarnet,[5,24,36,45,46] — long-term maintenance therapy is necessary to prevent recurrence of CMVR, which nevertheless occurs in 18% to 54% of patients.[4,46-48] It is likely that all patients will relapse if the survival is sufficiently long (49) though this generally responds to an increase in anti-CMV therapy. Both drugs are associated with toxic side effects, ganciclovir with bone marrow suppression and foscarnet with renal impairment, metabolic abnormalities and seizure. Foscarnet therapy is associated with an increased survival period,[24] however, patients with impaired renal function had a longer survival with ganciclovir.

Overall, ganciclovir was better tolerated than foscarnet which requires a prolonged infusion time and the maintenance of adequate hydration is often poorly tolerated. Minimum-dose maintenance regimens are daily infusions of ganciclovir 5 mg/kg daily or foscarnet 90 mg/kg for seven days a week. While induction treatment for CMVR is usually administered in a hospital setting, maintenance therapy can be carried out at home with the assistance of the GP, district nurse, partner, or friend. A central line facilitates maintenance treatment, though generalised septicaemia caused by indwelling central venous lines in AIDS patients is a life-threatening risk.[50] The use of positive pressure reservoirs for intravenous therapy, for example, the portable intermate R infusion delivery system, simplifies home maintenance therapy and allows the patient greater mobility during the infusions. Nursing and medical support in the community is necessary for effective domicilary treatment, otherwise problems such as central line infections and poor compliance may pass unnoticed.

In view of the practical difficulties in achieving adequate hydration with foscarnet, ganciclovir is still preferred for maintenance therapy. *In vitro* studies raise the possibility of synergism[51] between the two antiviral agents, and both ganciclovir and foscarnet may be used in combination, with the added advantage of preventing the development of CMV resistance.[52] This approach was examined in a multicentre, randomised clinical trial comparing maintenance monotherapy with dual agent therapy in treating recurrent CMVR.[53] Although retinitis control was significantly better with the latter regimen, the combination approach had a negative impact on quality-of-life scores, required a longer infusion time, and was more expensive than monotherapy.

Cidofovir

This is a nucleotide analogue with an *in vitro* potency ten-fold greater than ganciclovir,[54] and does not depend on phosphorylation for anti-CMV activity. The site of action is likely to be CMV DNA polymerase and this drug is indicated in patients who show recurrent disease or intolerance of other therapies. Although cidofovir shows activity against ganciclovir-resistant CMVR with UL97 mutations, "high-level" ganciclovir-resistant CMV strains will also show resistance to cidofovir. High-level resistance of CMV to ganciclovir is associated with alterations in both the UL97 and DNA polymerase genes.[55]

Cidofovir intravenous induction therapy is 5 mg/kg once weekly for two weeks, followed by 5 mg/kg every two weeks as maintenance. This dosing schedule permits peripheral intravenous line administration as an outpatient procedure without the need for a central line and provides a prolonged median time to CMVR progression of 120 days.[56] Unfortunately, cidofovir may induce renal tubular injury, characterised by degeneration and necrosis of the proximal convoluted tubule cell.[57] Prevention of cidofovir nephrotoxicity includes hydration and probenicid treatment which decreases the tubular secretion of cidofovir. Tubular toxicity may still occur despite these measures.[58] Probenicid-induced side effects include skin rash and nausea. Low intraocular pressure[59] and uveitis[60] have been reported as side effects of systemic cidofovir.

In the majority of individuals the likely reason for relapsing infection is subtherapeutic drug dosing to the retina rather than drug resistance. Increasing the dose and frequency of systemic treatment usually leads to infection control — switching monotherapy or alternating combination treatment are other options. However, complications of longer term intravenous therapy includes central line sepsis and systemic toxicity — both are serious and life threatening. Oral ganciclovir maintenance therapy obviates the need for a venous access catheter, but does not minimise the risk of neutropenia, a common sign of drug toxicity.

Oral ganciclovir

The introduction of oral ganciclovir at a dose of 3–4 g/day as maintenance therapy for CMVR[61] has allowed freedom from a central line, however, concerns over bioavailability and relapsing infection have limited its use. Currently, oral ganciclovir is used in patients who have peripheral CMVR rather than posterior retinal involvement, and at each clinic review close attention should be paid to the scar border which may show advancement despite minimally opaque borders.[62]

Treatment toxicity

In most centres in the UK, ganciclovir remains the first-line therapy, though toxicity is a common problem. Ganciclovir-associated netropenia was often associated with concomitant zidovudine administration. The use of alternative antiretroviral agents have led to a reduction in this side effect — the combination of indinavir, lamivudine and zidovudine is effective in reducing HIV RNA for as long as one year.[63] Therefore, ganciclovir-associated myelotoxicity is still likely to be encountered and may be managed by the following strategies: withholding or replacing zidovudine, using haematologic stimulating factors (G-CSF), replacing ganciclovir with foscarnet or cidofovir, using a combination of foscarnet, and ganciclovir or intravitreal therapy.

Antiretroviral Therapy

Preliminary data suggests that HAART may affect the natural history and treatment of CMVR. HAART regimens consist of an HIV protease-inhibitor combined with dideoxynucleoside agents — using a combination of drugs, dramatic increases in CD4 cell count and survival have been observed with a reduction in HIV load (see chapter 1). The recent finding of CMVR occurring more frequently at higher levels of CD4 cell count than before suggests that HAART may not provide sufficient protection to prevent CMVR, or suppress subclinical retinitis, if all anti-CMV CD4 T cell clones are lost prior to initiating HAART.[64] In contrast, the therapeutic effect of combination antiretroviral therapy for CMVR has been reported in patients who have stopped maintenance therapy for established retinitis,[65] or who have been treated with protease-inhibitors without anti-CMV therapy at the time of CMVR diagnosis.[66]

Intravitreal (Local) Therapy

Direct drug placement into the vitreous cavity achieves high intravitreal drug allowing direct diffusion to the target tissue. Local therapy may be employed as primary therapy at the time of diagnosis, or as salvage therapy when conventional systemic treatment fails. The decision to continue systemic therapy in addition to local treatment depends on the presence of extraocular disease, bilaterality of CMV retinitis, tolerance to systemic therapy, survival prognosis, patient preference, and drug availability. There is great interest in local therapy for CMVR particularly for patients who have problems with standard treatment regimens and in countries where health resources are restricted.

The combination of local and oral therapies aims to achieve optimal retinitis control whilst reducing the risk of extraocular CMV morbidity without the hazards associated with intravenous treatment. This section examines the efficacy of this strategy, the potential complications, and the evolving role of the intravitreal treatment option in CMV retinitis.

Intravitreal injection

Ganciclovir or foscarnet intravitreal injection is an established method for achieving control of CMV retinitis. In most UK centres this form of therapy is used when systemic maintenance fails or has unacceptable side effects. It is rarely used a primary therapy. Intravitreal ganciclovir has been reported to be effective in controlling CMVR in patients who cannot tolerate systemic therapy.[67-70]; this requires twice weekly injections of 200 µg of ganciclovir in 0.1 ml sterile water for two to three weeks, and weekly intravitreal injections are used as maintenance treatment. Increasing clinical experience with intravitreal injection has shown tolerance to higher drug doses than previously used without clinical signs of retinal toxicity. A weekly intravitreal injection of 400 µg/0.05 ml as maintenance therapy was used in a selected patient series as sole therapy with a median time to CMVR progression of approximately 14 weeks[71] — retinal detachment and endophthalmitis were noted complications. An intravitreal bolus injection of 2 mg/0.1 ml of ganciclovir provides therapeutic levels (above LD50) for up to seven days without clinical toxicity. There was no evidence of drug accumulation with weekly injections.[72] An alternative regimen has been described using intravitreal foscarnet 1200 µg/0.05 ml[73] or a higher dose 2400 µg.[74] Combination ganciclovir and foscarnet by sequential injections exploits the synergistic activity of these drugs,[75] however, the intraocular pressure increase from two bolus injections without "creating space" by paracentesis or other methods, is likely to compromise central retinal artery perfusion.

Intravitreal injections are given in a clinic setting with prior instillation of topical anaesthetic and subconjunctival infiltration of lignocaine either superotemporally or inferotemporally. If reconstituted, ganciclovir can be refrigerated for future intravitreal injections although care must be taken to allow the product to equilibrate with room temperature, otherwise crystallised material may be injected inadvertently[76] (see chapter 8 for more details).

The pharmacodynamics of bolus dose intravitreal ganciclovir or foscarnet mandates weekly injections as a maintenance regiment in order to maintain adequate intravitreal levels. This arduous schedule may be difficult to sustain for a prolonged period. Two new drugs with potent anti-CMV activity which are under investigation for intravitreal therapy are cidofovir[77,78] and Vitravene (Formiversen or Isis 2922).[79] Cidofovir has been licensed for systemic therapy (see above), and preliminary data available on intravitreal injection suggests a prolonged therapeutic response of six weeks or more after a single injection of 20 µg with co-administration of oral probenecid. Uveitis and hypotony are complications of intravitreal cidofovir and it appears that this drug has a relatively narrow therapeutic window, above which ciliary body toxicity occurs, unlike ganciclovir or foscarnet.

Formiversen inhibits transcription of CMV mRNA, thereby preventing viral replication. Like cidofovir, this drug shows a prolonged therapeutic effect after a single injection, however, uveitis and possible retinal pigment epithelial toxicity which are dose dependant have been observed. Formiversen has the advantage of a larger duration of action and may be given fortnightly for induction and monthly for maintenance therapy.

Ganciclovir-sustained release implant

This novel drug delivery system (Vitrasert R) is a non-erodible polymeric device holding a ganciclovir pellet which releases the drug over a seven-month period (see Fig. 6.5). The attraction of this system is the prolonged high intravitreal levels of drug achieved after a single operative procedure (see chapter 8).[80] This device is effective in controlling CMV retinitis as primary therapy[81] at the time of diagnosis, or as "salvage" when other forms of treatment have failed.[82] Complications include endophthalmitis, vitreous haemorrhage, and retinal

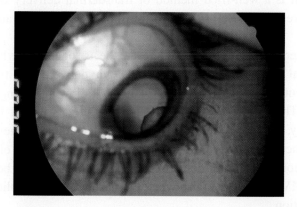

Fig. 6.5 Ganciclovir implant, sited inferotemporally at the pars plana shown against the red reflex.

detachment — the one-year cumulative risk of retinal detachment in CMV retinitis without surgery may be as high as 60%, though Vitrasert implantation may hasten the onset of this complication. This device is more effective than intravenous ganciclovir in sustaining CMVR control. However, patients treated with the implant and no systemic anti-CMV therapy run a higher risk of developing extraocular CMV disease.[83] Randomised controlled trials against standard therapy are underway to define their place in the management of CMVR.

The surgery should be carried out using peribulbar anaesthesia, with sedation if required, and can be planned as a day care procedure. In order to reduce the risk of vitreous haemorrhage, a platelet count should be checked and if low, a pre-/perioperative platelet transfusion is advisable. Asepsis and meticulous microsurgical technique should be employed to minimise the risk of complications (see chapter 8 for further details). The potential risk of HIV exposure to the surgeon and nursing staff should be minimised by following hospital infection control guidelines including the immediate disposal of needles and sharp instruments. In the event of inadvertent inoculation, antiviral chemoprophylaxis should be commenced immediately (see chapter 8)[85].

New Drug Delivery Systems

Iontophoresis

This is a less invasive drug delivery system compared to intravitreal implantation in which ions are driven across tissues and membranes by external electric potential, therefore, its use is restricted to ionisable drugs only. Factors influencing this process can be physicochemical such as pH, the strength of current ionic size, and concentration of the drug apart from some major physiological factors like tissue health. It is a well-tried method of transdermal delivery of protein-based drugs which are other wise difficult to transport across membranes due to their large size.

Recently, there has been renewed interest in the use of antivirals by iontophoresis in experimental animal eye studies. Ganciclovir delivered by this method has shown therapeutic vitreous levels for 24 hours following a single trans-scleral application.[86] There were no significant adverse effects except for mild retinal burn. Similarly, foscarnet delivery using this technique achieves intravitreal therapeutic concentration for 60 hours after its application, the elimination half-life being 24 hours.[87,88] Drug delivery with iontophoresis may be an alternative modality in CMV retinitis, though adverse effects on repeated applications requires further evaluation.

Liposomes and microspheres

This type of delivery system is designed to provide slow release of drug over a period of time and hence increases drug bioavailability while reducing drug toxicity. Liposomes are vesicles made up of phospholipids such as lecithin, phosphatidylglycerol, and phospatidylserine. Hydrophilic drugs remain entrapped within the liquid domains of the vesicles, whereas lipophilic drugs bind to the lipid layers. Liposomal preparations improve the efficacy of ganciclovir, foscarnet, and cidofovir, and may permit less frequent intravitreal injections, with sustained retinitis control.[89] The disadvantages of intravitreal liposomes include difficulties with sterilisation and storage and also transient media opacification on intravitreal injection.

Microspheres are similar to liposomes, with the drug remaining entrapped in polymer layers. The release rate can be controlled and prolonged by varying the molecular weights, proportions, and size of the polymers. The drug is released by degradation of the encapsulating polymer and concentration gradient diffusion. The polymers are polylactic and polyglycolic acid, and ganciclovir microspheres are made from polyorthoesters.[90] Microspheres overcome the disadvantages of liposomes, and in addition this delivery system can sustain therapeutic intravitreal drug levels of several months. Further investigations regarding biocompatability are underway.

It is likely that individualised therapy using a combination of local and systemic therapy through the course of CMV disease may offer the best hope.

Response to Therapy

Following the initiation of treatment of CMVR, ophthalmoscopic monitoring of both eyes is necessary. Changes in the appearance of the border infection usually accompanies a response to induction therapy, and patients should be examined weekly during this period. After the first week of treatment signs of active CMVR may still be present with oedematous, opaque, and variably haemorrhagic retina at the infected boundary. By the second or third week of induction, a healing response is seen with decreased opacification at the infected border, and a more granular appearance to the retina with resolution of the satellite spots; most importantly, failure of the borders to advance signifies infection control.

Cessation in centrifugal spread of CMVR is the major criterion used to assess a therapeutic response as altered border characteristics may not be a reliable sign of non-progression. Thereafter, the frequency of follow-up is determined by factors such as the site, laterality, control of infection (cessation of CMVR spread), and the appearance of the CMVR border. If the CMVR border is close to and threatening the macula/optic nerve, with signs of border activity and advancement frequent, follow-up every one to two weeks is necessary. If there is no sign of progression and the border looks inactive, follow-up might be lengthened to four to six weeks; patients with bilateral CMVR are more likely to relapse during maintenance therapy[28] and should be followed more frequently. A reduction in the frequency of ganciclovir or foscarnet maintenance treatment from seven to five days per week should only be considered for patients with stable and inactive CMVR. Further reduction is likely to lead to relapse.

A diagnosis of relapsing or breakthrough CMVR is made by serial examinations showing sequential creeping into previously unaffected retina, and is an indication for increased treatment. In the event of breakthrough injection, increasing the frequency of treatment from five to seven days per week may be sufficient to achieve control. If progression continues, repeat induction is indicated. "Smouldering" breakthrough CMVR must be distinguished from persistent white border opacification which does not advance, and is likely to represent atypical healing rather than active infection.[32] Failure to make this distinction may lead to unnecessary alterations in treatment. Conversely, it is important to recognise the "creeping" progression of CMVR which is associated with minimal border opacification.[91]

Prophylaxis for the Fellow Eye

Without therapy the likelihood of CMVR in the second eye of patients presenting with unilateral disease is estimated to be 60%, however, with intravenous anti-CMV treatment, this falls to zero to 15%.[46-48] A prospective evaluation of oral compared to intravenous ganciclovir as maintenance therapy for CMVR revealed a greater incidence of new bilateral lesions in previously uninvolved eyes in the oral-ganciclovir group (funduscopic assessment).[61] Daily intravenous maintenance therapy places major restrictions on the patient's mobility and carries the likelihood of toxic side effects. If all useful vision in one eye is lost, and the other is unaffected by CMVR, this raises the dilemma concerning prophylaxis for the unaffected eye.

In the absence of clinically manifest extraocular CMV disease, the response to HAART (see above) would influence the decision regarding second eye prophylaxis. Until prospective studies confirm the superior efficacy of maintenance therapy in preventing involvement of the second eye, an alternative is to simply observe the patient at four-weekly intervals and start treatment as soon as CMVR is detected. Three patients are reported who had no prophylaxis for the uninvolved eye and who remained free of CMVR when followed up to 35 weeks.[47]

Withholding systemic prophylaxis may lead to extraretinal CMV disease occurring in the gastrointestinal tract, adrenal glands, central nervous system, or lungs. 10% to 38% of patients receiving intravitreal ganciclovir and no systemic prophylaxis develop extraocular disease.[83,92,92] Disseminated CMV infection is a cause of death in patients with AIDS and postmortem studies reveal occult CMV infection in most patients.[94] The need for second eye and extraocular prophylaxis following CMVR diagnosis in one eye requires investigation by a randomised, controlled clinical trial and until then clinicians are likely to continue using oral ganciclovir[95] in this situation.

Retinal Detachment

This is discussed in detail in chapter 8.

Surveillance and Screening

CMVR is commonly asymptomatic and a prospective study showed that CMVR affected only the peripheral retina in 51% of AIDS patients.[5] Peripheral CMVR is not likely to be diagnosed until the disease advances into the posterior pole where the physician may detect it using direct ophthalmoscopy, or a fall in the visual acuity occurs. The degree of retinal scarring and visual morbidity is likely to be reduced if CMVR is detected and treated early. Until more data becomes available on the impact of screening protocols on visual outcome, ophthalmologists and attending physicians should devise sensible strategies for the early detection of CMVR. This may be achieved through a heightened awareness in the clinic setting, regular enquiry into visual symptoms, and ophthalmoscopy following pupillary dilatation. Encouraging self-testing of the vision in each eye in turn and emphasising the urgent need for reporting visual symptoms are likely to facilitate earlier CMVR detection.

The indications for ophthalmic referral include patients with visual symptoms, the presence of suspicious retinal lesions, a rapidly falling CD4 lymphocyte count, and evidence of extraretinal CMV disease. The findings of a recent study[96] supports screening when the CD4+ cell count falls to less than 50 cells/μl, or from 26% to 14% over a 12-month period, representing an overall risk reduction of 49%.[99] The drug-associated toxicity and cost of such an approach may make it impractical. In order to target the population at most risk of developing CMVR, quantitative PCR of CMV DNA from blood might allow CMV load to be assessed and correlated with retinitis risk. Maximising the sensitivity, specificity and predictive value of such laboratory-based techniques would allow targeted prophylaxis. The optimal drug and criteria for commencing therapy have yet to be identified. Drugs in development are cyclic-HPMPC, adefovir dipivoxil, lobucovir, and ganciclovir pro-drug. A humanised monoclonal antibody is also under investigation for the prevention or treatment of CMV infection.[100]

Although the use of HAART is likely to modify the incidence and natural history of CMVR, it is unlikely to eradicate the disease. Improved life survival following the diagnosis of CMVR may increase the likelihood and number of relapses which will ultimately lead to visual loss. At diagnosis of CMVR, CMV-viraemia has been linked to retinitis progression and increased mortality[101] and it may be appropriate to target this subgroup for more aggressive anti-CMV and antiretroviral therapies. CMV viral load data could be more informative in predicting recurrence, and allow treatment modification before progressive retinal destruction occurs. New approaches to therapy, including intravitreal drug placement and combination schedules of intravitreal/oral/intravenous modalities need to be fully evaluated with the aim of improving the visual outlook without compromising systemic well-being and life survival.

Outlook

CMVR is the most common intraocular infection encountered by ophthalmologists, though its incidence and prevalence is set to change in the coming years. The impression that CMVR is a late complication of AIDS is also changing as this disease is becoming a more common AIDS-defining illness.[102,103] In the more affluent parts of the world, life expectancy after diagnosis of CMVR has increased dramatically.[104] Until an effective and affordable prophylaxis strategy has been devised, ophthalmologists and physicians working in areas of the world with high rates of HIV infection, should be encouraged to develop local surveillance methods for detecting CMVR in order to prevent blindness among AIDS patients. At each routine visit the attending physician should enquire about visual symptoms. CMVR affecting the posterior retina may be asymptomatic, therefore, ophthalmoscopy, preferably after pupil dilation, should be part of any examination protocol.

Despite every effort to preserve vision and quality of life, progressive bilateral visual loss and increasing disability is likely to occur if the survival period is prolonged.[105] Although the survival outlook at this stage is poor, one should consider partially-sighted or blind registration. Counselling, home assessment, and even occupational therapy services can be especially helpful for these relatively young, sick patients and their families, and registration should be expedited. If all useful vision is lost in both eyes, or when the patient enters the terminal phase of their illness, treatment for CMVR should be withdrawn.

Although there is no cure for AIDS, patients who develop CMVR are strongly motivated to retain vision and maximise their quality of life. Although side effects of therapy are common, patients are motivated to comply with therapy and regular ophthalmic assessment until the terminal phase of their illness. Preservation of vision should remain a priority in the management of patients with AIDS, and is a responsibility shared by the ophthalmologist and attending physician.

References

1. Bankier A.T., Beck S., Bohni R. *et al.* "The DNA sequence of the human cytomegalovirus genoma," *DNA Seq.* **2** (1991), 1–12.

2. Peters B.S., Beck E.J., Anderson S. *et al.* "Cytomegalovirus infection in AIDS. Patterns of disease, response to therapy and trends in survival," *J. Infect.* **23** (1991), 123–125.

3. Ruger R., Bornkamm G.W., Fleckenstein B. "Human Cytomegalovirus DNA sequences with homologies to the cellular genome," *J. Gen. Virol.* **65** (1984), 1351–1364.

4. Jabs D.A., Enger C., Bartlett J.G. "Cytomegalovirus retinitis and acquired immunodeficiency syndrome," *Arch. Ophthalmol.* **107** (1989), 75–80.

5. Henderly D.E., Freeman W.R., Causey D.M. *et al.* "Cytomegalovirus retinitis and response to therapy with ganciclovir," *Ophthalmology* **94** (1987), 425–435.

6. Bloom P.A., Sandy C.J., Migdal C.S. *et al.* "Visual prognosis of AIDS patients with cytomegalovirus retinitis," *Eye* **9** (1995), 697–702.

7. Mathews R.E. "Third report of the international committee on taxonomy of viruses," *Intervirology* **12** (1979), 129–296.

8. Sonogyi T., Colimon R., Michelson S. "An illustrated guide to the structure of the human cytomegalovirus genome and a review of transcription data," *Prog. Med. Vir.* **33** (1986), 99–133.

9. Stinski M.F., Thomson D.R., Whaten M.W. *"Structure and Function of the Human Cytomegalovirus Genome."* The human herpesvirus, an interdisciplinary perspective, Elsevier, New York, (1980).

10. Mocarski E.S., Stinski M.F. "Persistence of the cytomegalovirus genome in human cells," *J. Virol.* **31** (1979), 761–771.

11. Marshall G.S., Stout G.G., Knights ME. *et al.* "Ontogeny of glycoprotein gB-specific antibody and neutralising activity during cytomegalovirus infection," *J. Med. Virol.* **43** (1994), 77–83.

12. Stinski M. "Molecular biology of cytomegalovirus replication," in: Ho M., (Ed.), *Cytomegalovirus: Biology and Function*, Plenum Press, New York (1991).

13. Spiller B.O., Hanna M.S., Devine D.V. *et al.* "Neutralisation of cytomegalovirus virions: the role of complement," *J. Infect. Dis.* **176** (1997), 339–347.

14. Rook A.H., Manishwitz, Fredrick W.R. *et al.* "Deficient, HLA-restricted, cytomegalovirus-specific cytotoxic T cells and natural killer cells in patients with the acquired immunodeficiency syndrome," *J. Infect. Dis.* **152** (1985), 627–630.

15. Engstrom R.E., Holland G.N., Hardy W.D. *et al.* "Hemorheologic abnormalities in patients with human immunodeficiency virus infection and ophthalmic microvasculopathy," *Am. J. Ophthalmol.* **109** (1990), 153–161.

16. Glasgow B.J., Weisberger A.K. "A quantitative and cartographic study of retinal microvasculopathy in acquired immunodeficiency syndrome," *Am. J. Ophthalmol.* **118** (1994), 46–56.

17. Palestine A.G., Rodrigues M.M., Macher A.M. *et al.* "Ophthalmic involvement in acquired immunodeficiency syndrome," *Ophthalmology* **91** (1984) 1092–1099.

18. Qavi H.B., Green M.T., Segall G.K. *et al.* "Demonstration of HIV-1 and HHV-6 in AIDS associated retinitis," *Curr. Eye Res.* **8** (1989), 379–387.

19. Skolnik P.R., Kosloff B.R., Hirsch M.S. "Bi-directional interactions between human immunodeficiency virus type 1 and cytomegalovirus," *J. Infect. Dis.* **157** (1988), 508–514.

20. Holland G.N., Sculer J.D. "Progression rates of cytomegalovirus retinopathy in ganciclovir-treated and untreated patients," *Arch. Ophthalmol.* **110** (1992), 1435–1442.

21. Holland G.N., Pepose J.S., Pettit T.H. *et al.* "Acquired immunodeficiency syndrome: Ocular manifestations," *Ophthalmology* **90** (1983), 859–873.

22. Pepose J.S., Holland G.N., Nestor M.S. *et al.* "Acquired immune deficiency syndrome. Pathogenic mechanisms of ocular disease," *Ophthalmology* **92** (1985), 472–484.

23. Jabs D.A., Bartlett J.G. (Editorial) "AIDS and ophthalmology: A period of transition," *Am. J. Ophthalmol.* **124** (1997), 227–233.

24. Studies of ocular complications of AIDS research group in collaboration with the AIDS clinical trial group. "Mortality in patients with the acquired immunodeficiency syndrome treated with eithes foscarnet or ganciclovir for cytomegalovirus retinitis," *N. Eng. J. Med.* **326** (1992), 213–220.

25. Chuang E.L., David J.L. "Management of retinal detachment associated with CMV retinitis in AIDS patients," *Eye* **6** (1992), 28–34.

26. Cheong I., Flegg P.J., Brettle R.P. *et al.* "CMV disease in AIDS: The Edinburgh Experience," *Int. J. STD AIDS* **3** (1992), 324–328.

27. Khadem M., Kalish S.B., Goldsmith J.A. *et al.* "Ophthalmologic findings in acquired immunodeficiency syndrome," *Arch. Ophthalmol.* **102** (1984), 201–204.

28. Dhillon B., Eddyshaw D., McLean H. *et al.* "Cytomegalovirus retinitis and AIDS in Edinburgh: Presentation, therapy, and visual outcome," *Int. J. STD AIDS* **3** (1993), 339–341.

29. Studies of ocular complications of AIDS research group in collaboration with the AIDS clinical trials group. "Foscarnet-Ganciclovir cytomegalovirus retinitis trial: 5. Clinical features of cytomegalovirus retinitis and diagnosis," *Am. J. Ophthalmol.* **124** (1997), 141–157.

30. Holland G.N., Sculer J.D. "Progression rates of cytomegalovirus retinopathy in ganciclovir-treated and untreated patients," *Arch. Ophthalmol.* **110** (1992), 1435–1442.

31. Spaide R.F., Vitale A.T., Toth I.R. *et al.* "Frosted branch angitis associated with cytomegalovirus retinitis," *Am. J. Ophthalmol.* **113** (1992), 522–528.

32. Keefe K.S., Freeman W.R., Peterson T.J. *et al.* "Atypical healing of cytomegalovirus retinitis" *Ophthalmology* **99** (1992) 1377–1388.

33. Jabs D.A., Enger C., Haller J. *et al.* "Retinal detachment in patients with cytomegalovirus retinitis," *Arch. Ophthalmol.* **109** (1991), 794–499.

34. Mueller A.J., Plummer D.J., Dua R. *et al.* "Analysis of visual dysfunctions in HIV-positive patients without retinitis," *Am. J. Ophthalmol.* **124** (1997), 158–167.

35. Bachman D.M., Bruni L.M., DiGioia R.A. *et al.* "Visual field testing in the management of cytomegalovirus retinitis," *Ophthalmology* **99** (1992), 1393–1399.

36. Holland G.N., Buhles W.C., Mastre B. *et al.* "A controlled retrospective study of ganciclovir treatment for cytomegalovirus retinitis. Use of a standardised system for the assessment of disease outcome," *Arch. Ophthalmol.* **107** (1989), 1759–1766.

37. Gass J.D.M. in: *Stereoscopic Atlas of Macular Diseases: Diagnosis and Treatment.* St Louis, Washington, Toronto, CV Mosby (1987), 496–497.

38. Cochereau-Massin I., LeHoang P., Lautier-Frau M. *et al.* "Ocular toxoplasmosis in human immunodeficiency virus infected patients," *Am. J. Ophthalmol.* **114** (1992), 130–135.

39. Holland G.N., Engstrom R.E., Glasgow B.J. *et al.* "Ocular toxoplasmosis and AIDS," *Am. J. Ophthalmol.* **106** (1988), 653–667.

40. Freeman W.R., Wiley C.A. "*In-situ* nucleic acid hybridisation," *Surv. Ophthalmol.* **34** (1989) 187–192.

41. Hennis H.L., Scott A.A., Apple D.J. "Cytomegalovirus retinitis," *Surv. Ophthalmol.* **34** (1989), 193–203.

42. Mitchell S.M., Fox J.D., Tedder R.S. *et al.* "Vitreous fluid sampling and viral genome detection for the diagnosis of viral retinitis in patients with AIDS," *J. Med. Vir.* **43** (1994), 336–340.

43. McCann J.D., Margolis T.P., Wong B.S. *et al.* "A sensitive and specific polymerase chain reaction-based assay for the diagnosis of cytomegalovirus retinitis," *Am. J. Ophthalmol.* **120** (1995), 219–226.

44. Doornenbal P., Baarsma G.S., Quint W.G. *et al.* "Diagnostic assays in cytomegalovirus retinitis: detection of herpes virus by simultaneous application of the polymerase chain reaction and local antibody analysis on ocular fluid," *Br. J. Ophthalmol.* **80** (1996), 235–240.

45. Palestine A.G., Polis M.A., de Smet M.D. *et al.* "A randomised, controlled trial of foscarnet in the treatment of cytomegalovirus retinitis in patients with AIDS," *Ann. Intern. Med.* **115** (1991), 665–673.

46. Gross J.G., Bouzette S.A. "Longitudinal study of cytomegalovirus retinitis in acquired immunodeficiency syndrome," *Ophthalmology* **97** (1990), 681–686.

47. Holland G.N., Sidikaro Y., Kreiger A.E. "Treatment of cytomegalovirus retinitis with gancicloir," *Ophthalmology* **94** (1987), 815–823.

48. Jabs D.A., Newman C., de Bustros S. *et al.* "Treatment of cytomegalovirus retinitis," *Ophthalmology* **94** (1987), 824–830.

49. Jabs D.A. "Treatment of cytomegalovirus retinitis — 1992," (Editorial) *Arch. Ophthalmol.* **11** (1992), 185–187.

50. Ravoglione M.C., Batten R., Pablos-Mendez A. *et al.* "Infections associated with Hickmans catheters in patients with acquired immunodeficiency syndrome," *Am. J. Med.* **86** (1989), 780–786.

51. Manischewitz J.F., Quinnan G.V., Jr, Lane H.C. *et al.* "Synergistic effect of ganciclovir and foscarnet on cytomegalovirus replication *in vitro*," *Antimicrob. Agents Chemother.* **34** (1990), 373–375.

52. Nelson M.R., Barter G., Hawkins D. *et al.* "Simultaneous treatment of cytomegalocirus retinitis with ganciclovir and foscarnet," *Lancet* **338** (1991), 250.

53. Studies of ocular complications of AIDS (SOCA) research group. "Combination foscarnet and ganciclovir therapy vs monotherapy for the treatment of relapsed cytomegalovirus retinitis in patients with AIDS: The cytomegalovirus retreatment trial," *Arch. Ophthalmol.* **114** (1996), 23–33.

54. Stals E.S., de Clerq W., Bruggman D. "Comparative activity of (2)-1-(3-hydroxy-2-phosphonylmethoxypropyl) cytosine and 9-(1,3 dihydroxy-2-propoxymethyl) guanine against rat cytomegalovirus infection *in vitro* and *in vivo*," *Antimicrob. Agents Chemother.* **35** (1991), 2262–2266.

55. Smith I.L., Cherrington J.M., Jiles R.E. *et al.* "High-level resistance of cytomegalovirus to ganciclovir is associated with alterations in both the UL97 and DNA polymerase genes," *J. Infect. Dis.* **126** (1997), 257–263.

56. Lalezari J.P., Stagy R.J., Kupperman B.D. *et al.* "Intravenous cidovofir for peripheral cytomegalovirus retinitis; a randomised clinical trial," *Ann. Intern. Med.* **126** (1997), 257–263.

57. Polis M.A., Spooner K.M., Baird B.F. *et al.* "Anti cytomegalovirus activity and safety of cidofovir in patients with human immunodeficiency virus infection and cytomegalovirus viruria," *Antimicrob. Agents Chemother.* **39** (1995), 882–886.

58. Vittecoq D., Dumitrescu L., Beaufils H. *et al.* "Fanconi syndrome associated with cidofovir therapy," *Antimicrob. Agents Chemother.* **41** (1997), 1846.

59. Friedberg D.N. "Hypotony and visual loss with intravenous cidofovir treatment of cytomegalovirus retinitis," *Arch. Ophthalmol.* **115** (1997), 801–802.

60. Palau L.A., Ives D., Lalezari J.P. *et al.* "Recurrent iritis after intravenous administration of cidofovir," *Clin. Infect. Dis.* **25** (1997), p. 337.

61. Drew W.L., Ives D., Lalezari J.P. *et al.* "Oral ganciclovir as maintenance treatment for cytomegalovirus retinitis in patients with AIDS," *N. Engl. J. Med.* **333** (1995), 615–620.

62. Holland G.N., Tufail A. "New therapies for cytomegalovirus retinitis," *N. Engl. J. Med.* **333** (1995), 658–659.

63. Gulick R.M., Mellors J.W., Havlir D. *et al.* "Treatment with indinavir, zidovudine, and Lamivudine in adults with human immunodeficiency," **739**.

64. Jacobson M.A., Zegans M., Pavan P.R. *et al.* "Cytomegalovirus retinitis after initiation of highly active antiretroviral therapy," *Lancet* **349** (1997), 1443–1445.

65. Whitcup S.M., Nussenblatt, Polis M.A. *et al.* "Therapeutic effect of combination antiretroviral therapy on cytomegalovirus retinitis," *JAMA* **277** p. 1519.

66. Reed B.J., Schwab I.R., Gordon J. *et al.* "Regression of cytomegalovirus retinitis associated with protease-inhibitor treatment in patients with AIDS," *Am. J. Ophthalmol.* **124** (1997), 199–205.

67. Ussery F.M. III, Gibson S.R., Conklin R.H. *et al.* "Intravitreal ganciclovir in the treatment of AIDS-associated cytomegalovirus retinitis," *Ophthalmology* **95** (1989), 640–648.

68. Henry K., Cantrill H.L., Fletcher C. *et al.* "Use of intravitreal ganciclovir (dihydroxy propoxy methy guanine) for cytomegalovirus retinitis in patients with AIDS," *Am. J. Ophthalmol.* **103** (1987), 17–23.

69. Cantrill H.L., Henry K., Melroe H. *et al.* "Treatment of cytomegalovirus retinitis with intravitreal ganciclovir: Long term results," *Ophthalmology* **96** (1989), 367–374.

70. Heinemann M.H. "Long term intravitreal ganciclovir for cytomegalovirus retinopathy," *Arch. Ophthalmol.* **107** (1989) 1767–1772.

71. Hodge W.G., Lalonde R.G., Sampalis J. *et al.* "Once weekly intra-ocular injections of ganciclovir for maintenance therapy of cytomegalovirus retinitis: Clinical and ocular outcome," *J. Infect. Dis.* **174** (1996), 393–395.

72. Morlet N., Young S., Graham G. *et al.* "High dose intravitreal ganciclovir injection provides a prolonged therapeutic intraocular concentration," *Br. J. Ophthalmol.* **80** (1996), 214–216.

73. Diaz-Liopis M., Chipont E., Sanchez S. *et al.* "Intravitreal foscarnet for cytomegalovirus retinitis in a patient with acquired immunodeficiency syndrome," *Am. J. Ophthalmol.* **114** (1992), 742–747.

74. Diaz-Liopos M., Espana E., Munoz G. *et al.* "High dose intravitreal foscarnet in the treatment of cytomegalovirus retinitis in AIDS," *Br. J.Ophthalmol.* **78** (1994), 120–124.

75. Desatnik H.R., Foster R.E., Lowder C.Y. "Treatment of clinically resistant cytomegalovirus retinitis with combined intravitreal injections of ganciclovir and foscarnet," *Am. J. Ophthalmol.* **122** (1996), 121–123,

76. Fiscella R.G., Goldstein D., Labib S. *et al.* "The formation of crystals in ganciclovir used for intraocular injection," *Arch. Ophthalmol.* **115** (1997), 945–946.

77. Rahhal F.M., Arevalo J.F., de la Paz E.C. *et al.* "Treatment of cytomegalovirus retinitis with intravenous cidofovir in patients with AIDS," *Ann. Intern. Med.* **125** (1996), 98–103.

78. Taskintuna I., Rahhal F.M., Arevalo J.F. *et al.* "Low dose intravitreal cidofovir (HPMC) therapy of cytomegalovirus retinitis in patients with acquired immune deficiency syndrome," *Ophthalmology* **104** (1997), 1049–1057.

79. Flore-Aguilar, Besen G., Wong C. *et al.* "Evaluation of retinal toxicity and efficiency of anti-cytomegalovirus and anti-herpes simplex virus antiviral phophorothioate ologonucleotides ISIS 2922 and ISIS 4015," *J. Infect. Dis.* **175** (1997) 1308–1316.

80. Canborn G.E., Anand R., Torti R.E. *et al.* "Sustained-release ganciclovir therapy for treatment of cytomegalovirus retinitis," *Arch. Ophthalmol.* **110** (1992), 188–195.

81. Martin D.F., Parks D.J., Mellow S.D. *et al.* "Treatment of cytomegalovirus retinitis with an intraocular sustained release implant," *Arch. Ophthalmol.* **112** (1994), 1531–1539.

82. Marx J.L., Kapsuta M.A., Patel S.S. *et al.* "Use of ganciclovir implant in the treatment of recurrent cytomegalovirus retinitis," *Arch. Ophthalmol.* **114** (1996), 815–820.

83. Musch D.C., Martin D.F., Gordon J.F. *et al.* "Treatment of cytomegalovirus retinitis with a sustained-release ganciclovir implant," *N. Engl. J. Med.* **337** (1997), 83–90.

84. Friedlander S.M., Goldstein D.A. "Early reactivation of cytomegalovirus retinitis following placement of a ganciclovir implant," *Arch. Ophthalmol.* **115** (1997), 802–803.

85. Landers III M.B., Fraser V.J. "Perspective. Antiviral chemoprophylaxis after occupational exposure to human immunodeficiency virus: Why, when, where, and what," *Am. J. Ophthalmol.* **124** (1997), 234–239.

86. Lam T.T., Fu J., Chu R. *et al.* "Intravitreal delivery of ganciclovir in rabbits by trans-scleral iontophoresis," *J. Ocular Pharmac.* **10** (1994), 571–575.

87. Sarraf D., Equi R.A., Holland G.N. *et al.* "Trans-scleral iontophoresis of forcarnet," *Am. J. Ophthalmol.* **115** (1993), 748–754.

88. Yoshizumi M.O., Roca J.A., Lee A.A. *et al.* "Ocular iontophoretic supplementation of intravenous foscarnet therapy," *Am. J. Ophthalmol.* **122** (1996), 86–90.

89. Akula S.J., Ma P.E., Payman G.A. "Treatment of cytomegalovirus retinitis with intravitreal injection of liposome encapsulated ganciclovir in a patient with AIDS," *Br. J. Ophthalmol.* **78** (1994), 667–680.

90. Gaynon M., Heller J., Wuthirch P. "Sustained release of ganciclovir from poly (orthoester) polymer," *(Abst) Invest. Ophthalmol. Vis. Sci.* **32** (1991), p. 883.

91. Dhillon B., Cacciatori M., Ling C. "'Creeping' cytomegalovirus retinitis in AIDS," *Br. J. Ophthalmol.* **8** (1996), 771–772.

92. Cochereau-Massin I., LeHoang P., Lautier-Frau M. *et al.* "Efficacy and tolerance of intravitreal ganciclovir in cytomegalovirus retinitis in acquired immune deficiency syndrome," *Ophthalmology* **98** (1991), 1348–1355.

93. Polsky B., Wolitz R., Cantrill H. *et al.* "Intravitreal ganciclovir salvage therapy for cytomegalovirus retinitis (ACTG 085): A preliminary report," (Abstracts) *7th International Conference on AIDS*, June 19–22, Florence, Italy, (1991), WB 2340.

94. Pepose J.S., Holland G.N., Nestor M.S. *et al.* "Acquired immune deficienty syndrome. Pathogenic mechanisms of ocular disease," *Ophthalmology* **92** (1985), p. 472.

95. DeArmond B. "Future directions in the management of cytomegalovirus infections," *J. AIDS* **4**(suppl) (1991), S53–S56.

96. Kupperman B.D., Petty J.G., Richman D.D. *et al.* "Correlation between CD4+ counts and prevalence of cytomegalovirus retinitis and human immunodeficiency virus related non infectious retinal vasculopathy in patients with AIDS," *Am. J. Ophthalmol.* **115** (1993), 575–582.

97. Hoover D.R., Peng Y., Saah A. *et al.* "Occurrence of cytomegalovirus retinitis after human immunodeficiency virus immunosuppression," *Arch. Ophthalmol.* **114** (1996), 821–827.

98. Gellrich M.M., Baumert E., Rump J.A. *et al.* "Clinical utility of cytomegalovirus urine cultures for ophthalmic care in patients with HIV," *Br. J. Ophthalmol.* **80** (1996), 818–822.

99. Spector S.A., McKinlay G.F., Lalezari J.P. *et al.* "Oral ganciclovir for the prevention of cytomegalovirus disease in persons with AIDS," *N. Engl. J. Med.* **334** (1996), 1491–1497.

100. Hamilton A.A., Manuel D.M., Grundy J.E. *et al.* "A humanised antibody against human cytomegalovius (CMV)gp UL75 (gH) for prophylaxis of treatment of CMV infections," *J. Infect. Dis.* **176** (1997), 59–68.

101. Studies of ocular complications of AIDS (SOCA) and the AIDS Clinical Trials Group. "Cytomegalovirus (CMV) culture results, drug resistance and clinical outcome in patients with AIDS and CMV retinitis treated with ganciclovir or foscarnet," *J. Infect. Dis.* **176** (1997), 50–58.

102. Porter K., Fairley C.K., Wall P.G. *et al.* "AIDS defining disease in the UK: The impact of PCP prophylaxis and twelve years of change," *Int. J. STD AIDS* **7**(4) (1996), 252–257.

103. Montaner J.S., Le T., Hogg R. "The changing spectum of AIDS index diseases in Canada," *AIDS* **8**(5) (1994), 693–696.

104. Courtright P. "The challenge of HIV/AIDS related eye disease," (Editorial) *Br. J. Ophthalmol.* **80** (1996), 496–497.

105. Roarty J.D., Fisher E.J., Muussbaum J.J. "Long term visual morbidity of cytomegalovirus retinitis in patients with acquired immune deficiency syndrome," *Ophthalmology* **100** (1993), 1685–1688.

CHAPTER 7

NEUROPHTHALMIC PROBLEMS IN HIV AND AIDS

Elizabeth M Graham and Rosalyn M Stanbury

Introduction

Clinical surveys show neurological disorders occur in 40% of adult AIDS patients[1] while postmortem studies reveal neuropathology in 70% to 80% of AIDS patients.[2] Of those with neurological manifestations 41% had an opportunistic infection,[3] the organisms most frequently involved are toxoplasma, cryptococcus, cytomegalovirus, and herpes zoster. CNS involvement is more usual in the late stages of HIV infection but in 10% it can be the initial manifestation.[4] 3% to 8% of HIV-positive patients have neurophthalmic complications.[5-7] Of 177 patients reviewed with AIDS or AIDS-related complex who had had an ocular examination, one study found no neurophthalmic problems in the AIDS-related complex group (50 patients) and ten affected patients in the AIDS group (127 patients).[6] HIV disease can be divided into different stages — acute seroconversion illness, early, middle, and late stages (see also chapter 2). In each stage the conditions that can cause neurophthalmic problems are discussed. The final section deals with the differential diagnosis of the various neurophthalmic clinical situations, which can present to the ophthalmologist.

Acute Seroconversion Illness

Clinical Features

Initial infection with HIV is usually asymptomatic, but in 30% to 50% an acute retroviral seroconversion syndrome develops.[8] The symptoms develop acutely two to six weeks after exposure to HIV and last up to 14 days. The illness is very much like glandular fever with fever, lethargy, pharyngitis, lymphadenopathy, arthralgia, myalgia, anorexia, nausea, vomiting, diarrhoea, and a maculopapular rash. Neurological involvement includes aseptic meningitis (CSF — raised protein and pleocytosis),[9] encephalitis,[10] cranial nerve palsies, particularly facial,[11] myelopathy, and radiculopathy. The Guillain-Barre syndrome has been described in association with seroconversion[12,13] but cases have not included any ocular involvement. The Miller Fisher syndrome (ophthalmoplegia, ataxia, and areflexia), which is thought to be a subgroup of the Guillain-Barre syndrome, has been described in one case.[14]

Investigations

Investigations at this stage show a raised ESR, thrombocytopenia, lymphopenia (CD4 and CD8) with atypical lymphocytes, followed by a lymphocytosis (CD8). The lymphocyte count then normalises but the CD4 count does not return to pre-infection levels. The serum aminotransferase may be raised. In most individuals HIV antibodies are detectable by two to three weeks from the start of the seroconversion illness. IgM antibodies peak at two to five weeks and disappear by three months; IgG antibodies follow the appearance of the IgM antibodies and persist. The acute seroconversion illness appears to coincide with the peak in plasma viraemia, therefore, if the antibodies are negative the cause of the condition can be confirmed by p24 antigen testing, HIV culture, or using the polymerase chain reaction.

Although neurophthalmological abnormalities are uncommon at this stage of the disease, the acute seroconversion illness should be considered in patients presenting with neurophthalmic complications of meningitis, encephalitis, and the Guillain-Barre syndrome in the setting of a glandular fever-like illness.

Treatment

Other causes should be excluded and if HIV infection is confirmed, antiretroviral triple therapy should be considered. It has been shown that rapid viral replication is occurring in lymphoid tissue from the moment the infection is acquired[15] and this is the basis for treating with antiretroviral drugs at this stage,[16] but this is not established practice as yet. The recent British HIV Association guidelines[17] does not specifically address this situation but the International AIDS Society — USA[18] recommendations suggest treating with the most potent combination available for at least six months, with further treatment being guided by clinical judgement dependant on viral load, CD4 counts, drug toxicity, patients acceptance, and cost.

Early Disease CD4 > 500 Cells/µl

During this phase of the disease the majority of patients have no symptoms relating to infection with the HIV. There may be lymphadenopathy, seborrhoeic dermatitis, folliculitis, aphthous ulcers, and autoimmune disease such as immune thrombocytopaenic purpura. Neurological conditions occurring at this stage include the Guillain-Barre syndrome, multiple sclerosis, and infections with the herpes zoster virus and herpes simplex virus.

Guillain-Barre Syndrome

GBS has been reported to occur in the early phase of HIV infection as well as part of the seroconversion illness.[13] The occurrence of this condition in the early phase of HIV disease may be related to seroconversion for such agents as campylobacter or cytomegalovirus. The clinical and electrophysiological features of the GBS are the same in HIV-positive and HIV-negative populations. An elevated CSF protein with normal white blood cells is the hallmark of the GBS in HIV-negative patients; in HIV-positive patients there may also be a CSF pleocytosis due to the HIV itself. Therefore, in a patient with the clinical characteristics of the GBS or Miller Fisher syndrome where the CSF shows a pleocytosis, HIV disease should be considered.

Multiple Sclerosis

There appears to be a relationship between multiple sclerosis (MS) and HIV infection which is more than a chance occurrence of the two conditions. Seven patients with "definite" MS and HIV disease have been described[19] and in four patients the MS predated the HIV infection by 3.5 to 18 years. No change in the pattern of their MS occurred following HIV infection. Three patients were described as having a relapsing remitting pattern of MS which first occurs at the time of or within three months of contracting HIV. In all three, optic neuritis (one bilateral) was part of the initial presentation and all had a relatively rapid neurological decline. A brain biopsy was performed on one of these cases and the features were characteristic of MS with no changes consistent with HIV encephalopathy. In a further report, a 33-year-old man developed MS ten months after becoming HIV positive.[20] During the course of his illness he developed an homonymous hemianopia and a brain biopsy was consistent with MS. A fulminant form of MS has been also described.[21] The first, a 66-year-old man, developed rapid, sequential bilateral optic neuritis followed by widespread neurological disease and died within two months. The second case was also rapidly fatal but had no ocular problems. The presence of HIV antibodies was found for the first time during their neurological illnesses. Postmortem examinations were characteristic of MS. All the patients described in these reports fulfilled the critieria for definite MS, in the majority optic neuritis was present, and in all the progression of the disease was rapid. Therefore, in patients with optic neuritis and a rapidly deteriorating neurological condition with an MRI scan compatible with MS, an HIV test should be considered.

Varicella-Zoster Virus Infection

The herpes zoster virus is an enveloped double-stranded DNA virus. Infection with this virus spans all stages of HIV infection. A San Francisco study comparing HIV-positive and HIV-negative homosexuals showed a relative risk of 17 for developing varicella-zoster virus (VZV) infection.[22] Descriptions of chicken pox in HIV-positive patients are limited and it is not known whether complications such as pneumonia or meningo-encephalitis occur with increased frequency. On the other hand shingles, including HZO, has been described by several authors as being more frequent, prolonged, and more often recurrent in HIV-positive patients. Neurological complications of VZV infection include radiculitis, myelitis, meningoencephalitis, and cerebral arteritis. The varicella-zoster meningoencephalitis is rare compared with herpes simplex encephalitis although its incidence may be underestimated as the diagnosis is difficult to establish. The cerebral arteritis typically occurs weeks to months after trigeminal or cervical shingles and presents as a contralateral stroke due to thrombotic occlusion of the ipsilateral middle cerebral artery.

The commonest neurophthalmic manifestation of VZV disease in HIV infection is optic neuritis (see Fig. 7.1) Optic nerve abnormalities at the time of diagnosis

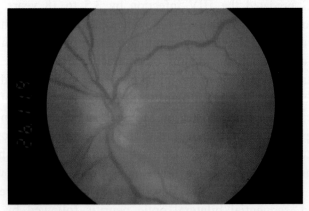

Fig. 7.1 Varicella-zoster optic neuropathy. A swollen optic disc with an area of retinal necrosis infero-temporally.

of progressive outer retinal necrosis syndrome have been described in 17%.[23] Their findings include disc swelling, hyperaemia and optic atrophy. In immunocompetent patients with acute retinal necrosis, optic nerve involvement has been thought to be secondary to the retinal involvement. Other authors have described optic nerve disease predating the onset of retinal necrosis in HIV-positive patients (see Table 7.1).

Table 7.1 Varicella-Zoster infection in AIDS.

Author	Shingles	Optic Neuritis	PORN
• Winward[24]	Left HZO Oral ACV	two weeks later Left ON	Simultaneous left peripheral PORN
• Litoff[25]	Right HZO Intravenous ACV three weeks later Left HZO Intravenous ACV	Simultaneous Left ON	six weeks later Left PORN
• Shayegani[26]	–	Left ON Intravenous foscarnet three weeks later Right ON	three days later Bilateral PORN
• Friedlander[27]	T4 shingles Oral ACV	two months later Left ON	one month later Left PORN
• Friedlander[27]	Thoracic shingles Famciclovir	two weeks later Right ON	three weeks later Right PORN
• Friedlander[27]	Thoracic shingles Oral ACV	three weeks later Bilateral ON	three days later Bilateral PORN

In all but one of the cases, where optic neuritis preceded PORN, there had been a recent episode of shingles which had been treated with either oral or intravenous antiviral agents. It is possible that this allowed for the selection of a more virulent strain of the VZV. In many of these cases the cause of the optic neuropathy was not apparent until the appearance of the PORN. The visual prognosis of PORN is extremely poor, therefore the occurrence of an optic neuropathy within weeks of an episode of shingles should alert the clinician to the possibility of herpes zoster optic neuropathy and allow early antiviral treatment in order to achieve the best possible visual outcome.

Herpes Simplex Virus Infection

The herpes simplex virus is an enveloped virus with double-stranded DNA. There are two antigenic types: HSV-1 and HSV-2. In the main, HSV-1 causes oral, ocular and CNS disease and HSV-2 causes genital disease, although the reverse can occur. HSV is the commonest cause of fatal encephalitis in the immunocompetent population and can occur as a result of the primary or a recurrent infection. The features include a combination of a change in mental state and conscious level with focal signs relating to cortical or brain stem involvement. Neurophthalmic signs may therefore include visual field defects and ocular motility abnormalities. Diagnosis is dependant on MRI changes (oedema and necrosis) and CSF abnormalities (pleocytosis, haemorrhage, and PCR identification of HSV). EEG changes are helpful but not diagnostic. Treatment is with intravenous aciclovir followed by oral maintenance therapy.

HSV encephalitis occurs in the immunocompetent as well as the immunocompromised. There is no clear evidence that it occurs more frequently in the immunosuppressed, but it should be included in the differential diagnosis of encephalitis, especially in the early stages of HIV infection.

Middle Stage Disease, CD4 200–500 Cells/μl

Many patients remain asymptomatic during this stage of their disease. Conditions present in the early stage continue and may worsen, for example recurrent herpes simplex and varicella zoster disease. Recurrent bacterial infections affecting sinus and lungs can occur. These infections suggest that early HIV-induced immunologic changes affect the host responses to pathogenic organisms before advanced immunodeficiency allows the development of an AIDS-defining illness. Syphilis and tuberculosis are two important infections that may be seen at this stage of the disease and although lymphoma may also be seen at this level of CD4 count, it occurs more commonly in later stages of the disease.

Syphilis

There is an increased incidence of syphilis in the HIV-positive population. Infection with this bacteria passes through three stages: primary, secondary, and tertiary. Secondary syphilis develops in 100% of patients after two weeks if the primary infection is not treated. At this stage CSF examination shows abnormalities in 50% and treponemal organisms in 25%, but only 1% to 2% develop a symptomatic meningitis. With no treatment the signs resolve over one to two months and the infection becomes latent. Humoral and cell-mediated immunity both play a role in achieving latency. In patients who receive no treatment, tertiary syphilis will develop in 33% (neurological 7%, cardiovascular 9%, parenchymal 17%). With adequate treatment of early syphilis, neurosyphilis almost never develops in the immunocompetent, but despite this viable treponemes can still be found in lymph nodes. Therefore, the host's immune system, with the help of penicillin, can contain the infection.

Syphilis in HIV infection

HIV infection does not appear to alter primary and secondary syphilis, but neurosyphilis occurs more commonly and earlier.[28] The cases of neurosyphilis seen in HIV disease are very like those cases of neurosyphilis which developed following inadequate treatment in the pre-penicillin era, i.e. the early neurosyphilis, meningovascular in type, rather than the late tabes dorsalis and general paresis of the insane.[29] In a review of the literature of 38 patients with neurosyphilis and HIV infection, 13 were HIV positive, seven had the AIDS-related complex, and 18 had AIDS.[30] In 40% HIV was first diagnosed when neurosyphilis presented and 16 patients had previously been treated with the recommended dose of penicillin. The neurological abnormalities found were as follows: five were classified as asymptomatic as they had abnormal CSF but no neurological signs, 23 had acute meningitis, 11 had meningovascular syphilis (presenting with signs of a cerebrovascular accident, especially in the basilar distribution), and one general paresis. In the group with meningitis, 13 had cranial nerve abnormalities: eight had optic nerve dysfunction, four had VIIIth nerve problems and one patient had III, IV and VIth abnormalities. The CSF was abnormal in some way in 36 out of 38 and 30 out of 37 had a positive CSF VDRL.

When the ocular findings in neurosyphilis were compared between HIV-positive and HIV-negative patients, ocular abnormalities were found with greater frequency in the HIV-infected group — ten patients (42%) of the HIV-positive group compared with three patients (14%) in the negative group. Optic neuritis was the most common abnormality, occurring in three members of the HIV-positive group.[31] On the other hand, in patients with ocular syphilis, neurosyphilis has been reported to occur in up to 85%.[32] In 15 eyes of nine patients with ocular syphilis, ocular findings include iridocyclitis in three, vitritis in one, neuroretinitis in five, papillitis in two, retrobulbar optic neuritis in two and optic perineuritis in two.[33] 66% of this group had neurosyphilis and all showed an excellent response to treatment.

Optic perineuritis is a syndrome characterised by normal visual acuity, an enlarged blind spot on visual field examination, optic disc oedema, and normal intracranial pressure.[24] It is thought to be due to inflammation of the optic nerve sheath. It is usually seen in association with syphilitic meningitis. One case of a gumma involving the optic nerve has been reported.[34]

Diagnosis

The definitive diagnosis of syphilis depends on dark-field examinations and direct fluorescent antibody tests on lesions or tissue. Presumptive diagnosis is possible with serological tests. Two types of serological tests are available: treponemal, i.e. FTA-ABS and MHATP, and non-treponemal, i.e. VDRL and RPR. Treponemal antibody tests, once positive, usually remain so for life despite treatment, and do not corelate with disease activity. In HIV disease, reactivity may be lost with the progression of HIV infection and so this test cannot be used to exclude syphilis in patients with HIV. Non-treponemal antibody tests do correlate with disease activity and should be reported quantitatively. The vast majority of HIV-infected individuals with syphilis have a positive VDRL or RPR. The titre is often very high reflecting polyclonal activation and because of this the prozone phenomenon may cause a false negative test; if this is suspected the laboratory should be requested to test diluted specimens. Most HIV-infected patients with neurosyphilis have positive serological tests. In view of the fact that negative serology has been documented in a patient with AIDS and syphilis,[35] a history of syphilis, in the presence of negative serology, cannot be ignored.

Interpretation of the CSF findings in a patient with HIV and syphilis poses specific problems. 65% of patients positive for HIV will have CSF abnormalities[36] which include lymphocytosis, and raised protein and IgG. These changes also occur in syphilis, but when syphilis and HIV infection coexist the changes are usually more marked than with HIV alone. The glucose is usually normal in HIV disease but reduced in syphilis. Nevertheless, unless the CSF VDRL is positive it is not possible to attribute the CSF abnormalities to syphilis. A false positive VDRL should not occur during a traumatic tap if the serum VDRL is 1:256 or less, unless the tap is very blood stained. The CSF FTA-ABS is less specific (i.e. more false positives) but is more sensitive. Therefore, a negative FTA-ABS is strongly against a diagnosis of neurosyphilis.

Radiological abnormalities include meningeal enhancement in meningitis and multifocal infarction and multiple white matter lucencies in meningovascular syphilis.

Treatment

Treatment of ocular syphilis should be the same as that recommended for neurosyphilis in HIV.[37] The recommended regime is aqueous crystalline penicillin G, 12–24 million units administered two to four million units every four hours intravenously for ten to 14 days. Follow-up for clinical response with a VDRL or RPR should be at one, two, three, six, nine and 12 months after treatment.

CSF examination should be repeated at six months. If antibody titres have not declined four-fold by six months or if the CSF cell count has not reduced by six months, retreatment should be considered.

Ophthalmologists are likely to see more ocular syphilis and it should be considered in all neurophthalmic cases that pose a diagnostic dilemma. HIV should be considered in all cases that test positive for syphilis. All patients with HIV and syphilis should be investigated for neurosyphilis and if neurosyphilis cannot be excluded, a trial of penicillin treatment is indicated. Ocular syphilis may be the earliest sign of neurosyphilis and HIV infection.

Tuberculosis

HIV-positive individuals are at increased risk of developing active TB and the degree of immunosuppression need not be severe. When HIV-positive[217] and negative[303] intravenous drug users who enrolled in a methadone programme were studied, there was no difference between the incidence of positive skin tests in the two groups at entry to the programme, but active TB developed in 14% of the HIV-positive and in none of the HIV-negative group.[38] The prevalence of TB in the HIV population depends not only on their immunosuppression but also on their exposure. In developed countries between 3% to 8% of HIV-positive people will develop active TB.[39] In HIV patients with TB, pulmonary involvement occurs in 70% to 90%, extra-pulmonary in 40% to 80%, with 5% to 10% having CNS involvement.

Clinical features

The most common manifestation of tuberculous infection of the CNS is a meningitis but acute abscess formation, chronic indolent tuberculomas and an endarteritis with ischaemic foci can develop. The presentation of tuberculous meningitis is the same in HIV-positive and negative patients. Most patients have fever, are in a state of confusion, and suffer from headaches. Neck stiffness is not always a feature, and focal signs may be present. The CSF shows predominantly a lymphocytosis, raised protein, low sugar with a positive culture for *Mycobacterium tuberculosis*. A normal cell count and protein level have been reported. CT and MRI scans may show meningeal enhancement, hydrocephalus, and single or multiple focal lesions which can have ring enhancement. The neurophthalmic manifestations of TB infection of the CNS include papilloedema, cranial nerve palsies leading to oculomotor abnormalities, and visual field defects resulting from tuberculous parenchymal lesions, including cortical blindness.[40]

Diagnosis

Diagnosis depends on a high index of suspicion, particularly in patients from areas with a high incidence of TB. The sensitivity of tuberculin skin testing is inversely related to the degree of immunosuppression, but some patients with severe immunosuppression will respond to tuberculin. The Centre for Disease Control and the American Thoracic Society recommend that in an HIV-positive patient a reaction of >5 mm should indicate MTB infection. A negative result does not exclude TB. The chest X-ray may be atypical and multiple sputum specimens should be obtained, induced with nebulised hypertonic saline if necessary. Blood and urine should be cultured and aspiration or biopsy of enlarged lymph nodes should be considered. TB is rapidly progressive in HIV infection, so, if initial investigations prove negative, more invasive procedures should be considered, for example a bone marrow or liver biopsy. Ring enhancing lesions on an MRI scan in a febrile, HIV-positive patient would usually be treated as toxoplasmosis if there is no evidence of TB. If there is no clinical response, a brain biopsy may be necessary in view of the fact that TB is a potentially curable disease.

Treatment

HIV immunosuppression does not interfere with the effectiveness of antituberculous therapy (see chapter 1). Treatment should be with a quadruple regime. A four-drug regime ensures that even if the organism is resistant to one, there is still adequate treatment to eliminate the organism. Mortality is greater in the HIV-positive population and is related to the degree of immunosuppression. These patients should be followed closely as their CD4 count falls. Failure of treatment is due to either poor compliance or drug resistance. Compliance may be the most important factor as patients feel well after a few weeks and may then stop treatment. Until recently the U.K. experienced low levels of drug resistance — between 1982 and 1991, 0.6% of isolates were resistant to isoniazid or rifampicin whereas in 1994, 2.8% of isolates in North Thames (London) were resistant.[41] In this situation the choice of drugs must include at least three to which the organism is sensitive, and treatment tends to be more toxic, expensive and less successful.

Late Stage CD4 < 200 Cells/µl

The revised CDCP classification of HIV infection defines all patients with CD4 counts < 200 cells/µl as having AIDS.[42] This group is at high risk of developing certain opportunistic infections and tumours and include PCP, cerebral toxoplasmosis

(CTP), lymphoma, Kaposi's Sarcoma (KS), and oesophageal candida. With more profound immunosuppression, as the CD4 count falls below 50 cells/μl, CMV disease, disseminated MAI, cryptococcal meningitis (CM), progressive multifocal leukoencephalopathy (PML), and HIV-associated dementia are also seen. With no treatment, patients in this group have a 50% to 70% chance of developing a new AIDS-related condition or dying within 18–24 months.[43] Therefore, at this stage prophylactic therapy for PCP is instituted and antiretroviral therapy is recommended.[17,18] Although PCP, KS, MAI, and candidal infection occur at this stage of the disease, associated neurological disease is rarely encountered.

Toxoplasma

Toxoplasma gondii (TG) is the commonest opportunistic pathogen of the brain in patients with AIDS, accounting for 40% of known CNS infections. CTP develops, usually, as the CD4 count falls below 100 cells/μl. In 95% of cases, this is due to reactivation of a latent infection as a consequence of loss of immune surveillance and prior to the AIDS epidemic, CTP was an extremely uncommon condition occurring in a few immunosuppressed patients. TG is found throughout the world and there is a geographical variation in seroprevalence[44] : UK and the US < 50% (London 20%), France, Germany and Central Africa 80%. The prevalence is higher in humid climates and varies with culinary habits. As CTP is a recrudescence of latent infection, its incidence is dependant on the underlying geographical variation. It is estimated that 30% of seropositive AIDS patients will develop CTP.[45] The reason that two-thirds escape is unclear but suggestions that a genetic predisposition exists or that organisms vary in virulence are possible explanations. Acute, primary infection can also occur and in a 28-month follow-up of 72 HIV-positive patients, there was a seroconversion rate of 5.5%.[46]

Pathological findings

The pathological findings of CTP are focal areas of encephalitis separated by normal brain tissue. Three zones can be identified: a central zone with necrosis and no organisms, an intermediate zone with scattered necrosis and tachyzoites, and an outer zone with very little necrosis and tissue cysts. Acute and chronic inflammatory cells are seen and also vascular proliferation and vasculitis. Multiple areas in the brain are involved and it is thought that reactivation is rapidly followed by haematogenous spread to other sites. Occasionally a diffuse encephalitis develops.

Clinical features

The clinical course of 115 patients with AIDS and CTP has been reported.[47] Symptoms develop sub-acutely over a period of a few days to two weeks with fever and malaise seen in about 50% of patients (see Table 7.1).

Table 7.1 Frequency of clinical signs in AIDS and CTP.

• Focal signs	69%
• Headache	55%
• Confusion	52%
• Fever	47%
• Abn. Conc. Level	42%
• Seizures	29%
• Meningism	10%

The focal neurological signs include hemipariesis, hemisensory loss, aphasia, visual field defect, or cranial nerve palsy, and very occasionally a posterior fossa syndrome with ataxia and dysarthria. TG infection can therefore involve the visual system in many ways including causing optic neuritis. CTP is an important cause of CNS morbidity, but in the eye, toxoplasma chorioretinitis (see chapter 5) is less common than CMV retinitis (see chapter 6). CMVR occurs in 20% to 30% of AIDS patients whereas toxoplasma chorioretinitis occurs in 1%.[5] In two small series of patients with AIDS and CTP, 10% to 20% had ocular involvement[48,49] and approximately one-third to half of patients with HIV infection and toxoplasma chorioretinitis will have CTP[50,51] and the visual symptoms may precede the CTP.[51] In some situations, distinguishing toxoplasma and CMV in the retina can be difficult[52,53] and toxoplasma can also involve the optic nerve.[54]

Visual field defects due to toxoplasma infection of the optic chiasm, tracts, radiation and cortex[55] can occur. Brain stem involvement with palsies of 3rd,[56] 4th and 6th cranial nerves and gaze palsies are well reported in CTP (see Fig. 7.2). Treatment may result in resolution of the lesion by imaging, but this is not necessarily accompanied by improvement of the palsies. Parinaud's syndrome with multiple ring enhancing lesions seen by MRI due to CTP has been reported as the initial manifestation of HIV.[57] Raised intracranial pressure with papilloedema and non-localising cranial nerve palsies can occur due to the mass effect that occurs in approximately half of cases of CTP (see Fig. 7.3).

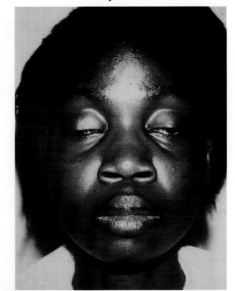

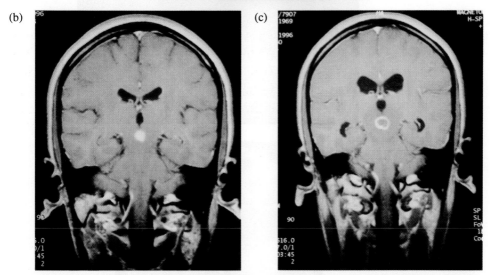

Fig. 7.2 Cerebral toxoplasmosis. (a) Bilateral ptosis due to third nerve palsies; (b) MRI T1 showing a uniformly enhancing lesion in the mid-brain; and (c) MRI T1 one week later, the lesion now shows ring enhancement.

Investigations

The clinical findings are not sufficiently distinctive to differentiate CTP from other intracranial mass lesions. Investigations include serological tests, brain scanning, and CSF examination. The presence of anti-toxoplasma antibodies indicates that CTP is possible and their absence indicates that it is unlikely,

(a)

(b)

(c)

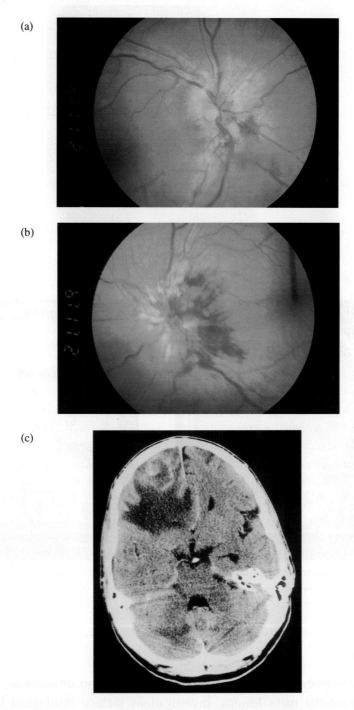

Fig. 7.3 Cerebral toxoplasmosis. (a) and (b) Bilateral papilloedema; and (c) CT scan showing a right frontal lobe lesion with ring enhancement, oedema and mass effect.

but false negatives can occur. The absolute level of antibodies or a change in the level is of no help and one in six cases of CTP have been reported to be seronegative.[47] Comparing results of the ELISA with immunofluorescence techniques, the results were discordant only at very low levels of antibody with the immunofluorescent technique being less sensitive than ELISA.[58]

CT scanning shows hypo-or iso-dense areas which enhance with contrast medium. T1 MRI shows a similar pattern to the CT and T2 MRI shows hyperdense areas with oedema. The MRI scan is more sensitive and often shows up more lesions than are visible on the CT, but the findings are not sufficiently distinctive to be diagnostic of CTP. The condition from which CTP has to be distinguished most frequently is CNS lymphoma. Certain features are suggestive of CTP as the lesions tend to be multiple, show ring enhancement (but can be diffuse when small) and there is usually marked surrounding oedema with a marked mass effect. All these features can occur with lymphoma, but a lymphoma is more likely to be single and to show heterogeneous enhancement. CTP lesions tend to be more spherical and lymphoma more elongated. In terms of location, CTP lesions were found in the basal ganglia in 48%, frontal lobe in 48%, parietal lobe in 37%, and occipital lobe in 19%.[47] Lymphomas are often periventricular in position and spread into the ventricle which is not a feature of toxoplasma.

The CSF can be normal but is usually abnormal with pleocytosis, slightly increased protein (this change could be due to HIV infection alone), but the glucose level is usually normal. Examination of the CSF is unlikely to help in establishing a diagnosis of CTP and a lumbar puncture may be hazardous due to the mass effect of the lesions. PCR on CSF may become a useful diagnostic tool but is not yet fully established.

At present the diagnosis of CTP depends on a compatible clinical picture and neuroimaging. Treatment is then commenced (see below) and after two weeks, if the diagnosis is CTP, 95% will have improved both clinically and on neuroimaging. Brain biopsy is reserved for those patients who fail to improve, who have atypical lesions, and who would be able to tolerate treatment if lymphoma was diagnosed.

Treatment

A combination of pyrimethamine and sulphadiazine (with folinic acid to prevent the bone marrow toxicity of pyrimethamine) is usually given. These agents both act on the folate metabolism of the organism and are synergistic. Treatment is continued for six to eight weeks and then the dose is reduced and continued indefinitely as secondary prophylaxis. With this regime approximately 10% will relapse. Hypersensitivity reactions are common, particularly to the sulphonamide drugs, in which case clindamycin can substituted; this drug has an inhibitory effect on the protein synthesis of the organism. Atovaquone may also be used. Steroids should be avoided if at all possible as they increase the immune suppression, but if there is significant mass effect, a short course of dexamethasone can be given (4–10 mg qds). If a therapeutic trial is being undertaken to distinguish between CTP and lymphoma, steroids can confuse the results by reducing the oedema and having a cytolytic effect on lymphoma cells.

Primary prophylaxis for patients with a CD4 count below 100 cells/µl and who are seropositive is advisable. Most of these patients are covered by their PCP prophylaxis. Up to 90% of patients with CTP respond to treatment with antiprotozoal agents. From presentation with CTP, the median survival was found to be 310 days (range 14 to 900 days) and the majority died from other AIDS-related illnesses.[59] Poorer survival was seen in patients with a temperature >38.4°C, an impaired level of consciousness, a history of KS or PCP, and a lymphocyte count of <25% of normal.

Lymphoma

Depletion of CD4 lymphocytes is associated with the development of NHL, particularly high-grade B cell types. In the HIV-positive population, this lymphoma frequently involves extranodal sites (brain, gastrointestinal tract, and bone marrow) and demonstrates a high degree of multiclonality. Latent infection with the Epstein-Barr virus appears to be important in the aetiology. The incidence of lymphoma is increasing both in the AIDS and non-AIDS groups; in the AIDS population it is becoming more common as the life-span is increasing. In those patients treated with zidovudine, there appears to be an increased risk of developing lymphoma at approximately two years after treatment. The estimated probability of developing NHL is 8% at two years after treatment and 19% at three years. Patients tend to develop NHL when their CD4 count has been below 50 cells/µl for at least one year. NHL is the second commonest malignancy (after KS) and the second commonest CNS mass lesion after toxoplasmosis and it is from this that it needs distinguishing clinically.

Clinical features

There are two clinical types of NHL: systemic and CNS. Clinically, 80% with systemic and 90% with CNS AIDS-associated NHL complain of systemic symptoms, i.e. fever, night sweats and weight loss of >10% of normal body weight, which is much higher than in the non-AIDS group. The presentation of systemic NHL is very varied because of the range of extranodal involvement. 50% of systemic

NHLs have secondary CNS involvement which is usually infiltration of the meninges rather than solid parenchymal masses, although cerebral metastases can occur. There may be signs of meningitis with cranial neuropathies, infiltration of the cavernous sinus has been seen as well as raised intracranial pressure. Neoplastic cells may be found in the CSF on cytological examination and often, more than one specimen needs to be taken to find these.

20% of AIDS-associated NHL are primary CNS lymphomas and these lesions are usually parenchymal rather than meningeal. These patients are more severely immunosuppressed and have more HIV-related illnesses than those with systemic NHL. Patients may present with memory loss and confusion (53%), focal signs (31%), fits (20%), and cranial nerve palsies (18%)[60] with the history being over weeks to months.

Neurophthalmic abnormalities can arise in a number of ways in NHL. Systemic NHL can cause neurophthalmic signs as a result of orbital spread[61-63] which, depending on the location of the lymphoma within the orbit, can lead to ocular motility problems, optic nerve compression, and proptosis. Orbital lymphoma has been reported in association with intraocular lymphoma.[64] When a systemic lymphoma spreads to the intraocular tissues, it usually infiltrates the uvea in contrast to the CNS lymphoma where the retinal pigment epithelium, the retina and the vitreous are the main sites of involvement.[65,66] The fundal signs can be confused with other causes of retinitis (see chapter 5). Horner's syndrome has been reported due to involvement in a pulmonary apex lymphoma.[7] Meningeal infiltration and parenchymal CNS metastases cause the main neurophthalmic abnormalities in systemic lymphoma and primary CNS lymphomas present with parenchymal lesions. Reported series do not always distinguish between systemic and CNS lymphoma. In 50 patients with AIDS and neurophthalmic signs, 13 had lymphoma (12 confirmed histologically), eight of whom also had meningitis.[7] Cranial nerve abnormalities were the most common finding with three unilateral and one bilateral VI nerve palsies, three unilateral and one bilateral III nerve palsies, one IV, one V, and two VII nerve palsies. In addition, there was one internuclear ophthalmoplegia, four pretectal syndromes and three patients with nystagmus. Three patients had a homonymous hemianopia, one an optic neuritis, and supranuclear ophthalmoplegia has also been reported.[67]

In primary CNS lymphoma the lesions can be single or multiple, and most commonly found in the cerebrum, basal ganglia or periventricular regions rather than in the posterior fossa. On CT the lesions are of low or less commonly high density, show oedema and a mass effect, and usually enhance. The pattern of enhancement can be ring or homogeneous. On the MRI T1 the lesions are of low intensity with peripheral enhancement (see Fig 7.4). These radiological

(a)

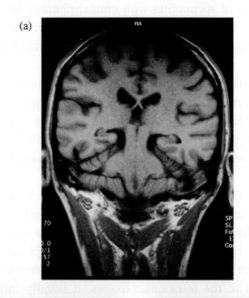

(b)   (c)

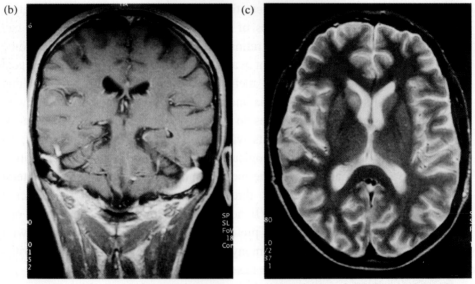

Fig. 7.4 CNS lymphoma. (a) MRI T1 and (b) MRI T2 with contrast medium showing small lesion in the right temporal lobe with central enhancement; (c) MRI T2 showing increased signal in the head of the right caudate nucleus of same patient.

(d)

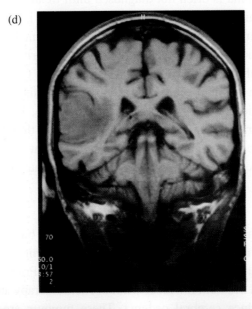

(e)

(f)

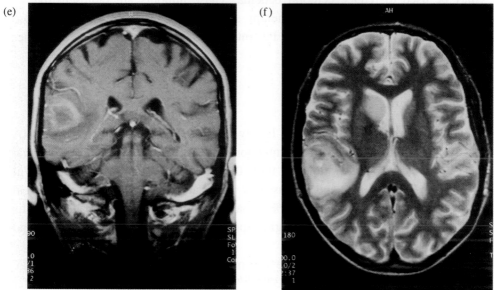

Fig. 7.4 (d) MRI T1 and (e) MRI T1 with contrast medium three weeks later, the lesion has markedly increased in size with peripheral enhancement; (f) MRI T2 showing increased signal in the right temporal lobe and caudate nucleus.

characteristics make it difficult to distinguish it from cerebral toxoplasmosis (see above). Lymphoma is often not diagnosed until treatment for toxoplasmosis has failed and a brain biopsy has been performed. CSF is often unhelpful only showing a mild lymphocytosis and elevation in protein, but lymphoma cells are seen more commonly in systemic lymphoma than in primary CNS lymphoma. A brain biopsy is the only definitive way to diagnose CNS lymphoma using either a stereotactic technique or via a craniotomy. This investigation should be reserved for patients who have an accessible lesion, have failed a trial of anti-toxoplasma therapy, who have no immediately life-threatening illness, and who would agree to treatment. Many patients present at a very late stage and have a poor prognosis so that aggressive treatment may not be appropriate.

Treatment

Treatment of systemic lymphoma is with chemotherapy, but this is often limited by poor bone marrow reserves and CNS involvement requires intrathecal methotrexate. Median survival is poor at five to 11 months. Primary CNS lymphoma requires whole brain irradiation with or without chemotherapy and dexamethasone may be used to reduce cerebral oedema. These tumours are radiosensitive as those patients treated with radiotherapy survive a mean of 134 days and those not treated surviving only 42 days. Patients died of opportunistic infections rather than tumour progression.[60]

Cytomegalovirus Infections

CMV is a member of the herpes family and is a large, double-stranded DNA virus. 90% of patients with HIV infection have antibodies to CMV, but clinical disease does not usually develop until the CD4 cell count falls below 100/μl (especially below 50/μl) and is caused by reactivation of the latent virus. Clinical disease due to CMV is seen in 40% of patients with AIDS. It can cause retinitis (see chapter 6), colitis, oesophagitis, pneumonitis, hepatitis, adrenalitis, and neurological disease.

Although CMV retinitis is the commonest clinical manifestation of CMV infection (see chapter 6), 14% to 32%[68,69] of patients with CMV retinitis suffer visual loss from involvement of the optic nerve head. The optic nerve head appears oedematous with haemorrhage and there is often peripapillary retinitis, (see Fig. 7.5). CMV papillitis should be included in the differential diagnosis of a swollen optic nerve head in AIDS. Although in most patients with CMV papillitis, it occurrs with contiguous CMV retinitis, retrobulbar optic neuropathy

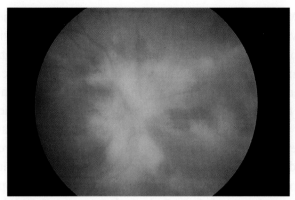

Fig. 7.5 CMV papillitis. Swollen optic nerve head with peripapillary retinal necrosis.

can also be seen which may represent an independent focus of infection.[69] Pathological evidence for direct involvement of the optic nerve by CMV is sparse but "owl's eye" inclusions have been described in the optic nerve with associated mononuclear infiltration extending posterior to the lamina cribrosa.[70]

Optic nerve involvement has been classified into two types.[68] In type I, there is spread of retinitis up to the disc margin with maintenance of good central acuity, but with altitudinal or arcuate field defects. In type II, there is primary involvement of the optic nerve head with secondary spread to the peripapillary retina and visual acuity rapidly deteriorates despite prompt and prolonged use of ganciclovir and frequently foscarnet.[71]

CMV encephalopathy

Autopsy findings indicate that neurological disease due to CMV is relatively common, occurring in 16% of patients,[72] and second only to HIV encephalopathy. On the other hand, symptomatic disease is uncommon and is likely to be underestimated because of the difficulties in establishing the diagnosis during life. Descriptions of CMV neurological disease are also difficult to interpret as there are often coincident conditions, e.g. cerebral toxoplasmosis or progressive multifocal leucoencephalopathy. CMV neurological disease usually occurs in the setting of CMV disease affecting multiple organs — 86% of patients with CMV encephalitis were found to have evidence of CMV in an extra-neural site.[73] Recognition of CMV retinitis may be of assistance in establishing the cause of co-existent neurological abnormalities — of 47 postmortems where the eye and the brain had been examined, 23% had CMV encephalitis and 91% of these had CMV retinitis. Of 51% who had CMV retinitis, 42% of these had CMV encephalitis. Of those patients with peripapillary retinitis, 75% had evidence of CMV encephalitis. The extent of retinitis and whether or not it was bilateral, was not associated with an increased association with encephalitis but CMV encephalitis has also been reported to occur during treatment for CMV retinitis.[75] From these results there appears to be a strong association between CMV retinitis and CMV encephalitis, and in patients with CNS symptoms without CMV retinitis, their nervous system disease is unlikely to be due to CMV. The mechanism by which the CMV spreads from the eye to the brain is not clear, but a haematogenous route is considered most likely given that there is no evidence for direct spread along the optic nerve at present. 86% of those with peripapillary retinitis had no evidence of CMV in the optic nerve at autopsy.

There are four characteristic pathological features of CMV encephalitis.[76] The commonest are microglial nodules — dense aggregates of macrophages and red blood cells found mainly in the gray matter. Isolated cytomegalic cells with no microglial nodules or inflammation have been seen but their clinical significance is doubtful. Areas of focal parenchymal necrosis with cytomegalic cells are seen in approximately 16% of patients. In one-third a ventriculoencephalitis is found where there is destruction of the ependymal lining and periventricular parenchyma with many cytomegalic cells present. This resembles the congenital CMV infection of the CNS. Vasculitis and demyelination have also been described.

A correlation of the various pathological findings with the clinical picture has not been obvious. No association was found with isolated cytomegalic cells, focal parenchymal necrosis, or microglial nodules.[73] It has been suggested that the microglial form causes a dementia and that CMV is aetiologically important in HIV dementia. At present, the relationship between the two is not clear. However, in 32 patients with a ventriculoencephalitis there was a subacute presentation with confusion and lethargy which rapidly progressed, over days and weeks, to coma and death. 90% of this group had CMV disease elsewhere and 62% had CMV retinitis. 59% were receiving ganciclovir or foscarnet when their neurological disease presented. Focal neurologic signs were present in 50% and 40% had cranial nerve palsies, particularly involving III and VII. The clinical presentations can be diverse — for example, one patient had hemiplegia, hemisensory loss, right sixth nerve palsy, right gaze palsy, and left lower motor neurone seventh nerve palsy,[77] another an inter-nuclear ophthalmoplegia, and a third, had tetraparesis with a sixth nerve palsy[78] — to present but a few.

The diagnosis of CMV encephalitis is difficult in life. A subacute encephalitis in the setting of advanced immunosuppression and CMV disease elsewhere is suggestive. A variety of changes on CT scanning have been reported varying from normal, or showing atrophy, ventricular enlargement and periventricular enhancement.[73] MRI scanning is more sensitive with a greater proportion showing periventricular enhancement with or without ventricular enlargement. The CSF findings are often non-specific with a raised protein level, reduced sugar, and lymphocyte pleocytosis. CMV was cultured in only one of 12 specimens. At present PCR for CMV in the CSF is the most helpful investigation with a sensitivity of 79% and specificity of 95%.[73] The studies included had a range of sensitivities from 79% to 100% with one at 33%. It has been suggested that CMV may be detected by PCR, but not be clinically significant, and that only high concentrations of CMV DNA are important diagnostically. The significance of low concentrations of CMV is at present unknown.

Treatment

The treatment of CMV encephalitis involves the use of ganciclovir and/or foscarnet and both drugs have been shown to penetrate into the CSF. There are few studies on the treatment of CMV encephalitis and in general, the response is poor in those patients with ventriculoencephalitis having a median survival from onset of neurological symptoms to death of 42 days.[73]

Progressive Multifocal Leukoencephalopathy

PML is a demyelinating disease of the CNS due to infection of oligodendrocytes by the JC virus. The JC virus is a Papova virus and has been named after the initials of the patient from whom the virus was initially grown. It is a non-enveloped, double-stranded DNA virus which is neurotropic. It exclusively infects glial cells, but not neurons. Almost all adults have antibodies to the JC virus, but no acute disease has been associated with infection. The mode of spread is thought to be respiratory. Current evidence suggests that the JC virus remains latent in lymphocytes, particularly B-lymphocytes and during immunosuppression these cells enter peripheral blood and from there infect the CNS. The incidence of PML is approximately 4% of AIDS patients.[72]

Pathological findings

The pathological findings include demyelination with enlarged oligodendroglial nuclei and large, bizarre astrocytes. It is usually multifocal and is frequently observed in the parieto-occipital region but can involve other cortical areas, the cerebellum and brain stem. Lesions first appear at the junction of the gray and white matter and affected areas can be several centimetres in diameter.

Clinical features

Clinical presentation is usually with a focal neurological deficit that progresses over weeks and months. Progressive limb weakness occurs in a half and visual field defects in one-third of patients.[79] In ten patients with PML, a homonymous hemianopia or quadrantanopia was found in seven and cortical blindness in one. Cranial nerve lesions were found in three; one patient had left V, VI and VII palsies, one patient had bilateral V and right VI palsies with an upgaze palsy, and the third patient had left V and VI palsy. Horizontal nystagmus was detected in four. Nine had other CNS signs and the remaining patient had a homonymous hemianopia with no other neurological abnormality.[80] Patients with brain stem signs had a worse prognosis than those with cortical signs. To date there have been no reports of direct involvement of the optic nerves or chiasm. There are rarely signs of any mass effect, eg. headache, but occasionally there are symptoms of gray matter involvement such as fits. The clinical course is frequently one of relentless progression with dementia and death occurring within a few months, although spontaneous remission has been reported.

Investigations

A definitive diagnosis can really only be made by biopsy, but the clinical and radiological features can be sufficiently characteristic to allow distinction from toxoplasmosis, lymphoma, and infarction. The CT scan shows hypodense white matter lesions which do not enhance. The MRI T1 weighted images are of low signal and enhancement is rare, faint and peripheral if it occurs. The T2 weighted image is hyperintense, homogeneous with indistinct margins and has a scalloped subcortical appearance. The lesions can be single or multiple and show no mass effect. The lobes involved in descending order of frequency are: parietal, occipital, frontal and temporal, with the brain stem and cerebellum less commonly involved (see Fig. 7.6). The CSF can be normal or show non-specific changes. PCR for JC virus has a low specificity at present but evidence of local synthesis of antibodies can be helpful.

Treatment

There is no established treatment for PML. There are case reports of stabilisation of the disease with subcutaneous interferon alpha and intravenous or intrathecal cytosine arabinoside (Ara C). At present, the most useful approach appears to be maximising the antiretroviral therapy for the underlying HIV infection when the resulting reduction of immunosuppression may allow for stabilisation or improvement of the PML.[81]

(a) (b)

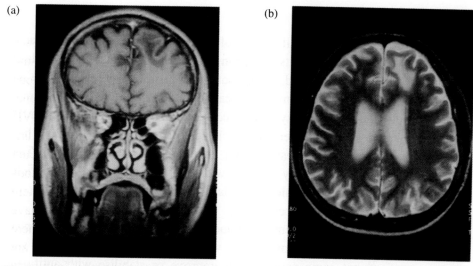

Fig. 7.6 PML. (a) MRI T1 showing left frontal low signal lesion with no enhancement or oedema; and (b) MRI T2 showing an increased signal in the lesion.

Cryptococcal Meningitis

Cryptococcus neoformans is an encapsulated yeast-like fungus. It is found widely in the environment, particularly in the droppings of pigeons and other birds. Disease due to cryptococcus is thought to be a result of a primary infection rather than reactivation of latent organisms. 6% to 10% of patients with AIDS develop cryptococcal meningitis (CM) and it is seen more commonly in African patients where the organism is frequently found in the environment (see chapter 9). The organism enters via the respiratory tract and although pulmonary infection is usually asymptomatic, there may be cough, dyspnoea and hypoxaemia with bilateral changes of interstitial pneumonitis on the chest X-ray. Cutaneous involvement may also be seen and papules, nodules, and ulcers have all been described. These lesions can resemble those of molluscum contagiosum, a common condition seen in AIDS patients (see chapter 2).

Pathological features

Large numbers of budding yeasts can be seen invading the meninges with very little evidence of an inflammatory response. As the infection progresses, the yeast spreads along the Virchow-Robin spaces and lesions may coalesce in the parenchyma to form cryptococcomas, often seen in the basal ganglia. Diffuse brain swelling can occur causing raised intracranial pressure, which can also be caused by reduced CSF absorption and the mass effect of any cryptococcomas.

Clinical features

Clinically, the commonest manifestation of cryptococcal infection is a subacute meningitis with 75% of patients presenting with fever, malaise, and headache over a two to four week period.[82] Signs of meningism are present in 25% and 40% experienced nausea and vomiting. Focal deficits and fits are very uncommon. Approximately one-third have symptoms compatible with an encephalitis in that they show altered mentation, personality change, or lethargy. 10% to 20% have signs of raised intracranial pressure with papilloedema, (see Fig. 7.7). Visual loss in this situation is usually gradual with constriction of the visual fields and preservation of central vision until late in the course of the disease, but occasionally rapid loss can occur.

Direct optic nerve involvement in cryptococcal meningitis is well documented. It can be part of a fulminant meningitis with rapid loss of vision and a very poor prognosis,[24] but some patients will improve or stabilise with antifungal treatment.[83] However, they may relapse.

(a)

(b)

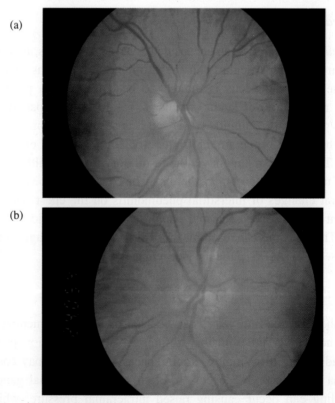

Fig. 7.7 Cryptococcal meningitis. (a) and (b) showing bilateral papilloedema.

The mechanism of the visual loss in CM is considered to be due either to direct invasion of the optic nerves by the organism, which may cause necrosis,[84] or to a restrictive arachnoiditis.[85] In 80 HIV-positive patients with cryptococcal infection, papilloedema was found in 32.5%, visual loss in 9%, sixth nerve palsy in 9%, and optic atrophy in 2.5%.[86] one patient had a chorioretinal cryptococcoma. Coincident HIV microvasculopathy was seen in 49% and CMV retinitis in 5%. Of the seven patients who suffered visual loss four were blind in both eyes — two secondary to optic atrophy, one due to optic neuropathy and one had cortical blindness. The three with unilateral loss consisted of one with a central vein occlusion secondary to papilloedema and two with an optic neuropathy. Optic neuropathy and atrophy were less frequent in the group of patients treated with oral conazoles raising the possibility that in some cases amphotericin B may be toxic to the optic nerve[87] although improved visual function has been seen in others.[83] On the other hand, the group of patients that did not receive amphotericin B may have been less severely affected and therefore less likely to have ophthalmic complications. When the figures for visual involvement in cryptococcal meningitis in AIDS patients are compared with non-AIDS patients,[88] there are fewer cases of optic atrophy (2% vs. 8%) and visual loss (9% vs. 22%) in the AIDS group. This may be due to the reduced inflammatory response in those patients and hence a reduced number of cases of a restrictive arachnoiditis.

Investigations

Cases of cryptococcal meningitis invariably have a positive serum cryptococcal antigen[89] and false positives are uncommon. The CT and MRI scans may be unremarkable, but enhancement may be seen in the meninges. T2 weighted MRI may show small hyperintensities thought to represent organisms in the Virchow-Robin spaces. Very occasionally cryptococcomas are seen, especially in the basal ganglia and hydrocephalus is rare. Examination of the CSF is the main diagnostic investigation and should be done as soon as possible as early treatment is very important. The opening pressure is elevated in two-thirds of patients, although papilloedema is present in only one-third. The constituents are normal in one-fifth. Elevated protein, pleocytosis, and reduced sugar may be seen. Cryptococcal antigen is detected in 95%,[89] positive India ink staining in 75%, and positive cultures in greater than 85%.

Treatment

The complete cure of CM in AIDS patients is unlikely. The aim of treatment is to reverse the symptoms and for the CSF to become culture-negative. Clinical trials on the optimum treatment have been inconclusive. The bulk of evidence favours treatment of severe CM, particularly if there is raised intracranial pressure or cranial nerve involvement, with amphotericin B and flucytosine. Both drugs are toxic and require careful monitoring. Amphotericin B is nephrotoxic and can cause fever, nausea, and vomiting. Flucytosine can cause bone marrow suppression and diarrhoea. It cannot be tolerated in some AIDS patients because of the myelosuppression. Fluconazole has been successful in milder cases of CM. The failure rate of treatment is between 15% and 30% with abnormal mental status, extraneural sites of infection, and hyponatraemia being poor prognostic signs.[82]

The management of the raised intracranial pressure can cause considerable problems in this group.[90] Symptomatic or progressive hydrocephalus requires ventricular shunting. Raised intracranial pressure which is symptomatic or > 350 mm water with no evidence of hydrocephalus on scanning, can be managed by daily lumbar punctures to remove CSF. Acetazolamide or a lumbar Ommaya reservoir may be necessary. Steroids should be avoided if possible as they may worsen the meningitis. They may have a place in the management of cerebral oedema with imminent herniation. In patients with raised intracranial pressure and papilloedema with progressive visual failure, optic nerve sheath fenestrations may stabilise or improve visual function, with resolution of the disc oedema. Visual function can remain stable despite intracranial pressures up to 500 mm water.[91] In patients with raised intracranial pressure, visual loss may result from this elevated pressure or be due to direct infiltration of the optic nerve by cryptococcal organisms or be due to a restrictive arachnoiditis. The time course and pattern of visual field loss are helpful in distinguishing these three causes. If the raised intracranial pressure is considered to be the principle cause, other means of reducing it should probably be used before an optic nerve sheath fenestration is considered.

If no further treatment is given approximately 50% of patients will relapse. Fluconazole is the treatment of choice for maintenance and on this, relapse rates of approximately 2% have been recorded.[92] Routine measurement of serum cryptococcal antigen is not useful in predicting relapse.

Histoplasmosis

Histoplasma capsulatum is a dimorphic yeast present in soil. Most infections occur in endemic areas such as Central America where 2% to 5% of AIDS patients have histoplasmosis. Clinically, in AIDS patients, it is a severe, disseminated infection with half of patients having respiratory involvement and one-fifth CNS disease.[93] CNS involvement includes meningitis, encephalitis, and abscesses. Cerebral infarcts secondary to arteritis or emboli from histoplasma endocarditis can occur. Viable fungal spores have been found in a biopsy of the optic nerve sheath of a patient with disseminated infection who presented with a retrobulbar optic neuritis which progressed to papillitis.[94] In general, diagnosis involves culture of the organism and detection of histoplasma polysaccharide antigen in body fluids. CT and MRI scanning may show ring enhancing lesions and infarction. Treatment is with amphotericin B with ketoconazole as maintenance therapy.

Cerebrovascular Disease

Clinical cerebrovascular disease in AIDS has a prevalence greater than expected for the age of the group (0.5% to 1.6%) and the findings in neuropathological series shows a frequency of 11% to 34%. In an autopsy study comparing patients who had died of AIDS with an age-matched population who had died of other causes, there was no increase in vascular lesions in the AIDS patients.[95] It appears that cerebrovascular disease is not a direct complication of HIV infection but an event that is associated with serious systemic illness. Haemorrhage usually occurs as a result of thrombocytopaenia and is much less common than infarction. The presentation of the cerebrovascular disease may be that of a stroke or transient ischaemic attacks, including amaurosis fugax. The aetiology, as in the non-HIV-positive population, may include hypertension, diabetes mellitius, raised serum lipids, smoking, an abnormal clotting profile, cardiac abnormalities such as atrial fibrillation, prolapsed mitral valve and infective endocarditis, or be associated with the oral contraceptive pill. In the HIV-positive group other aetiologies for cerebrovascular disease need consideration.[96] Opportunistic infections can be associated with vasculitis and these include: herpes zoster, syphilis, tuberculosis, CMV, *Candida albicans*, *Aspergillus fumigatus*, *Cryptococcus neoformans* and possibly HIV itself. Lymphoma can also cause a vasculitis. Substance abuse with amphetamine and cocaine may cause a vasculitis and can also induce a hypertensive episode with resultant haemorrhage. The injections may contain particles which can act as emboli.

Arterial dissection should be suspected if a patient has a stroke in the carotid territory with an ipsilateral Horner's syndrome. Arteries in the neck can also be injured, eg. when a noose is used to induce near asphyxiation. The diagnosis can be made by CT or MRI scanning and in this situation, anticoagulation is recommended to limit further thrombosis.

HIV-Associated Dementia Complex

This condition is thought to be due to the HIV itself. The dementia complex occurs mainly in late HIV infection and data from the Multicentre AIDS cohort study[97] show incidence rates for AIDS dementia over a five-year period of 7.3 cases/100 person years for individuals with a CD4 count of 100 cells/µl or less and three for CD4 counts between 101–200 cells/µl.

Clinical features

Clinically, the patients experience cognitive difficulties with poor concentration, loss of memory, and behavioural changes with social withdrawal. Motor slowing also occurs and early in the process, ocular motor abnormalities have been demonstrated to occur. The ocular motor performance of 47 HIV-positive patients, at all stages of the disease including AIDS dementia, were compared to 25 control subjects and saccades, anti-saccades (making a movement away from fixation in a direction equal and opposite to a presented stimulus), fixation, and smooth pursuit were all examined.[98] The results showed that saccades were hypometric with poor accuracy in all HIV groups when compared to the controls. Anti-saccades, which are a means of testing suppression of the "visual grasp reflex", were delayed and inaccurate in all groups but particularly in the AIDS dementia group. In another study, only the AIDS dementia group showed this abnormality.[99] Fixation stability was also significantly worse in the AIDS dementia group whereas smooth pursuit gain was decreased in all groups. It appears that a range of eye movement disorders exist at all stages of HIV infection with fixation and anti-saccade problems particularly occurring in AIDS dementia. However, it is not clear at present whether ocular motor problems occurring early in the course of HIV infection predict the later onset of dementia.

In addition to motor slowing, the patient becomes hyper-reflexic and may be spastic, ataxic and develop a grasp reflex. The condition may plateau or progress to a near-vegetative state.

Investigations

These are undertaken largely to exclude other treatable pathology. Neuroimaging shows atrophy and the MRI T2 weighted image, in severe cases, may show focal or diffuse hyperintense signals in the basal ganglia or white matter. The CSF shows no specific changes, but usually contains markers of immune activation such as β2-microglobulin and neopterin.

Pathology

The pathological findings have not been clearly correlated with the clinical symptoms but four main groups have been described.[100] The first is HIV encephalitis with foci of microglia, macrophages, and multinucleated giant cells; the second, HIV leucoencephalopathy with diffuse myelin pallor and astrocytosis, activated macrophages and multinucleated giant cells; the third, diffuse poliodystrophy with reduced cortical thickness, neuronal loss, astrocytosis and microglial proliferation; and the fourth, vacuolar myelopathy with vacuolar myelin changes in the spinal cord. This last group is, however, associated with a spastic, ataxic gait. In a recent clinical pathological study, multinucleated giant cells and myelin pallor were found only in patients with dementia, but only 50% of patients with dementia had these changes.[101]

Treatment

This is directed against the HIV infection. Zidovudine crosses the blood-brain barrier and there is evidence that zidovudine treatment protects against dementia. When dementia is present, high-dose zidovudine has been shown to be beneficial and careful monitoring for myelosuppression is necessary. Trials showing efficacy of other nucleoside analogues, non-nucleoside reverse transcriptase inhibitors, and protease inhibitors are not yet available.

The response of patients with dementia to antiretroviral treatment is very variable; in some it can be dramatic and last many months. Untreated, their life expectancy is approximately six months.

HIV-Associated Optic Neuropathy

There is evidence that the HIV itself can produce an optic neuropathy. There are a few reported cases of optic neuropathy apparently due to direct HIV infection of the nerve, but in all cases, this has been a diagnosis of exclusion.

Axonal loss has been reported in the optic nerves of AIDS patients without secondary infection. In the 12 optic nerves that were studied (eight AIDS patients, four age-matched controls), there was a 40% loss of axons in the AIDS group. Mean axonal diameter was unchanged indicating that all classes of axon were affected and the degeneration affected the optic nerve diffusely.[102] It is possible that this nerve fibre loss is a consequence of HIV retinal microvasculopathy (see chapters 2 and 5) with multiple cotton wool spots. Over the course of the disease, it is likely that all patients will have cotton wool spots at some time.[103] If this axonal loss was due to this, more clustering of the degenerated axons would be expected. Alternatively, the degenerative process could be occurring in the optic nerve itself.

In another study, light microscopy showed thickened meninges, axonal degeneration with various stages occurring in each optic nerve, degeneration of oligodendrocytes, and activated microglia.[104] PCR studies showed HIV DNA to be present in four of the five optic nerves examined. Previous studies have found that HIV tends to infect the mononuclear phagocyte series of cells, multinucleated giant cells, and microglia rather than directly infecting neurons. Similarly, in this study viral particles were not found within the axons of the optic nerves. It is proposed that the optic nerve degeneration is mediated by the HIV-infected mononuclear phagocyte series of cells via cytokines. TNF-α and lymphotoxin have been implicated in oligodendrocyte degeneration and in the activation of astrocytes.

Clinical features

However, it is recognised that visual acuity can remain normal despite marked axonal loss. To assess whether sub-clinical visual dysfunction existed in HIV-positive patients without obvious ocular abnormalities, contrast sensitivity, colour vision, visual fields and electro-diagnostic tests have been examined. Seventy eight patients with no clinical ocular complaint, divided equally between HIV-negative, asymptomatic HIV-positive, AIDS-related complex and AIDS, were examined using contrast sensitivity testing and the Farnsworth-Munsell 100 hue colour vision test.[105] A significant increase in error scores on the Farnsworth-Munsell test was detected in the AIDS group with no specific axis being affected. A tritan defect has also been reported.[106] There were also significant abnormalities in the contrast sensitivity test in all but the lowest spacial frequencies, affecting both the AIDS-related complex and the AIDS groups. These findings can be explained either by a primary optic neuropathy or macular damage.

Visual field examinations have been performed in HIV-positive groups with no clinical ocular problems. In 74 eyes of 37 patients with HIV infection and 143 controls examined with the Humphrey field analyser 640, there was an overall loss of visual sensitivity in the HIV-positive group[107] and these results have been confirmed as well as detecting localised defects.[108] Both groups felt the findings to be consistent with neuroretinal dysfunction.

Visual evoked potentials (VEP) in 100 HIV-positive patients and 40 age-matched controls, were determined in patients with no detectable neurological or ophthalmological abnormality.[109] The latency of the P100 in foveal (f-VEP) and full field (c-VEP) pattern shift VEPs was increased in the HIV-positive group, and those with CD4 < 100 cells/μl had an additional delay in the f-VEP.

f-VEP amplitude was the same in all groups, but the c-VEP amplitude was significantly lower in patients with advanced HIV infection when compared to early disease and controls. The abnormality in the f-VEP P100 latency suggests demyelination and the reduction in c-VEP amplitude indicates axonal loss. There was a 33% reduction in mean amplitude which, it was felt, corresponded with the 40% loss of optic nerve axons previously demonstrated.[102] There was a trend towards higher c-VEP amplitudes and lower f-VEP latencies in the zidovudine-treated groups, independent of CD4 counts, indicating that inhibition of viral replication may preserve visual function. It is not possible to exclude the possibility that dysfunction of the visual cortex may be contributing to these abnormal VEPs.

Most of the data described above indicates that evidence exists for a subclinical optic neuropathy. Evidence for a clinical optic neuropathy due to direct HIV infection is less clear. Two patients presented with bilateral retrobulbar optic neuropathies where all recognised causes of optic neuropathy in HIV-infected patients were excluded.[110] One patient improved with AZT and the other with corticosteroids. Another patient is reported who lost vision to no perception of light in one eye over a 15-day period and in whom the fundus examination was normal.[111] MRI showed enhancement of the retro-bulbar portion of the optic nerve and optic chiasm. After 18 days spontaneous improvement began to occur and the eye returned to near normal with a normal MRI. Ten weeks after the initial eye problem, he developed lesions in the cerebellum with mass effect seen on the MRI. Toxoplasma antibodies were negative; he did not respond to antitoxoplasma therapy and died. This picture is most compatible with CNS lymphoma. It is possible that this optic neuropathy was due directly to the HIV as spontaneous remission of an optic neuropathy in association with lymphoma is very unusual, but has been reported.

A clinical diagnosis of anterior ischaemic optic neuropathy was made in one patient who presented with sudden deterioration of vision and an inferior altitudinal field defect with a pale swollen optic nerve. No other cause was found over a ten-month follow-up.[112]

Cases of optic neuropathy in AIDS require careful investigation in order to identify any infective or malignant cause before ascribing them to direct HIV infection of the optic nerves. If this diagnosis is made optimal antiretroviral therapy would be the treatment of choice.

Differential Diagnosis and Investigation of Clinical Problems

This section discusses various neurophthalmic abnormalities which may present to the ophthalmologist. For each of these situations, a differential diagnosis is given with the results from two small series.[6,7] Tables 7.2–7.6 summarise the typical history, systemic and neurological findings (Table 7.2), additional ocular findings (Table 7.3), specific blood tests (Table 7.4), neuroimaging (Table 7.5) and CSF results (Table 7.6) which will help in establishing a diagnosis.

Papilloedema

Papilloedema is the swelling of the optic discs secondary to raised intracranial pressure. Visual function is generally good with only an enlarged blind spot on visual field testing. Patients characteristically present with headache and may exhibit non-localising signs of raised intracranial pressure, eg. IIIrd and VIth nerve palsies.

Differential Diagnosis

Meningitis	Middle stage	• tuberculous
		• syphilis
	Late stage	• cryptococcal
		• systemic lymphoma
		• histoplasmosis
Intracranial mass lesions	Late stage	• cerebral toxoplasmosis
		• CNS lymphoma

Results of Surveys

Mansour[6]	two cases	• one cerebral toxoplasmosis
		• one cryptococcal meningitis
Keane[7]	eight cases	• four cerebral toxoplasmosis
		• four cryptococcal meningitis

Comments

The two most frequent causes of papilloedema are cerebral toxoplasmosis and cryptococcal meningitis. In general, these are not difficult to distinguish from each other. If the cause of the papilloedema is an intracranial mass lesion, the main differential is between CTP and lymphoma and these can be very difficult to distinguish from each other (see above). The appearances on neuroimaging are not sufficiently distinctive to make a definite diagnosis, but cerebral toxoplasmosis has a greater tendency to have multiple lesions which are ring enhancing and spherical. These features can all occur with lymphoma but a single, heterogeneously enhancing lesion is more likely to be lymphoma. Lymphomas also tend to grow along the ventricles which is not a feature of toxoplasmosis. In general, if the clinical picture and neuroimaging are compatible with cerebral toxoplasmosis, a two week therapeutic trial should be given. No response indicates that toxoplasmosis is unlikely and a brain biopsy may need to be considered.

Table 7.2 History, systemic involvement and typical neurological features.

	History	Fever	Systems	Headache	Meningitis	Cognitive decline	Depressed conscious level	Focal neurology	Fits
• Cerebral toxoplasmosis	Days/ weeks	+	−	+	−	+/−	+	+	+
• CNS lymphoma	Weeks/ months	+	−	+	−	+/−	+/−	+	+
• Systemic lymphoma	Weeks/ months	+	LN GIT	+	+	−	+/−	+/−	+/−
• PML	Weeks/ months	−	−	−	−	+	−	+	−
• Cryptococcal meningitis	Days/ weeks	+	Lung Skin	+	+	+/−	+/−	+/−	−
• HIV dementia	Months	−	−	−	−	+	+/−	+/−	−
• CMV encephalitis	Days/ weeks	+	Pneumon -itis Colitis	+/−	−	+	+	+	+/−
• Meningeal syphilis	Days/ weeks	+	Secondary syphilis	+	+	−	−	−	−
• Meningo- vascular syphilis	Sudden	−	−	−	−	−	−	+	+/−
• TB	Days/	+	LN	+	+	+/−	+/−	+/−	+/−

Table 7.3 Additional ocular findings.

Condition	Ocular Findings
• Cerebral toxoplasmosis	Chorioretinitis
• CNS lymphoma	Uveitis, infiltration of the retina and retinal pigment epithelium, retinal vasculitis
• Systemic lymphoma	Uveitis, choroidal infiltration
• Progressive multifocal leukoencephalopathy	–
• Cryptococcal meningitis	Cryptococcoma, choroidal infiltration
• HIV-associated dementia	–
• CMV encephalitis	CMV retinitis
• Syphilis	Uveitis, chorioretinitis
• TB meningitis	Uveitis, choroidal granulomata, retinal vasculitis
• Herpes simplex	Keratitis, uveitis, retinal necrosis
• Varicella-zoster	Keratitis, uveitis, retinal necrosis

Table 7.4 Specific blood tests.

Condition	Blood Tests
• Cerebral toxoplasmosis	IgG and IgM anti-toxoplasma antibodies
• CNS lymphoma	–
• Systemic lymphoma	–
• Progressive multifocal leukoencephalopathy	–
• Cryptococcal meningitis	Cryptococcal antigen
• HIV-associated dementia	–
• CMV encephalitis	CMV antigen tests
• Syphilitic meningitis	VDRL or RPR and FTA-ABS
• Meningovascular syphilis	VDRL or RPR and FTA-ABS
• TB meningitis	Blood culture

Table 7.5 Typical findings on neuroimaging.

Condition	CT	MRI-T1	MRI-T2	Comments
• Cerebral toxoplasmosis	Low density ring enhancing	Low signal ring enhancing	High signal centre Low signal capsule High signal oedema	Multiple lesions with oedema and mass effect
• CNS lymphoma	Low density irregular/ring enhancing	Low signal irregular/ring enhancing	Variable signal High signal oedema	Single or multiple lesions with oedema and mass effect
• Systemic lymphoma	Normal meningeal enhancement Metastases	Normal meningeal enhancemant Metastases	Normal Metastases	Hydrocephalus
• Progressive multifocal leuko-encephalopathy	Low density No enhancement	Low signal No enhancement	High signal Homogeneous	White matter lesions with no oedema or mass effect
• Cryptococcal meningitis Cryptococcomas	Normal meningeal enhancement Low density +/− Enhancing	Normal meningeal enhancement Low density Non-enhancing	Normal High intensity in VR spaces and basal ganglia	Occasional hydrocephalus
• HIV-associated dementia	Normal/atrophy Low density No enhancement	Normal/atrophy	Normal/atrophy High density Poorly defined	Subcortical lesions with no oedema or mass effect
• CMV encephalitis	Normal periventricular low density areas with enhancement	Normal periventricular low signal with enhancement	Normal periventricular high signal	Ventricular enlargement
• Syphilitic meningitis	Normal meningeal enhancement	Normal meningeal enhancement	Normal	–
• Meningovascular syphilis	Infarct	Infarct	Infarct	Especially basilar artery territory
• TB meningitis Tuberculoma	Normal meningeal enhancement High density enhancing	Normal meningeal enhancement Low signal solid/ring enhancing	Normal High signal oedema	Occasional hydrocephalus Multiple lesions with oedema, may have central calcification

Table 7.6 Special investigations on CSF.

Condition	CSF Investigation
• Cerebral toxoplasmosis	(PCR)
• CNS lymphoma	Cytology
• Systemic lymphoma	Cytology
• Progressive multifocal leukoencephalopathy	PCR for JC virus Local antibody synthesis
• Cryptococcal meningitis	India ink stain Cryptococcal antigen Culture
• HIV-associated dementia	–
• CMV encephalitis	PCR
• Syphilitic meningitis	VDRL, FTA-ABS
• Meningovascular syphilis	VDRL, FTA-ABS
• TB meningitis	Microscopy and culture (PCR)

Optic Neuropathy

The signs of optic neuropathy include reduced visual acuity, poor colour vision, a relative afferent pupillary defect (if unilateral or asymmetrical), and visual field abnormalities. The optic disc may be swollen or normal in appearance, and optic atrophy occurs as the condition progresses.

Differential Diagnosis

Seroconversion	• multiple sclerosis
Early/middle stage	• syphilis • varicella-zoster • ethambutol toxicity
Late stage	• cytomegalovirus • toxoplasmosis
	• cryptococcosis • lymphoma • histoplasmosis • HIV

Results of Surveys

Mansour[6]	• two cases of CMV papillitis
Keane[7]	• two cryptococcal, one syphilis, one lymphoma

When CMV involves the optic nerve it usually causes a papillitis which is associated with peripapillary retintitis and the observation of this assists in making the diagnosis. A possible case of retrobulbar optic neuritis due to CMV has been described.[69] In the cases of multiple sclerosis described, in addition to the optic neuritis, they have all shown rapid neurological decline. In HIV-positive patients syphilis cannot be excluded on negative serological tests, so in the presence of a positive history, a therapeutic trial of penicillin should be considered.

Swollen optic discs in cryptococcal meningitis can be due to raised intracranial pressure when central vision is preserved, and to direct invasion of the optic nerve by the organism or a restrictive arachnoiditis when visual acuity is extremely poor. Optic nerve involvement is unusual in toxoplasmosis and not always associated with a chorioretinitis, but can be associated with cerebral toxoplasmosis. Neuroimaging will be helpful in establishing the diagnosis. Varicella zoster optic neuropathy has almost always been reported in patients with a history of shingles in the recent past and may herald the onset of retinitis.

HIV optic neuropathy is a diagnosis of exclusion and the search for other causes should be continued in follow-up.

Homonymous Hemianopia

The finding of a homonymous hemianopia indicates involvement of the post-chiasmal visual pathways.

Differential diagnosis

Early stage	• herpes simplex encephalitis
	• varicella-zoster virus arteritis
Middle stage	• meningovascular syphilis
Late stage	• cerebral toxoplasmosis
	• lymphoma
	• progressive multifocal leucoencephalophy
	• CMV encephalopathy
	• cerebrovascular disease
	• cryptococcal meningitis
	• HIV — associated dementia symmetry

Results of Surveys

Mansour[6]	• three cerebral toxoplasmosis, three lymphoma
Keane[7]	• one cerebral toxoplasmosis, one cryptococcal meningitis

---

Again the difficulty of distinguishing cerebral toxoplasmosis from lymphoma occurs (see above). PML can usually be differentiated from CTP and lymphoma by neuroimaging as it does not enhance and displays no mass effect. However, the neuroimaging can be confused with HIV-associated dementia. Lesions of PML involve the subcortical U fibres which are spared in HIV-associated dementia. The lesions seen on the scan in HIV-associated dementia are rarely associated with focal neurological deficit in contrast to PML. Cerebral infarction which occur in meningovascular syphilis and cerebrovascular disease can be distinguished by their sudden onset.

Ocular Motor Deficits

Ocular motor deficits can result from involvement of the cranial nerves, from brain stem involvement, and from abnormalities in supranuclear control.

Differential Diagnosis

Radiculitis	Early stage	• varicella-zoster virus
	Late stage	• cytomegalovirus
Meningitis	Middle stage	• tuberculous • syphilis
	Late stage	• cryptococcal • lymphoma • histoplasmosis
Brain stem	Early stage	• herpes simplex encephalitis
	Middle stage	• meningovascular syphilis
	Late stage	• cerebral toxoplasmosis • lymphoma • PML • CMV encephalitis • cerebrovascular disease

Results of Surveys

	Mansour[6]	Keane[7]
IIIrd nerve	one CT	• two CT, four lymphoma • three CM
IVth nerve	one CT, one lymphoma	• one lymphoma

VIth nerve	one CT	• three CT, four lymphoma
		• four CM, one syphilis
		• meningitis
		• three viral encephilitis
Gaze palsy	one CT	• one CT, one CM,
		• three viral encephalitis
INO	-	• one lymphoma,
		• one viral encephalitis
Pretectal syndrome	-	• four CT, four lymphoma
		• one viral encephalitis
		• one histoplasmosis
Skew deviation	-	• one CT, one viral encephalits

Again the commonest causes are CT and lymphoma with 15 cases each. The patients in Keane's group who are labelled as viral encephalitis include herpes, PML, CMV, and HIV-associated dementia. These were not separated as the exact diagnosis was difficult to establish.

Some patients may present with specific patterns of ocular motor abnormality associated with orbital disease or cavernous sinus involvement. With orbital involvement other signs will be present to localise the disease, such as proptosis (see chapter 4). Opportunistic infections of the orbit have been reported in eight patients.[113] They included invasive *aspergillosis* (four patients), *proprionibacterium acnes* (one patient), *pseudomonas aeruginosa* (one patient), *Staphlococcus aureus* (one patient) and syphilitic periostitis (one patient). In six patients orbital infection was associated with contiguous sinus infection and in the staphylococcal case with an endophthalmitis. Lymphoma has also been reported as involving the orbit.[64] Cavernous sinus involvement is rare but has been seen with lymphoma, and a patient with an eosinophilic granuloma has been reported.[114]

References

1. Levy R.M., Bredesen D.E., Rosenblum M.L. "Neurological manifestations of AIDS: Experience at UCSF and a review of the literature," *J. Neurosurg.* **62** (1985), 475–495.

2. Petito C.K., Cho E.S., Lemann W. *et al.* "Neuropathology of AIDS: An autopsy review," *J. Neuropathol Exp. Neurol.* **45** (1986), 635–646.

3. Guiloff R.J. AIDS: Neurological opportunistic infection in Central London," *JRSM* **82** (1989), 278–280.

4. Levy R.M., Breseden D.E. "CNS dysfunction in AIDS," *J. AIDS* **1** (1986), 41–64.

5. Jabs D.A., Green W.R., Fox R. *et al.* "Ocular manifestations of AIDS," *Ophthalmology* **96** (1989), 1092–1099.

6. Mansour A.M. "Neurophthalmic findings in AIDS," *J. Clin. Neuro-ophthalmol.* **10** (1990), 167–174.

7. Keane J.R. "Neuro-ophthalmologic signs of AIDS: 50 patients," *Neurology* **41** (1991), 841–845.

8. Cooper D.A., Maclean P., Finlayson R. *et al.* "Acute AIDS retrovirus infection," *Lancet* **I** (1985), 537–540.

9. Ho D.D., Rota T.R., Schooley R.T. *et al.* "Isolation of HTLV III from CSF and neural tissues of patients with nurologic syndromes related to AIDS," *NEJM* **313** (1985), 1493–1497.

10. Carne C.A., Smith A., Elkington S.G. *et al.* "Acute encephalopathy coincident with seroconversion for anti-HTLV III antibodies," *Lancet* **II** (1985), 1206–1208.

11. Piette A.M., Tusseau F., Vignon D. *et al.* "Acute neuropathy coincident with seroconversion for anti-LAV/HTLV-III," *Lancet* **I** (1986), p. 852.

12. Vendrell J., Heredia C., Pujol M. *et al.* "Guillain-Barre syndrome associated with sero-conversion for anti-HTLV-III," *Neurology* **37**(1987), p. 544.

13. Cornblath D.R., McArthur J.C., Kennedy P.G.E. *et al.* "Inflammatory demyelinating peripheral neuropathies associated with human T-cell lymphotropic virus type-III infection," *Ann. Neurol.* **21** (1987), 32–40.

14. Sillevis Smitt P.A.E., Portegies P. "Fisher's syndrome associated with HIV infection," *Clin. Neurol. Neurosurg.* **92** (1990), 353–355.

15. Ho D.D., Neumann A.U., Perelson A.S. *et al.* "Rapid turnover of plasma virions and CD4 lymphocytes in HIV-1 infection" *Nature* **373** (1995), 123–126.

16. Ho D.D. "Time to hit HIV, early and hard," *NEJM* **333** (1995), 450–451.

17. "British HIV Association guidelines for antiretroviral treatment of HIV seropositive individuals," *Lancet* **349** (1997), 1086–1092.

18. Carpenter C.C.J., Fischl M.A., Hammer S.M. *et al.* "Antiretroviral therapy for HIV infection in 1996," *JAMA* **276** (1996), 146–154.

19. Berger J.R., Sheremata W.A., Resnick L. *et al.* "Multiple sclerosis-like illness occurring with human immunodeficiency virus infection," *Neurology* **39** (1989), 324–329.

20. Berger J.R., Tornatore C., Major E.O. *et al.* "Relapsing remitting human immunodeficiency virus-associated leukoencephalomyelopathy," *Ann. Neurol.* **31** (1992), 34–38.

21. Gray F., Chimelli L., Mohr M. *et al.* "Fulminating multiple sclerosis-like leukoencephalopathy revealing human immunodeficiency virus infection," *Neurology* **41** (1991), 105–109.

22. Buchbinder S.P., Katz M.H., Hessol N.A. *et al.* "Herpes zoster and HIV infection," *J. Infect. Dis.* **166** (1992), 1153–1156.

23. Engstrom R.E., Holland G.N., Margolis T.P. *et al.* "Progressive Outer Retinal Necrosis Syndrome," *Ophthalmology* **101**(9) (1994), 1488–1502.

24. Winward K.E., Latif M.H., Glaser J.S. "The spectrum of optic nerve disease in human immunodeficiency virus infection," *Am. J. Ophthalmol.* **107** (1989), 373–380.

25. Litoff D., Catalano R.A. "Herpes zoster optic neuritis in human immunodeficiency virus infection," *Arch. Ophthalmol.* **108** (1990), 782–783.

26. Shayegani A., Odel J.G., Kazim M. *et al.* "Varicella-zoster virus retrobulbar optic neuritis in a patient with human immunodeficiency virus," *Am. J. Ophthalmol.* **122** (1996), 586–588.

27. Friedlander S.M., Rahhal F.M., Ericson L. *et al.* "Optic neuropathy preceding acute retinal necrosis in acquired immunodeficiency syndrome," *Arch. Ophthalmol.* **114** (1996), 1481–1485.

28. Johns D.R., Tierney M., Felsenstein D. "Alteration in the natural history of neurosyphilis by concurrent infection with HIV," *NEJM* **316** (1987), 1569–1572.

29. Musher D.M. "Syphilis, neurosyphilis, penicillin and AIDS," *J. Infect. Dis.* **163** (1991), 1201–1206.

30. Musher D.M., Hamill R.J., Baughn R.E. "The effect of HIV infection on the course of syphilis and response to treatment,:" *Ann. Intern. Med.* **113** (1990), 872–881.

31. Katz D.A., Berger J.R., Duncan R.C. "Neurosyphilis. A comparative study of the effects of infection with HIV," *Arch. Neurol.* **50** (1993), 243–249.

32. Levy J.H., Liss R.A., Maguire A.M. "Neurosyphilis and ocular syphilis in patients with concurrent HIV infection," *Retina* **9** (1989), 175–180.

33. McLeish W.M., Pulido J.S., Holland S. *et al.* "The ocular manifestations of syphilis in the HIV type 1 infected host," *Ophthalmology* **97** (1990), 196–203.

34. Lawton Smith J., Frazier Byrne S., Cambron C.R. "Syphiloma/Gumma of the optic nerve and HIV seropositivity," *J. Clin. Neuro-ophthalmol.* **10** (1990), 175–184.

35. Hicks C.B., Benson P.M., Lupton G.P. *et al.* "Seronegative secondary syphilis in a patient infected with the HIV with Kaposi sarcoma," *Ann. Int. Med.* **107** (1987), 492–495.

36. Mc.Arthur J.C., Cohen B.A., Farzedegan H. *et al.* "Cerebrospinal fluid abnormalities in homosexual men with and without neuropsychiatric findings," *Ann. Neurol.* **23** (1988), S34–S37.

37. Centers for Disease Control, "Sexually transmitted disease treatment guidelines," *MMWR* **38**(suppl 8) (1989), 1–13.

38. Selwin P.A., Hartel D., Lewis V.A. *et al.* "A prospective study of the risk of tuberculosis among intravenous drug users with HIV infection," *N. Engl. J. Med.* **320** (1989), 545–550.

39. Barnes P.F., Bloch A.B., Davidson P.T. *et al.* "Tuberculosis in patients with acquired immunodeficiency virus infection," *N. Engl. J. Med.* **324** (1991), 1644–1650.

40. Bishburg E., Sunderam G., Reichman L.B. *et al.* "Central nervous system tuberculosis with the acquired immunodeficiency syndrome and its related complex," *Ann. Intern. Med.* **105** (1986), 210–213.

41. Coker R., Miller R. "HIV associated tuberculosis," *Brit. Med. J.* **314** (1997), p. 1847.

42. CDC. "1993 revised classification system for HIV infection and expanded surveillance case definition for AIDS among adolescents and adults," *MMWR* **41** (No. RR-17) (1992).

43. Mac Donnell K.B., Chimiel J.S., Poggensee L. *et al.* "Predicting progression to AIDS: Combined usefulness of CD4 lymphocyte counts and p24 antigenaemia," *Am. J. Med.* **89** (1990), 706–712.

44. Holliman RE. "Serological study of prevalence of toxoplasmosis in asymptomatic patients infected with HIV," *Epidemiol. Infect.* **105** (1990), 415–418.

45. Grant I.H., Gold J.M.W., Rosenblum M. *et al.* "*Toxoplasma gondii* serology in HIV infected patients: The development of central nervous system toxoplasmosis in AIDS," *AIDS* **4** (1990), 519–521.

46. Partisani M., Candolfi H., de Mautort E. *et al.* "Seroprevalence of latent *Toxoplasma gondii* infection in HIV-infected individuals and long-term follow-up of toxoplasma sero-negative subjects (abstract no.WB 2294)," in: *Program and abstracts of the VII International Conference on AIDS,* Florence, (1991).

47. Porter S.B., Sande M. "Toxoplasmosis of the central nervous system in AIDS," *NEJM* **327** (1992), 1643–1648.

48. Snider W.D., Simpson D.M., Nielsen S. *et al.* "Neurological complications of AIDS. Analysis of 50 patients," *Ann. Neurol.* **14** (1983), p. 403.

49. Luft B.J., Conley F., Remington J.S. *et al.* "Outbreak of central nervous system toxoplasmosis in Western Europe and North America," *Lancet* **1** (1983), p. 783.

50. Cochereau-Massin I., LeHoang P., Lautier-Frau M. *et al.* "Ocular toxoplasmosis in HIV infected patients," *Am. J. Ophthalmol.* **114** (1992), 130–135.

51. Holland G.N., Engstrom R.E., Glasgow B.J. *et al.* "Ocular toxoplasmosis in patients with AIDS," *Am. J. Ophthalmol.* **106** (1988), 653–667.

52. Grossniklaus H.E., Specht C.S., Allaire G. *et al.* "*Toxoplasma gondii* retinochoroiditis and optic neuritis in AIDS," *Ophthalmology.* **97** (1990), 1342–1346.

53. Falcone P.M., Notis C., Merhige K. "Toxoplasmic papillitis as the initial manifestation of AIDS," *Ann. Ophthalmol.* **25** (1993), 56–57.

54. Wei M.E., Campbell S.H., Taylor C. "Precipitous visual loss secondary to optic nerve toxoplasmosis as an unusual presentation of AIDS," *Aust. and NZ J. Ophthalmol.* **24** (1996), 75–77.

55. Sue C.M., Morris J.G.L., Leicester J. *et al.* "Confusion, cortical blindness and fever," *Med. J. Aust.* **162** (1995), 527–531.

56. Antworth M.V., Beck R.W. "Third nerve palsy as a presenting sign of AIDS," *J. Clin. Neuro-ophthalmol.* **7** (1987), 125–128.

57. Griffin D.K., Shriver M.E., Hauser R. "Parinaud's symdrome as the initial manifestation of AIDS," *J. Neuroimaging* **4** (1994), 113–114.

58. Miller C.N., Sugai K., Yajko D.M. *et al.* "Evaluation of serologic kits for IgG toxoplasma antibodies. in: *Program and Abstracts of the 30th Interscience Conference on Antimicrobial agents and chemotherapy, Atlanta*, Washington DC," American Society for Microbiology (*abstract*), (1990).

59. Renold C., Sugar A., Chave J.-P. *et al.* "Toxoplasma encephalitis in patients with AIDS," *Medicine* **71** (1992), 224–239.

60. Baumgartner J.E., Rachlin J.R., Beckstead J.H. *et al.* "Primary central nervous system lymphomas: Natural history and response to radiation therapy in 55 patients with AIDS," *J .Neurosurg.* **73** (1990), 206–211.

61. Turok D.I., Meyer D.R. "Orbital lymphoma associated with AIDS," *Arch. Ophthalmol.* **110** (1992), 610–611.

62. Antle C.M., White V.A., Horsman D.E. *et al.* "Large cell orbital lymphoma in a patient with AIDS. Case report and review," *Ophthalmology* **97** (1990), 1494–1498.

63. Mansour A.M. "Orbital findings in AIDS," *Am. J. Ophthalmol.* **110** (1990), 706–707.

64. Matzkin D.C., Slamovits T.L., Rosenbaum P.S. "Simultaneous intraocular and orbital non-Hodgkin lymphoma in AIDS," *Ophthalmology* **101** (1994), 850–855.

65. Stanton C.A., Sloan B. III, Slusher M.M. *et al.* "AIDS related primary intraocular lymphoma," *Arch. Ophthalmol.* **110** (1992) 1614–1617.

66. Schanzer M.C., Font R.L., O'Malley R.E. "Primary ocular malignant lymphoma associated with AIDS," *Ophthalmology* **98** (1991), 88–91.

67. Guiloff R.J., Fuller G.N. "Clinical aspects of other neurological diseases, in: Rudge P. (ed.), Bailliere's Clinical Neurology, Neurological Aspects of Human Retroviruses," **1** (1992), 175–182.

68. Gross J.G., Sadun A.A., Wiley C.A. *et al.* "Severe visual loss related to isolated peripapillary retinal and optic nerve head cytomegalovirus infection," *Am. J. Ophthalmol.* **108** (1989), 691–698.

69. Roarty J.D., Fisher E.J., Nussbaum J.J. "Long-term visual morbidity of cytomegalovirus retinitis in patients with AIDS," *Ophthalmology.* **100** (1993), 1685–1688.

70. Grossniklaus H.E., Frank K.E., Tomsak R.L. "Cytomegalovirus retinitis and optic neuritis in AIDS," *Ophthalmology* **94** (1987), 1601–1604.

71. Patel S.S., Rutzen A.R., Marx J.L. *et al.* "Cytomegalovirus papillitis in patients with AIDS," *Ophthalmology* **103** (1996), 1476–1482.

72. Kure K., Llena J.F., Lyman W.D. *et al.* "HIV-1 infection of the nervous system: An autopsy study of 268 adult, pediatric and fetal brains," *Hum. Pathol.* **22** (1991), 700–710.

73. Arribas J.R., Storch G.A., Clifford D.B. *et al.* "Cytomegalovirus encephalitis," *Ann. Intern. Med.* **125** (1996), 577–587.

74. Bylsma S.S., Achim C.L., Wiley C.A. *et al.* "The predictive value of cytomegalovirus retinitis for cytomegalovirus encephalitis in AIDS," *Arch. Ophthalmol.* **113** (1995), 89–95.

75. Schwarz T.F., Loeschke K., Hanus I. *et al.* "CMV encephalitis during ganciclovir therapy of CMV retinitis," *Infection* **18** (1990), 289–290.

76. Morgello S., Cho E.S., Nielsen S. *et al.* "Cytomegalovirus encephalitis in patients with AIDS an autopsy study of 30 cases and review of the literature," *Hum. Pathol.* **18** (1987), 289–297.

77. Masdeu J.C., Small C.B., Weiss L. *et al.* "Multifocal cytomegalovirus encephalitis in AIDS," *Ann. Neurol.* **23** (1988), 97–99.

78. Fuller G.N., Guiloff R J., Scaravilli F. *et al.* "Combined HIV-CMV encephalitis presenting with brain stem signs," *J. Neurol. Neurosurg. Psych.* **52** (1989), 975–979.

79. Berger J.R., Kaszovitz B., Post M.J. *et al.* "Progressive multifocal leukoencephalopathy associated with HIV. A review of the literature with a report of sixteen cases," *Ann. Intern. Med.* **107** (1987), 78–87.

80. Ormerod L.D., Rhodes R.H., Gross S.A. *et al.* "Ophthalmic manifestations of AIDS associated progressive multifocal leukoencephalopathy," *Ophthalmology* **103** (1996), 899–906.

81. Conway B., Halliday W.C., Brunham R.C. "HIV associated progressive multifocal leukoencephalopathy: apparent response to 3-azido-3-deoxythymidine," *Rev. Infect. Dis.* **12** (1990), 479–482.

82. Chuck S.L., Sande M.A. "Infections with *cryptococcus neoformans* in AIDS," *N. Engl. J. Med.* **321** (1989), 794–799.

83. Golnik K.C., Newman S.A., Wispelway B. "Cryptococcal optic neuropathy in the AIDS," *J. Clin. Neuro-ophthalmol.* **11** (1991), 96–103.

84. Cohen D.B., Glasgow B.J. "Bilateral optic nerve cryptococcosis in sudden blindness in patients with AIDS," *Ophthalmology.* **100** (1993), 1689–1694.

85. Lipson B.K., Freeman W.R., Beniz J. *et al.* "Optic neuropathy associated with cryptococcal arachnoiditis in AIDS patients," *Am. J. Ophthalmol.* **107** (1989), 523–527.

86. Kestelyn P., Taelman H., Bogaerts J. *et al.* "Ophthalmic manifestations of infections with *cryptococcus neoformans* in patients with AIDS," *Am. J. Ophthalmol.* **116** (1993), 721–727.

87. Li P.K.T., Lai K.N. "Amphotericin B induced ocular toxicity in cryptococcal meningitis," *Br. J. Ophthalmol.* **73** (1989), 397–398.

88. Okun B., Butler W.T. "Ophthalmologic complications of cryptococcal meningitis," *Arch. Ophthalmol.* **71** (1964), p. 52.

89. Nelson M.R., Bower M., Smith D. *et al.* "The value of serum cryptococcal antigen in the diagnosis of cryptococcal infections in patients infected with the HIV," *J. Infect. Dis.* **21** (1990), 175–181.

90. Harrison M.J.G., McArthur J.C. "Opportunistic infections - fungii," In: *AIDS and Neurology*, Churchill Livingstone, (1995), 119–128.

91. Garrity J.A., Herman D.C., Imes R. *et al.* "Optic nerve sheath decompression for visual loss in patients with AIDS and cryptococcal meningitis with papilledema," *Am. J. Ophthalmol.* **116** (1993), 472–478.

92. Powderly W.G., Saag M.S., Cloud G.A. *et al.* "A randomised, controlled trial of fluconazole versus amphotericin B as maintenance therapy for prevention of relapse of cryptococcal meningitis in patients with AIDS," *N. Engl. J. Med.* **326** (1992), p. 793.

93. Wheat L.J., Connolly-Stringfield P.A., Baker R.L. *et al.* "Disseminated histoplasmosis in AIDS: clinical findings, diagnosis and treatment and review of the literature," *Medicine* **69** (1990), 361–374.

94. Yau T.H., Rivera-Velazquez P.M., Mark A.S. *et al.* "Unilateral optic neuritis caused by *histoplasma capsulatum* in a patient with AIDS," *Am. J. Ophthalmol.* **121** (1996), 324–326.

95. Berger J.R., Harris J.O., Gregorius J. *et al.* "Cerebrovascular disease in AIDS: a case control study," *AIDS*, **4** (1990), 239–244.

96. Harrison M.J.G., McArthur J.C. "Cerebrovascular disease," in: *AIDS and Neurology*, Churchill Livingstone (1995), 197–206.

97. Bacellar H., Munoz A., Miller E. *et al.* "Temporal trends in the incidence of HIV-1-related neurologic disease: Multicentre AIDS cohort study, 1985–1992," *Neurology* **44** (1994), 1892–1900.

98. Merrill P.T., Paige G.D., Abrams R.A. *et al.* "Ocular motor abnormalities in HIV infection," *Ann. Neurol.* **30** (1991), 130–138.

99. Currie J., Benson E., Ramsden. *et al.* "Eye movement abnormalities as a predictor of the AIDS dementia complex," *Arch. Neurol.* **45** (1988), 949–953.

100. Budka H., Wiley C.A., Kleihues P. *et al.* "HIV- associated disease of the nervous system: review of nomenclature and proposal for neuro-pathology based terminology," *Brain. Pathol.* **1** (1991), 143–152.

101. Glass J.D., Wesselingh S.L., Selnes O.A. *et al.* "Clinical-neuropathologic correlation in HIV - associated dementia," *Neurology* **43** (1993), 2230–2237.

102. Tenhula W.N., Xu S., Madigan M.C. *et al.* "Morphometric comparisons of optic nerve axon loss in AIDS," *Am. J. Ophthalmol.* **113** (1992), 14–20.

103. Holland G.N., Gottlieb M.S., Foos R.Y. "Retinal cotton-wool patches in AIDS," *N. Engl. J. Med.* **307** (1982) 1704–1705.

104. Sadun A.A., Pepose J.S., Madigan M.C. *et al.* "AIDS-related optic neuropathy: A histological, virological and ultrastructural study," *Graefe's Arch. Clin. Exp. Ophthalmol.* **233** (1995), 387–398.

105. Quiceno J.I., Caparelli E., Sadun A.A. *et al.* "Visual dysfunction without retinitis in patients with AIDS," *Am. J. Ophthalmol.* **113** (1992), 8–13.

106. Geier S.A., Kronawitter U., Bogner J.R. *et al.* "Impairment of color contrast sensitivity and neuroretinal dysfunction in patients with symptomatic HIV-infection or AIDS," *Br. J. Ophthalmol.* **77** (1993), 716–720.

107. Geier S.A., Nohmeier C., Lachenmayr B.J. *et al.* "Deficits in perimetric performance in patients with symptomatic HIV infection or AIDS," *Am. J. Ophthalmol.* **119** (1995), 335–344.

108. Plummer D.J., Sample P.A., Arevalo J.F. *et al.* "Visual field loss in HIV-positive patients without infectious retinopathy," *Am. J. Ophthalmol.* **122** (1996), 542–549.

109. Malessa R., Agelink M.W., Diener H-C. "Dysfunction of visual pathways in HIV-1 infection," *J. Neurol. Sci.* **130** (1995), 82–97.

110. Newman N.J., Lessell S. "Bilateral optic neuropathies with remission in 2 HIV positive men," *J. Clin. Neuro-Ophthalmol.* **12** (1992), 1–5.

111. Sweeney B.J., Manji H., Gilson R.J.C. *et al.* "Optic neuritis and HIV-1 infection," *J. Neurol. Neurosurg. Psych.* **56** (1993), 705–707.

112. Brack M.J., Cleland P.G., Owen R.I. *et al.* "Anterior ischaemic optic neuropathy in AIDS," *Brit. Med. J.* **295** (1987), 696–697.

113. Kronish J.W., Johnson T.E., Gilberg S.M. *et al.* "Orbital infections in patients with HIV infection," *Ophthalmology* **103** (1996), 1483–1492.

114. Gross F.J., Waxman J.S., Rosenblatt M.A. *et al.* "Eosinophilic granuloma of the cavernous sinus and orbital apex in an HIV positive patient," *Ophthalmology* **96** (1988), 462–467.

CHAPTER 8

OCULAR SURGERY IN HIV/AIDS PATIENTS

Steve D Schwartz and Adnan Tufail

Introduction

Surgical procedures in HIV-infected individuals may be identical to that performed in immunocompetent patients, for example cataract surgery. They may also be a modified standard technique to match the particular disease processes that can occur, as in the case of CMV-related retinal detachments, or a procedure unique to HIV-infected individuals, such as the insertion of intraocular drug release devices. The changing pattern of disease and the emergence of new therapies in HIV-infected individuals means that surgical approaches are constantly evolving.

This chapter will concentrate mainly on the management of retinal detachment and the insertion of intravitreous drug release implants, which are the most commonly performed ophthalmic surgical procedures in the setting of HIV-related disease. Cataract surgery may, however, become more commonly performed as a result of prolonged survival after retinal surgery or secondary uveitis, induced by drugs or immune recovery. Adnexal surgery, local therapy and other vitreoretinal procedures, as well as precautions for health care workers in the surgical setting are also covered.

Retinal Detachments

Retinal detachment secondary to necrotising herpes virus retinitis in patients with HIV infection represents a unique challenge to the vitreoretinal surgeon. The choice of procedure should not be just dictated by that most likely to be successful over the short term, in terms of an anatomical correction and visual rehabilitation, but must also consider the wider range of issues specific to the

201

patients with multiple systemic infections and limited life expectancy. As the length of survival of patients with AIDS increases especially with the advent of HAART, attention has been focused not just on the appropriate management of retinal detachments, but also on the complications associated with particular techniques of retinal detachment repair, such as the use of silicone oil, which in the long term may impair vision in its own right, from a variety of mechanisms.

Rhegmatogenous Retinal Detachment Associated with CMV Retinitis

Epidemiology

Prior to the AIDS epidemic, rhegmatogenous retinal detachments were considered to be a late complication of the disease. They occurred as oedema resolved and retinal holes developed in the healing process.[1,2] The reported prevalence of rhegmatogenous retinal detachments in patients with AIDS and CMV retinitis ranges widely, partly depending on the time interval studied, from approximately 15% to 35%.[3–7,8] The reported intervals from diagnosis of CMV retinitis to retinal detachment have ranged from medians of approximately four months[9,10] to a mean of approximately seven months.[11] The risk of retinal detachment increases over time. It has been estimated that there is a cumulative risk of 50% for retinal detachment at one year,[4,9,12] and the SOCA Research Group reported risks of 18.9% at six months rising to 37.9% at one year with patients on intravenous therapy.[8] Another study found a smaller risk among their patients: 11% at six months and 24% at one year.[13]

In addition to duration of disease, the rate of retinal detachment is related to a number of disease characteristics, including the location of the lesions and extent of infection. Several studies have confirmed an increased risk of retinal detachments in patients with infection extending to the ora serrata.[5,9] Lesions in the anterior portion of the retina underlie the vitreous base, where the vitreous body is normally adherent to the retina. Any traction of the vitreous body on the infected retina can result in the formation of retinal tears, and can facilitate movement of fluid to the subretinal space. In patients whose CMV retinitis lesions involved more than 50% of the retina at diagnosis, an increased rate of retinal detachment was reported, but a relationship between lesion size at baseline and detachment rates for patients with lesions smaller than 50% was not established[9] whereas other studies have reported the opposite.[13]

Multiple studies have suggested that patients with active retinitis are more likely to have retinal detachments,[13,14] although others have not found such a relationship.[8,9] With completely inactive lesions there may be sufficient chorioretinal scarring to prevent retinal detachment.[14] The number of disease progressions at the time of retinal detachment has also been associated with an increase risk of detachment.[8]

Initially when antiviral agents became available for the treatment of CMV retinitis, there was some concern that use of these drugs was associated with increased rates of retinal detachment.[5,6] It had been suggested that antiviral drugs hasten the development of rhegmatogenous retinal detachments by accelerating the healing of lesions, at which time retinal holes are more likely to develop,[6] and by reducing adhesive scar formation.[5] In another study, antiviral therapy was found to delay detachments by unclear mechanisms unrelated to either lesion size or location.[9] The increased number of retinal detachments seen after the introduction of anti-CMV therapies may just reflect the increasing survival of patients that was occurring at the same time. The effect of prolonged patient survival after diagnosis of CMV retinitis in patients on HAART on the prevalence of CMV-related retinal detachment is unknown. In addition, HAART may precipitate intraocular inflammation as the CD4 T-lymphocyte count rises[15,16] and whether this will increase the risk of retinal detachment or of developing proliferative vitreoretinopathy has not yet been established.

A majority of patients in several studies have had retinal detachments in both eyes,[14,17] but the SOCA Group found that in only 13 of 68 patients were the detachments bilateral.[8] The presence of a retinal detachment in the opposite eye is not an independent risk factor for rhegmatogenous retinal detachment.[13,8] This observation suggests that patients with bilateral disease have similar extents of disease and location of lesions in each eye, or that host factors may influence the risk of retinal detachment. Myopia has been reported to be a risk factor in patients who developed retinal detachments,[10] although this was not confirmed statistically by the SOCA Research Group.[8] In addition, age has been associated with the risk of developing retinal detachment presumably due to changes in the vitreous that occur with age that may allow the passage of liquid vitreous to the necrotic area in CMV retinitis.[8,11]

The increasing use of invasive local therapies for the treatment of CMV retinitis, such as intravitreous drug injections or implantation of intraocular devices for sustained release of ganciclovir, has led to concern about the possibility of an increased of rate of retinal detachment. Retinal detachments may develop sooner in eyes that are treated with intraocular devices as shown in one study where retinal detachment or tear occurred in 18% of eyes, but five of the seven retinal detachments occurred sooner than 65 days after implant of the intraocular device.[18] An increased rate of early retinal detachments in short-term studies may ultimately be balanced by a reduced rate of late retinal detachment. The replacement of devices after they are exhausted of drug may increase the risk of retinal detachment.

Pathophysiology

In the acute stage of disease, there may be subretinal fluid with exudative retinal detachment.[19] In the later stages of CMV retinitis, the necrotic retina thins with formation of multiple retinal holes, which predispose patients to retinal detachment. Eventually the necrotic retina is replaced by a thin gliotic membrane.

Lesions in the anterior portion of the retina underlie the vitreous base, where the vitreous body is normally adherent to the retina. Any traction of the vitreous body on the infected retina can result in the formation of retinal tears and facilitate movement of fluid to the subretinal space.

Clinical features

Symptoms of retinal detachment include increased floaters, photopsia, new scotomata or sudden enlargement of existing scotomata, the sensation of a curtain over one's vision, or sudden blurring of vision. Small peripheral retinal detachments can be asymptomatic, however.

Examination may reveal the presence of vitreous cells, the release of pigment into the vitreous cavity, and retinal elevation. CMV retinitis alone is not usually associated with marked vitreous cells and pigmentation in patients with low CD4 counts, and so if noted, a careful search should be made for the presence of retinal detachment. As retinal detachments in AIDS may present with only very shallow elevation of thin, translucent retina, cursory examination with a 20 dioptre lens may miss it and, therefore, careful examination should be performed with higher magnification should retinal detachment be suspected. An exudative detachment related to active retinitis should be excluded as it will settle with medical therapy alone. The examination should also attempt to determine the activity of the CMV retinitis which may require if active, re-induction therapy either systemically or locally, or insertion of a ganciclovir implant at the time of detachment repair.

Treatment

(A) Laser

Laser retinopexy for retinal detachment

Initial studies looking at the role of laser retinopexy in the treatment of CMV-related retinal detachments did not show it to be effective in preventing retinal detachments.[11] However, later studies have suggested a role for laser retinopexy in selected detachments either as definitive or temporising therapy.[20,21] Laser treatment to prevent retinal detachment extension posteriorly should consist of a double or triple row of burns surrounding all areas of active (see Fig. 8.1) or healed retinitis. If an area of healed retinitis cannot be adequately surrounded, such as when it is adjacent to the optic nerve head, grid laser treatment in that area should be considered.[22] Direct laser treatment of active retinitis can cause retinal breaks and should be avoided.

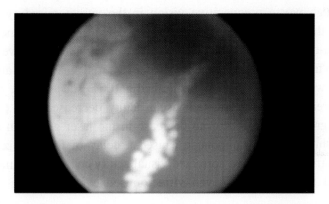

Fig. 8.1 Argon laser treatment surrounding area of active retinitis to prevent RD extension posteriorly (RD not shown).

The technique to apply laser photocoagulation is briefly as follows. With a slit-lamp mounted laser system or laser indirect ophthalmoscope, spots should be 200 to 500 μm in size and placed no more than one burn width apart and preferably, in a confluent triple concentric surround pattern. A duration of 0.1 seconds for a slit lamp-mounted laser or 0.2 seconds for a laser indirect ophthalmoscope is typical. The power setting should be enough to achieve moderate whitening of the retina. Wavelength selection has no impact on the success of the resultant chorioretinal adhesion, although longer wavelengths may be needed in cases of cataract or vitreous haemorrhage. Indirect laser retinopexy may be particularly helpful in carrying out treatment to the ora serata.

Of 22 peripheral, quadrantic retinal detachments with argon laser retinopexy, a 77% success rate was reported.[20] A space of 500μ between the burns and the edge of active lesions was recommended and a scatter laser treatment pattern was also placed in shallowly detached areas. Direct laser treatment of active retinitis, however, can cause retinal breaks and should be avoided. Others have reported successful treatment of most quadrantic peripheral detachments with barrier photocoagulation alone.[21] In another study of five macula-on detachments treated with prophylactic laser, three failed.[10] The area of detachment was found to have crossed the treatment borders two to four weeks later, at a time when one might have expected chorioretinal adhesions to have developed.

Laser treatment has also been reported to delay progression of detachments when compared to observation. This delay in progression led to fewer vitrectomies being required — 30% in the laser-treated group versus 56% of observed eyes. Visual results were also better in laser-treated eyes compared to vitrectomised eyes, although worse preoperative vision in the vitrectomised eyes confounds analysis of this outcome. Another study evaluated visual outcomes in patients with macula-on detachments treated with laser or vitrectomy.[23] Five of the seven detachments treated with laser resolved and one recurred nine months after treatment. Vitrectomy with silicone oil tamponade had a 100% success rate. Nevertheless, early post-treatment best corrected visual acuity decreased by 1.6 lines in the vitrectomy group, compared to no decrease in the laser group. In addition, the hyperopic shift after oil tamponade caused a delay of four to six weeks until spectacle correction and best corrected visual acuity could be obtained. Cataracts also formed in five of the seven vitrectomised eyes, requiring extraction in three.

Studies on the role of photocoagulation in treatment of CMV-related retinal detachments are difficult to interpret because of variable selection criteria of those patients subjected to laser rather than surgical treatment, variable length of follow-up, and variable control of retinitis (which may cross the zone of retinopexy if active). Despite the variable reported results, barrier photocoagulation of macula-on retinal detachments appears to be a useful therapeutic consideration which can improve quality of life by delaying or eliminating the need for vitrectomy surgery in selected patients with limited areas of CMV-related retinal detachments. Patient survival prospects and their general health should be taken into account when deciding on the modality of therapy.

Laser retinopexy for retinal tears

In nine eyes with CMV retinitis and flap tears, the tears were treated prophylactically with laser retinopexy.[22] Two of these eyes went on to develop retinal detachment. This 22% failure rate is higher than might be expected in the general population. The sample size is small, however, and the detachment rate is consistent with that seen in patients with CMV retinitis. It is therefore difficult to attribute any added risk to the presence of a flap tear in this group of patients.

Laser retinopexy for preventing retinal detachment

Prophylactic laser retinopexy surrounding areas of active retinitis was undertaken in two patients in an effort to prevent the development and spread of retinal detachment.[24] Both subsequently went on to develop RD. In another study, prophylactic laser was performed in five fellow eyes of patients with CMV-related RD.[11] Three of these eyes subsequently detached, with detachment progressing through the treated areas. However, more promising results have also been reported.[25] Prophylactic laser was used on nine eyes to surround areas of retinitis if they involved more than 25% of the retina. Three of these eyes developed detachments, but they were contained by the barrier photocoagulation. A limitation of this approach is that repeat laser may be necessary to contain moving borders of retinitis or detachment. These studies all have a relatively high rate of detachment, and often the barrier areas were ineffective at containing detachments. Nevertheless, this approach may be revisited in future in patients with extensive areas of inactive retinitis who are expected to remain inactive for a long time, after commencement of HAART with a good response, in whom the entire involved area may be comfortably surrounded.

Laser retinopexy for preventing progression of active retinitis

As early experience was gained with CMV retinitis, photocoagulation surrounding active retinitis was attempted with the hopes of limiting its spread. These attempts were unsuccessful.[26] With further understanding of the multifocal nature of the disease and the realisation that CMV is present in areas of apparently normal retina, it has become clear why barrier photocoagulation is an ill-fated approach to retinitis control.

(B) Surgical Management of Retinal Detachments

Surgery for CMV-related rhegmatogenous retinal detachment is typically performed under local anaesthesia without difficulty, although general anaesthesia may also be used. Most authors advocate standard three port pars plana vitrectomy and silicone oil internal tamponade in the repair of CMV-related retinal detachments (see Fig. 8.2 and 8.3).[5,10,11,14,17,24,27-29] The addition of ganciclovir (30 μg/ml) to the infusion bottle has been described.[30] As this group of patients is relatively young, the vitreous gel is often well formed and attached.[11,31] Posterior vitreous detachment is more common (65% at time of surgery),[11, 27] however, probably because of previous inflammation. Preoperative ultrasonography is useful in determining the status of the posterior hyaloid if it is not evident clinically.

Dissection of the posterior cortical gel from the retina is pivotal, but is often difficult in areas of thin, atrophic retina. A disposable soft-tipped extrusion cannula has been employed for this purpose,[11,11,27,32] along with membrane picks and intraocular scissors. Some authors perform a more conservative peeling in atrophic areas, only removing hyaloid or membranes that come away spontaneously,[33] while others perform retinectomies in areas of vitreous adherence to necrotic retina (see Fig. 8.4).[34] Internal drainage of subretinal fluid may be performed through pre-existing breaks or through a retinotomy, which should be made in the superior hemiretina[27] to ensure adequate tamponade in case of incomplete oil fill. If possible, the retinotomy should be within or next to an area of necrotic retina, and nasal to the optic nerve.[27] The retinotomy is surrounded with endolaser if located within a healthy retina.[10]

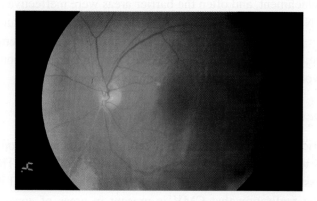

Fig. 8.2 CMV-associated RD with macula off. Note CMV retinitis in inferior quadrant.

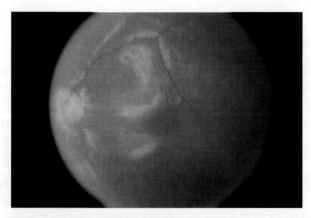

Fig. 8.3 The same eye as in Fig. 8.2. Retina now attached under silicone oil with visual acuity of 6/24 (Photograph courtesy of Dr. R. Engstrom).

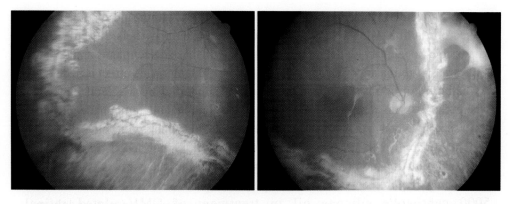

Fig. 8.4 The same eye as in Fig. 8.3, showing attached retina following excision of necrotic retina, silicone oil tamponade and endolaser photocoagulation. Visual acuity 6/18.

Some surgeons have suggested adding ganciclovir to the infusion fluid,[35] although no controlled study in humans has looked at whether this is beneficial. After initial air-fluid exchange, it is useful to wait several minutes to allow further desiccation of the vitreous base. During this waiting period, we do not allow any air flow through the sclerostomies, which has been suggested to be a potential cause of nerve fibre layer damage resulting in visual field changes after pars plana vitrectomy for macular hole surgery.[36] Direct fluid-oil exchange may alternatively be performed,[28,30,34] though this is a more technically difficult approach and is often hampered by problems with visualisation of the interface and incomplete evacuation of the aqueous layer.

Many authors also perform endolaser after air-fluid exchange. A triple row of laser should surround each break with or without laser surrounding the necrotic.[17,24,30,32] Scatter treatment may be used to cover necrotic retina in the inferior,[11,17,32,37] applied 360°.[38] Another suggested pattern intended to prevent recurrent inferior detachments from entering the macula, consists of a barrier of laser treatment along the inferior temporal vascular arcade, extending anteriorly above the horizontal meridian nasal to the optic disc and temporal to the macula.[33] None of these photocoagulation patterns has been proven to affect the outcome of surgery.

Vitrectomy without internal tamponade has been performed in some patients.[38] It has the advantage of rapid visual recovery without the complications of silicone oil, but has a poor success rate. Internal tamponade is therefore recommended by most surgeons. Silicone oil has become the standard agent used to achieve tamponade after pars plana vitrectomy for CMV-related retinal detachment. The permanent tamponade achieved with silicone oil is most appropriate in these patients, considering the presence of multiple holes within and at the borders of necrotic retina, which may be located quite posteriorly. It is difficult, if not impossible, to identify all the holes associated with these detachments and because large areas of retina are often necrotic, a widespread tamponade effect is necessary. As active retinitis may progress to areas not supported by a scleral buckle or where there is no tamponade effect of a gas bubble, oil tamponade provides more security when detachment repair is performed in patients with active disease.[20] Patients repaired with silicone oil also benefit from a much more rapid recovery of visual function compared to gas tamponade, and they are not limited by positioning requirements. There is reported experience with 1000, 1300, and 5000 centistoke silicone oil in treatment of CMV-related retinal detachments.[10,11,17,28,30] No differences in outcome for these different viscosity levels have been detected or suggested. The primary advantage of 1000-cs silicone oil over 5000-cs silicone oil is the ease and speed with which it can be injected into and removed from the eye. This corresponds to a lower infusion pressure, which might limit optic atrophy related to intraocular pressure elevations. Lower viscosity oils, however, are more likely to undergo emulsification.

Prior to infusion of silicone oil, sutures may be passed through the sclerostomy sites to expedite closure once a fill is achieved. A cannula may be introduced through the superior sclerostomy opposite the infusion port to facilitate removal of air from the vitreous cavity. The eye should be rotated so that the infusion is inferior and the air is evacuated superiorly such that all air bubbles are evacuated as the oil is infused. Postoperatively, patients should maintain face-down positioning for at least the first night after surgery,[31] although some advocate as much as a week of this.[39]

A two-stage surgical approach in CMV-related detachments has been suggested, which may more completely evacuate the aqueous fluid from the posterior segment, thus allowing for a better oil fill. At the time of vitrectomy, the eye is filled with an expansile concentration of SF6 or C3F8. As the gas expands over the next two to three days, any residual fluid in the subretinal space or vitreous cavity disappears. The patient is then brought back to the operating theatre, and an oil-gas exchange is performed. This technique has the obvious disadvantage of taking the patient to the operating theatre for a second time, and may also be more likely to lead to optic nerve and retinal perfusion problems due to elevated intraocular pressure in this susceptible group of patients.

In most patients with CMV-related retinal detachment, the removal of oil from the eye has not been performed. This is because of the previously short life expectancy of patients with advanced acquired immune deficiency syndrome. With the advent of HAART, the survival of many AIDS patients has been prolonged dramatically. It remains to be seen whether removal of silicone oil will be commonly performed in this group of patients.

Other tamponade agents

Long acting gases have also been used to achieve retinal tamponade after vitrectomy for CMV-related retinal detachment.[11,14,17,20,24] 20% sulfurhexafluoride was used in three eyes, one of which redetached and was subsequently repaired with silicone oil tamponade. In addition, two failures after vitrectomy with perfluorocarbon gas infusion were then successfully repaired with silicone oil tamponade.[24] Intraocular gas tamponade also demands prolonged postoperative positioning and is associated with a period of very poor vision until the gas bubble is reabsorbed sufficiently to clear the visual axis. These limitations are often significant in this group of patients with poor health, short life expectancy, and often bilateral disease.[24]

Pneumatic retinopexy was been unsuccessful in several reports,[14,27] but may be useful in patients in whom more extensive surgery cannot safely be performed and who have a detachment associated with a small area of hole formation in the superior retina. Otherwise, this is not a frequently used modality in the treatment of CMV-related retinal detachments.

The role of scleral buckle placement in the repair of CMV-associated retinal detachment

Scleral buckling has frequently been performed in conjunction with pars plana vitrectomy in reports of CMV-related detachment repair.[5,10,11,17,21,27,28,30,37,39-41] More recently, however, it has been proposed that buckling is perhaps not necessary in most cases,[17,24,37,39] and it is not felt to improve outcome in the majority of patients.[11,30,37,39] In 68 eyes with CMV-related retinal detachment repaired with vitrectomy and silicone oil tamponade,[39] 56 also had a 360° encircling scleral buckle placement. There was no significant difference in success or visual outcome between the two groups. Reattachment rates were 86% with buckling and 84% without buckling, with macular attachment rates of 91% in both groups. The mean best postoperative visual acuity was 20/66 with and 20/67 without buckling. However, in another large series, higher rates of reattachment and better visual outcome were reported when vitrectomy and silicone oil tamponade were combined with scleral buckle placement.[28] The lack of control for risk factors such as the extent of retinitis in the existing studies, and of a randomised prospective study investigating the role of scleral buckles in these patients, limit our ability to conclusively define when or if they are of benefit in combination with vitrectomy and silicone oil tamponade.

Most frequently, redetachments are shallow and located inferiorly, particularly when there is necrotic retina inferiorly. An inferior buckle may allow for more complete oil-retinal contact inferiorly, particularly when there is an incomplete oil fill.[27] The reflection from the oil interface on the surface of an inferior buckle is also more easily visualised, and allows one to better assess the completeness of the oil fill postoperatively. On the other hand, others have argued that the buckle effect may decrease with time during the postoperative period, allowing for accumulation of aqueous fluid in the posterior segment and leading to recurrent inferior detachment.[10]

When a scleral buckle is used in conjunction with vitrectomy, a solid silicone encircling element is typically chosen.[5,17,21,27,29,39] With encircling, there is the additional benefit of reducing the acquired hyperopia seen in oil-filled eyes. In one study, the anisometropia in patients repaired with oil averaged 5.5 diopters when no buckle was placed, compared to 3.7 diopters when buckling was performed.[27] Another study also found a decrease of hyperopic shift by one to four diopters when buckling was performed.[10] In addition, 56 oil-filled eyes with encircling bands were found to be on average 1.0 dioptres less hyperopic than 22 oil-filled eyes with buckles.[39] If a scleral buckle is desired, it should be placed prior to silicone oil infusion, typically under air.

In summary, scleral buckle placement has not been convincingly shown to be of significant additive benefit in patients undergoing pars plana vitrectomy with silicone oil tamponade for CMV-related rhegmatogenous retinal detachment, though some studies have suggested that this may be true. The reduction of induced hyperopia is advantageous, but must be weighed against the increased risk to the operating staff, operative time, and postoperative morbidity. In addition, the surgery becomes more difficult to perform under local anaesthesia, and is more likely to be associated with elevations of intraocular pressure which have been suspected of contributing to optic atrophy in these patients.

Scleral buckling alone has been attempted and in most,[27,42] but not all,[20,38] reports is not successful.[27,40] If it can be avoided, cryotherapy is not favoured as an adjunct to surgery.[20,27] Indirect photocoagulation is less likely to encite excessive inflammation and proliferative vitreoretinopathy.

Lensectomy in conjunction with pars plana vitrectomy

Lensectomy at the time of surgery is performed when lenticular opacity prevents adequate visualisation of the posterior segment.[24] The completion of surgery in as little time as possible will help to avoid problems with feathering of the lens capsule which can impair the view. If the view does degrade, indirect air-fluid exchange and endolaser may be useful in completing the case while preserving the lens. Avoiding lens removal will allow for a near 100% silicone oil fill and minimise anterior segment complications.

Lens removal may be associated with more silicone oil-related complications by allowing oil to enter the anterior chamber. If lensectomy is to be performed, it is best to maintain an intact posterior capsule for segregating oil to the posterior segment. If the posterior capsule is ruptured during surgery, or if there is zonular dehiscence allowing forward migration of silicone oil, it is important to perform an inferior iridectomy.[28] This is true even if an intraocular lens is implanted. If silicone oil is allowed into the anterior segment, the oil interface may cause pupillary block with anterior chamber angle closure and severe intraocular pressure elevation.

When lensectomy is performed, the immediate placement of an intraocular lens is the best course of action. A plano-convex PMMA optic is most appropriate for the silicone-filled eye. Other lens materials are associated with deposits of oil on the lens surface which may degrade the vision significantly. This is particularly true with silicone lenses. Silicone oil adheres to silicone lenses very tenaciously, forming a coating that is essentially impossible to remove and which alters the optical performance of the lens. Acrylic lenses are better, but still may develop oil droplets on their surfaces. This problem is essentially not encountered with solid PMMA optics.

The refractive surface formed by the anterior silicone oil interface is a very important component of the optical system in a silicone oil-filled eye. The refractive index of silicone oil is greater than that of aqueous. The most appropriate intraocular lens would actually have a concave posterior surface to match the convex anterior surface of the oil, and a convex anterior surface.

In binocular patients with a limited life expectancy and some degree of lens opacity at the time of retinal detachment, a case has been made to perform cataract extraction and lens implant at the time of detachment surgery, to allow early visual rehabilitation by reducing the anisometropia induced by silicone oil.

Complications

The use of intraocular silicone oil has several side effects that can affect a patient's vision. It alters a patient's refractive status by causing a marked hyperopic shift.[10,11,42] Silicone oil has also been observed to reduce a patient's accommodative amplitudes.[10] There is also a high rate of silicone oil-induced cataract formation. Early reports documented poor visual acuity[9,14] and progressive decline in vision[10,14,31] after retinal detachment repair. A variety of factors may contribute to poor vision, for example progression of CMV and the high rate of optic atrophy seen in patients after surgery.[31] Optic atrophy may be due to increased intraocular pressure during and after surgery.[31] Also, patients with AIDS are known to have alterations in blood flow;[43] as a result, there may be poor retinal and/or optic disc perfusion during surgery when fluid infusions elevate intraocular pressure. Silicone oil toxicity is not thought to be a cause of optic atrophy,[31] but could be related to the extent of retinitis in the affected eye.[17] Cataracts can contribute to decreased vision, but despite the high rate of cataract formation with the use of silicone oil, cataract was not the factor that limited vision for most patients in several series.[10,14,17]

Whether or not the macula has detached before surgical repair did not influence final vision in one study.[17] The best visual outcomes were related to good preoperative visual acuity, early surgical intervention, absence of preoperative optic atrophy, and lack of macular CMV infection.[37] Visual outcomes have been improving[11,37] with 71% of patients having visual acuity of 20/200 or better at last follow-up.[37] The factors contributing to the improvement in outcomes probably include patient selection, earlier intervention, improved surgical techniques, and earlier diagnosis and medical treatment of CMV infection.[37] Despite the fact that final visual results have been modest in many patients, the results are much better than those for eyes with retinal detachments that do not undergo surgery, which are invariably hand-motion level or worse.[9,14]

Patients undergoing surgical repair of a retinal detachment should be informed that the use of silicone oil makes visual rehabilitation of repaired eyes difficult, and that best corrected vision may be worse after surgery. In cases where vision is better in the opposite eye, they should be informed that good binocular vision after surgery may not be possible, but that the procedure is being performed to preserve some vision in the involved eye, in case vision is eventually lost in the other eye. Several reports have suggested that ultimately vision in an eye that has undergone retinal detachment repair may be better than in the opposite eye, due to the high rate of bilateral disease and bilateral detachments.[10,17,37]

Prognosis

Retinal detachments associated with CMV retinitis may be difficult to repair, because of extensive retinal necrosis, multiple hole formation, and possible associated proliferative vitreoretinopathy.[5,14] Studies have documented good anatomical success rates with these procedures with a final total retinal reattachment rate of 64% to 82% and a final macular reattachment rate of 86% to 92%.[17,37]

When detachments recur, they usually involve the inferior retina,[10] which may be due to inadequate silicone oil fill.

Visual success rates

Initially few patients obtained ambulatory vision,[9,31] but more promising results were found later by others.[14,17,33,37,40] In a study of retinal detachment repair in 65 eyes of 51 patients, a mean best postoperative visual acuity of 6/18 was reported, obtained at a mean of 6.5 weeks postoperatively, and a mean final visual acuity of 6/30.[17] In several studies mean visual acuity dropped after the first one to two months.[14,17,31] CMV optic neuritis, progressive smoldering retinitis, recurrent detachment, cataract, and anterior segment complications of silicone oil may explain some of the decline in vision. Alternatively, silicone oil toxicity, a controversal entity, has been proposed.[33]

Preoperative macular detachment had no impact on final visual outcome[17] and no difference in visual outcome was found if the retinal detachments were repaired before or during the first week after macular detachment[10,30] The presence of macular or papillomacular retinitis, in contrast, is more clearly associated with a worse mean best postoperative visual acuity, to a level of 6/60 in one study.[17] None of the patients recovered ambulatory vision when the visual acuity was hand motions or worse at the time of surgery.[24] Ambulatory vision was preserved, however, in 80% of eyes with CMV-related detachment and 67% of non-CMV necrotising retinitis eyes. Other studies have also shown that worse preoperative vision is associated with worse visual outcome.[14]

Survival

Reported survival rates after the diagnosis of CMVR and CMV-related retinal detachment vary to some degree, but are generally poor. A median survival of 17 weeks following diagnosis of retinal detachment has been reported,[14] whereas others found it to be nine months.[9] With the success of HAART, the postoperative survival of patients with AIDS-related retinal detachments has likely increased and this may affect our choice of procedure in the future.

Retinal Detachment Secondary to Non-CMV Infections

Necrotising herpetic retinopathies

Acute retinal necrosis leading to rhegmatogenous retinal detachment has been described in a number of patients with AIDS[14] as well as PORN[44-46] (see chapter 5). In the largest reported series of PORN patients, retinal detachments developed in 70% of eyes.[47] Both ARN-and PORN-related retinal detachments require vitrectomy with silicone oil tamponade,[14,24,28] but 25% of retinal detachments in 16 eyes of patients with PORN redetached.[47] The visual prognosis is not good, but in ARN patients ambulatory vision may be preserved whereas in PORN, all went on to no light perception vision.[14] In another study, there was no statistical difference in visual outcome of PORN patients who underwent surgical repair of retinal detachment compared to untreated patients.[47]

Other infections

Although exudative retinal detachments are more commonly observed in patients with syphilitic retinitis,[48] rhegmatogenous detachments also occur.[49,50] Pars plana vitrectomy with internal tamponade with or without scleral buckling is usually required in these patients because of the potential for multiple small breaks in the atrophic retina. Case reports have also described retinal detachment in association with toxoplasmic retinochoroiditis,[14] and candidal endophthalmitis.[21]

Epiretinal Membranes

With the advent of HAART, an immune recovery vitritis may develop along with the development of associated epiretinal membranes (see Fig. 8.5).[15,16] There has been some limited improvement in vision in attempting surgical peeling of these membranes (see Fig. 8.6), but there is a high risk of precipitating retinal detachment.

Diagnostic Procedures

Ocular Fluid Sampling

PCR-based assays of vitreous specimens has been found useful in the diagnostic evaluation of patients with infectious retinitis where the diagnosis is unclear on clinical evaluation alone,[51,52] and in checking for resistant isolates of CMV. Aqueous sampling has also been found useful in providing samples suitable for PCR testing.[53,54]

Aqueous tap

This may be undertaken at the slit lamp or under operating microscope control. Topical anaesthesia is applied and the conjunctival sac is cleaned with povidone-

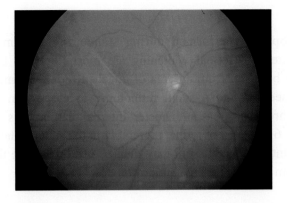

Fig. 8.5 Epiretinal membrane occurring in patient on HAART (Photograph courtesy of Dr. B. Dhillon).

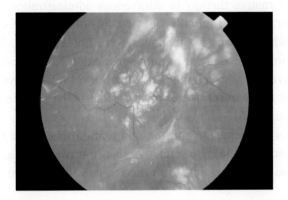

Fig. 8.6 Attempted removal of epiretinal membranes with silicone oil now *in situ* (Photograph courtesy of Dr. B. Dhillon).

iodine solution. The needle of an insulin syringe in inserted via the limbus into the anterior chamber and 100 ml to 200 μl of aqueous is aspirated.

Vitreous tap

To perform a vitreous tap 0.25 ml of subconjunctival lignocaine is injected into the quadrant to be tapped after cleaning the conjunctival sac with povidone-iodine solution. A 23-g gauge attached to a 1 ml or 2 ml volume syringe is inserted 4 mm behind the limbus and directed into the mid vitreous. Between 200 μl and 400 μl of vitreous is then aspirated. Many surgeons prefer to take vitreous specimens using an automated vitrectomy cutter.

Retinal biopsy

Endoretinal biopsy is performed during standard vitrectomy with internal tamponade.[32] Areas of retinal whitening are most likely to be diagnostic. If the biopsy is to be taken from an area of attached retina, balanced salt solution should be infused through a small retinotomy to elevate an area of interest approximately three disc areas in diameter. Internal diathermy is used to delineate a 2–4 mm by 3–6 mm area of retina, preferably in the superior hemiretina outside of the macula. Intraocular scissors may then be used to excise the retina, which is removed from the eye with a microforceps.

Administration of Local Therapy

Direct placement of ganciclovir, foscarnet, or cidofovir into the eye has been studied as an alternative therapy to intravenous administration of drug. Interest in this local therapy arose initially out of concern about the systemic toxicity of ganciclovir when alternative therapies were not available. It has also been advocated by some investigators as supplementation to systemic therapy, either following reactivation and enlargement of lesions[55] to improve the efficacy of intravenous drug at the onset of treatment,[56,57] or as the sole treatment for CMV retinitis (see chapter 6).

The desire for convenience and the observation that direct delivery of drug to the eye may actually be more effective than intravenously administered drug for delaying time to progression[18] are the reasons that interest in local therapy continues.

Supplementation of local drug levels in which patients receiving oral formulation of anti-CMV drugs (which may have low bioavailability) is viewed by many as the most promising future role for local therapy. There are a number of factors that must be taken into account when deciding between local and systemic therapies, including efficacy, toxicity, complications of the delivery method, risk of fellow eye or extraocular disease, and patient survival.[58,59]

Intravitreous Injection

The procedure is generally performed in a clean area or a minor procedure room. The eye in which the injection is to be given should be dilated beforehand. In order to prevent intraocular pressure rise post-injection, premedication with oral or intravenous acetazolamide has been reported,[55,60] as has mercury bag decompression.[61] Sterile lyophilised ganciclovir powder is reconstituted in balanced salt solution. The solution is filtered through a 22-μm filter into a tuberculin syringe, which is then capped with a 0.5-inch 27 to 30 gauge needle. After administration of a drop of topical anaesthetic agent, a cotton-tipped applicator soaked with topical anaesthetic is placed under the upper eyelid superotemporally for a few minutes. The drug-soaked pledget is then removed and an eyelid speculum is placed in the eye. The patient is instructed to look down at all times, and a few drops of 5% povidone-iodine solution are placed in the eye. 2% lignocaine with adrenaline can then be injected beneath the superotemporal conjunctiva posterior to the limbus, raising a small bleb although the procedure may be well tolerated with topical anaesthetic alone.[60] Retrobulbar anesthesia has been used but is generally not necessary.[55] The procedure is also performed in the inferotemporal quadrant by many surgeons, which facilitates injection under direct visualisation with an indirect ophthalmoscope,[55,62] usually aiming to avoid injecting directly anterior to an area of retinal necrosis, as this might be more prone to cause an iatrogenic tear.

0.1 ml of the ganciclovir solution is injected in the anaesthetised region, 3.5 mm to 4.0 mm posterior to the limbus. The needle is directed towards the mid-vitreous and inserted almost to the hub prior to injection. After injection, as the needle is withdrawn, a sterile cotton-tipped applicator soaked with balanced salt solution is placed with a slight pressure over the injection site for a few seconds. Indirect ophthalmoscopy is then performed to look for perfusion of the optic nerve head, vitreous haemorrhage, or retinal injury or detachment. If perfusion is absent and does not return within one to two minutes, a paracentesis is immediately performed. If not, the intraocular pressure is checked. A drop of topical antibiotic solution is then placed in the eye and the lid speculum is removed. There is no need to patch the eye. If the intraocular pressure is significantly elevated, topical aqueous suppressants may be administered and the pressure rechecked in one hour. The patient is placed on a topical antibiotics for a few days after injection.

Complications

Complications of intravitreous injection may be general, those related to pars plana injection procedure, and those specific for the compound injected.

Reported complications of local therapy include scleral induration, mild to moderate vitreous humor haze, iritis, mild to severe vitreous haemorrhage,[60] and infectious endophthalmitis.[18,60,62–67] The risk of endophthalmitis has been estimated at between 0.14% to 0.29% per injection,[58,66] or 2.6% per eye.[66] However, bacterial endophthalmitis may also be a complication of intravenous therapy.[68]

Conjunctival scarring and scleral induration at the injection site may occur with repeated injections.[60,65] Cataract is also uncommon unless direct lens trauma occurs at the time of injection. Subconjunctival hemorrhage associated with injection is a frequent but minor complication.[60] Keratitis occurred in 8% of patients in one study[60] and has been attributed to intensive use of topical anaesthetic drops.

Invasion of the vitreous base results in development of localised granulation tissue and vitreous body traction which can lead to retinal detachment, even after a single needle perforation of the pars plana.[69] Retinal detachment have been reported to occur at between 0.6% to 9% of patients receiving intravitreous injections.[60,63,66,67] Retinal detachments are common in patients with CMV retinitis, so some such cases may be simply the natural course of the disease. A controlled study has not been performed to look at the relative risks of detachment between intravitreous and systemic therapy.

Proliferative vitreoretinopathy may also occur secondary to pars plana injection.[69] Granulation tissue was found spreading from the injection site onto the pars plana and peripheral retina associated with a localised retinal detachment.

The development of optic atrophy has been reported to occur in 8% of patients undergoing repeated intravitreous injections of ganciclovir.[60] Optic atrophy may be occuring as a result of CMV retinitis, although concern has been raised that it may be secondary to acute elevation in intraocular pressure associated with intravitreous injections. The injection of smaller volumes of more concentrated ganciclovir has been advocated by some authors to avoid problems with retinal and optic nerve nonperfusion.[66,67] Prophylactic paracentesis, acetazolamide therapy, and mercury bag decompression have also been used to prevent a marked rise in ocular pressure.[55,60,61]

Specific Intravitreous Drugs

See chapter 6 for details of these drugs.

Intravitreous Injection in Silicone-Oil Filled Eyes

Intravitreous ganciclovir injection has safely been performed in the silicone oil-filled eye.[30,41] Some surgeons have also injected intracameral ganciclovir after oil infusion if there is active retinitis at the time of CMV-related retinal detachment repair.[29] A particular drug will distribute to different degrees in both the oil and aqueous phases filling the vitreous cavity. Ganciclovir is not felt to distribute into the oil phase significantly so the dose of drug injected is reduced by 50%, or in proportion to the oil fill.

Intraocular Drug Release Devices

The problems associated with once or twice weekly intravitreous injections stimulated interest in an intraocular device for sustained release of ganciclovir, which was introduced in 1992.[70] Intraocular devices offer the additional advantage of drug release at a steady rate, thereby avoiding the fluctuating drug levels associated with intermittent dosing, which might affect efficacy and facilitate the emergence of resistant virus strains.

The first generation implant was composed of a disc-shaped, 6-mg pellet of ganciclovir coated with 10% polyvinyl alcohol (PVA), which is permeable to ganciclovir.[70-72] This pellet is then covered on all but one face with ethylene vinyl acetate, which is impermeable to ganciclovir. This is again entirely coated with PVA. An anchoring tab of polyvinyl alcohol holds the pellet in position. The newer commercially available implant contains at least 4.5 mg of ganciclovir and releases the drug at adequate intraocular levels for about eight months. With the increased longevity of many of those afflicted with AIDS with the advent of HAART, however, it is not uncommon for patients to undergo more than one implantation procedure with the available eight-month device. To minimise the need for reimplantation, a sustained-release intravitreous ganciclovir implant with a life span of approximately two years is currently under development.

Surgical technique – insertion of intraocular devices

The device can implanted under local anaesthesia. The conjunctival incision is typically made in the inferotemporal quadrant at the limbus, and haemostasis is achieved using bipolar diathermy. The device is prepared by passing a double armed 8-0 nylon suture through the base of the anchoring strut of the device, and the excessive strut is trimmed to reduce the chance of it protruding through the sclera.[72] A microvitreoretinal blade is used to enter the inferotemporal sclera 4 mm from the limbus. The incision is then enlarged to 4 mm to 5 mm circumferentially. Using an automated vitrectomy device, or by simple excision, any prolapsed vitreous is removed.

The edge of the sclerostomy incision is opened to confirm that a full-thickness incision of the underlying pars plana has been made. The strut of the device is grasped with forceps and inserted into the eye with the drug pellet facing the front of the eye, avoiding damage to the membrane surrounding the drug pellet. The supporting suture passing through the strut is used to anchor the device by passing it through either side of the scleral incision, and is then tied with burial of the suture ends. The scleral incision is also closed with 8-0 nylon and balanced salt solution is injected, if necessary, through the wound to restore intraocular pressure. Indirect ophthalmoscopy is performed to verify correct intravitreous placement (see Fig. 8.7). The conjunctival is closed with absorbable sutures and, finally, sub-conjunctival antibiotics and steroid injections are administered.

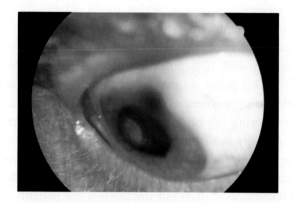

Fig. 8.7 Ganciclovir implant *in situ.*

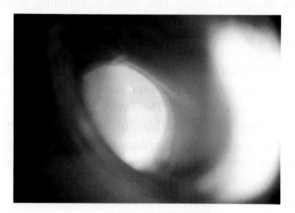

Fig. 8.8 Empty ganciclovir implant *in situ* — note colour (Photograph courtesy of Dr. B. Dhillon).

The implant can be scheduled for exchange at 32 weeks, or be exchanged earlier if progression of CMV retinitis has occurred. The implant may be examined clinically to determine if it is empty if progression has occurred at an earlier time than expected. Instead of the original orange colour of the device, it will appear reddish-brown (see Fig. 8.8).[73] Although some authors have reported removing and replacing implants as the device becomes empty of drug,[73] others place subsequent implants in other quadrants rather than remove the primary implant. The surgery to remove the empty device and anchor a fresh one in the same site may be more difficult and complicated. Vitreous haemorrhage is a more prominent complication of implant exchange than primary implantation, especially if the same entry site is used repeatedly.[18, 74] The old implants tend to be well tolerated, though there is a risk of erosion, migration into the vitreous, and lens touch with cataract formation.[75] In patients successfully treated with HAART, it is possible now to consider allowing implants to run out rather than performing scheduled replacements, particularly when there is non sight-threatening zone 2/3 involvement, as the improved immune system itself may control the retinitis.[76]

Clinical experience

Twenty-six patients with untreated CMV retinitis in zones 2 and/or 3 were randomised to receive an intraocular device or to have therapy deferred until there was progression of disease.[18] The median time to disease progression in the group receiving intraocular devices was 226 days compared to 15 days for the deferral group. Many factors can influence the study results, and different studies should be compared with caution. Nevertheless, the very large difference between the median time to disease progression in this study and the 47-day median time to progression reported from the SOCA Research Group for patients receiving intravenous ganciclovir probably represent a real difference in the ability to prevent spread of disease between drug administered by intraocular devices and drug delivered intravenously at maintenance therapy doses, especially since the results were determined by the same fundus photograph reading centre.[18,77]

This study did not address the efficacy of intraocular devices for treatment of progressive disease in patients who have already received intravenously administered drug, and who may have strains of virus that are already relatively resistant to ganciclovir.[18] Earlier studies by others, however, suggest that there may be a role for the use of intraocular devices in such salvage therapy.[73]

The ability of intraocular devices to prevent enlargement of lesions must be weighed against the risk of new bilateral disease, non-ocular CMV disease, and early retinal detachments. 50% of patients with unilateral disease who were treated with an intraocular device in the one study, had developed bilateral disease at six months.[18] In contrast, the cumulative risk of bilateral disease in the SOCA Research Group study was only 27% at six months in patients receiving intravenous ganciclovir.[77] Once an eye develops CMV retinopathy, it is at risk for retinal detachment, regardless of the success with which it is controlled medically.

The fact that local therapy does not treat non-ocular disease has also been viewed as a major disadvantage. All patients with untreated CMV retinopathy have evidence of non-ocular tissue-invasive CMV infections at autopsy,[19] although the rate with which these infections cause clinically apparent disease is hard to determine. Non-ocular, clinically apparent CMV disease occurred in eight of 26 patients (31%) with intraocular devices, and in at least one patient, death was attributed to CMV infection.[18] Systemic therapy for CMV retinitis has been shown to decrease the incidence of non-ocular infections,[78] but in the absence of non-ocular CMV disease, the need to administer systemic anti-CMV therapy has not been well established. Although systemic therapy appears to prolong patient survival,[79,80] it has never been shown that early treatment of non-ocular CMV infection is any more beneficial than treating the clinical manifestations of infections when they develop.

Complications

A transient reduction in vision for several weeks after surgery commonly occurs due to vitreous haemorrhage[18,73,75,81] and astigmatism, that usually resolves within a month.[18,87] Patients must also realise that there is the possibility of a potentially visually devastating result, such as endophthalmitis or retinal detachment. Disease progression may be noted for the first two weeks after implantation,[18] and does not necessarily indicate failure. Deferral of clinical assessment of the response to the implant up to one month postoperatively has therefore been advocated.[82] Beyond that time, retinitis should be stable. If it is not, then failure of local therapy is likely. This was noted in two of 30 eyes in the phase I study of the device, and later in up to 24% of eyes.[82] Glaucoma secondary to hyphaema can further complicate the postoperative course.[82]

Although bacterial endophthalmitis may occur, it is uncommon in most reported series[73,75] although one group reported a rate of 1.7% of eyes treated.[81] A sterile vitritis was noted in eight eyes[75] and was attributed to residual ethylene oxide in implants related to the sterilisation process. This is not a complication with the commercially available devices currently in use.

Confirmation of the position of the device intraoperatively is necessary as occasionally suprachoroidal placement of the device has occurred.[71,82] If this complication occurs, the device should be repositioned. Other complications include implant migration or extrusion, corneal dellen,[73] wound dehiscence,[82] and hypotony.[18] Invasive procedures may increase the rate of retinal detachment, but this association during local treatment of CMV retinitis is difficult to establish, since retinal detachment is a well-known complication of all necrotising infectious retinopathies, even if disease is medically controlled. Retinal detachments may develop sooner when eyes are treated with intraocular devices, however. The SOCA Research Group identified the risk of retinal detachment among patients receiving intravenous ganciclovir to be 27% at six months[77]; in another study of 38 patients with retinal detachment who had been treated with systemic therapy, the median time to detachment was four months.[9] In another study, retinal detachment or a retinal tear occurred in 18% of eyes, but five of seven retinal detachments occurred sooner than 65 days after implantation of the intraocular device.[18]

As with other CMV-related retinal detachments, the favoured approach to surgical repair is pars plana vitrectomy with silicone oil tamponade.[18,71,73,82] As ganciclovir is released from the intravitreal implant at a steady rate based on the concentration gradient, the device may be left in place when silicone oil tamponade is performed. Ganciclovir will not redistribute into the oil phase, and it is presumed that the drug will be distributed in the aqueous compartment of an oil-filled eye. Leaving the implant surrounded by an aqueous fluid phase in the vitreous cavity whenever possible[82] has been suggested, but such an underfill might be less effective in cases of inferior retinitis or detachment.

Cataract Surgery in AIDS Patients

When cataract extraction is required in the non-vitrectomised eye of an AIDS patient, the approach and management are essentially no different than with other types of cataract. As noted at the beginning of this chapter, however, the operating staff must be conscious of the risk of transmission of HIV with contaminated percutaneous injuries. Sutureless incisions and conjunctival closures are most appropriate in this setting, as they eliminate the risk associated with the suture needles. Although a patient may have no evidence of CMV retinitis or other AIDS-defining conditions, it is best to implant a lens that will not cause problems if a vitrectomy and oil fill are needed in the future. Silicone oil adheres to the surface of foldable silicone and acrylic lenses, causing refractive aberrations which may limit vision. Polymethylmethacrylate is the most appropriate intraocular lens material.

The management of cataracts in the eyes of AIDS patients who have undergone vitrectomy with silicone oil tamponade is not a simple matter. The procedure is more difficult due to the increased tendency for the posterior capsule to move anteriorly when it is not tethered to the vitreous body. In addition, these lenses tend to be quite dense. Intraocular lens power calculation is problematic due to the alteration in axial length measurement caused by silicone and also to characteristics of the oil-lens interface. A three-step modification of intraocular lens calculation has been suggested using specific sound velocities to calculate axial length, using convexoplano lenses, and adding a constant to the lens power to compensate for the refractive index of silicone oil.[83] Removal of the lens from a silicone oil-filled eye may leave the eye with a silicone underfill. Therefore, 0.3 ml to 0.7 ml of oil should be added to the vitreous cavity in conjunction with cataract extraction in order to maintain a complete fill.[32]

Adnexal Surgery

Molluscum Contagiosum

The periocular skin around the lash roots and occasionally the ocular surface are common sites for molluscum lesions (see chapters 2 and 4). Lid lesions may cause a secondary irritative keratitis and follicular conjunctivitis by the shedding of viral infected cells. The large molluscum lesions that may occur in HIV-infected patients may lead to difficulty in differentiating it from basal cell carcinoma and cryptococcal cutaneous infection. A biopsy should be therefore be considered in atypical lesions.

Molluscum lesions in the immunosuppressed do not resolve spontaneously. Lid lesions may be treated with incision, excision, laser, or cryotherapy, and epibulbar lesions with excision.[84] Although individual lesions are easy to treat, with AIDS patients the lesions usually recur and spread and often become refractory to treatment.

Kaposi's Sarcoma

Ocular KS is the initial site of presentation of the disease in an estimated 14% of patients. Ocular KS tends not to be aggressive and causes visual loss or pain infrequently. Symptoms are usually due to a mass effect that may result in ptosis, altered lid position, or ocular surface irritation. Many KS lesions can be observed until they cause local symptoms (see chapter 4).

Treatment is not curative but is aimed at alleviating symptoms. It may be local or systemic depending on the number, site, and size of the lesion(s).[85,86] Cryotherapy is the usual treatment of choice for lid or peribulbar lesions. Radiotherapy has been advocated for the use of large lesions greater than 3 mm in height.[86] Multiple and visceral KS can be treated with systemic chemotherapy.[87] Complications of radiotherapy and cryotherapy include skin depigmentation and, in addition, radiotherapy may cause lash loss, conjunctivitis, dermatitis, and potentially optic neuropathy.[87] In the orbit, KS lesions are relatively benign although they tend to recur after treatment in up to 60% of cases.

Squamous Cell Carcinoma

In Africa, HIV infection is strongly associated with an increase in the incidence of conjunctival carcinoma (see chapter 9).[105,106] Treatment depends on the size and location of the tumour. Carcinoma in HIV-infected patients may be more aggressive early globe invasion, and may require frequent follow-up examination, even after complete excision of the tumour.[107]

Precautions for Health Care Workers in the Surgical Setting

The risk of transmission of HIV from the infected patient to health care personnel by percutaneous exposure to infected blood has been estimated at up to 0.3%.[91,92] It has been estimated that the life-time risk of surgeons to acquire HIV infection is between 0.5%[93] and 5%,[83] although the figure is probably considerably lower for ophthalmic surgeons, with use of effective precautions and with post-exposure prophylaxis. The risk of HIV infection after percutaneous exposure increases with a larger volume of blood and, probably, a higher titre of HIV in the source patient's blood.[94]

Although post-exposure prophylaxis with antiretroviral drugs appears to be protective, its use cannot eliminate the chance of disease transmission and so universal precautions should be carefully heeded when performing surgery. Double-gloving is standard practice,[10,31,38,40] although the current data on such protection derive exclusively from studies that use glove leak and contamination as outcome measures. There are no data that measure protection in terms of actual disease transmission.[95] Shoes should be worn by the surgeon at all times.[38] Minimising the risk of injury to the surgeon and operative staff by limiting passage of needles or sharp instruments between personnel has been advocated by many.[10,38] Some surgeons advocate the use of disposable instruments,[31] and blunt-tipped suture scissors,[83] or of guarding of instruments such as a microvitreoretinal blade.[96] Never reloading the same suture needle, using a new suture for every pass, and never leaving needles dangling in the surgical field have also been suggested. Some surgeons use an intermediate instrument stand or a basin positioned between the surgeon and scrub nurse where needles and instruments can be put down, rather than handing them directly back and forth, the so-called "hands-free" or "no-touch" technique.[38,83] These protocols may be inconvenient when performing vitrectomy or other procedures during which the surgeon is using the operating microscope. The surgeon must recognise potential risks of contamination and develop a personalised regular protocol in such cases.

Deep percutaneous injury with a needle contaminated by blood portends the highest risk of viral transmission. In particular, hollow needles with large bores may carry a relatively large volume of contaminated blood.[91] Any such needles used during the operative procedure should be deposited directly into a sharp disposal container immediately after use without recapping. After a retrobulbar anaesthetic injection, for example, someone other than the person giving the block should be present to apply pressure to the globe, so that the needle and syringe may be disposed of by the person who gave the block. All intraocular and periocular fluids should be strictly isolated.[31] Appropriate labelling of specimens sent for pathologic examination or diagnostic testing, to indicate that they are an infection hazard, should occur and the samples should be placed in a sturdy container with a secure lid to prevent leakage during transport.

In case of exposure to contaminated fluids or tissues, the exposed area should immediately be flushed with water, disinfectant such as topical 10% povidone-iodine, or other suitable solutions.[97] Post-exposure chemoprophylaxis (PEP) for health care workers is effective in reducing the chance of HIV transmission and should be readily available, as treatment should be initiated preferably within one to two hours of exposure,[98] and should be continued for four weeks, although the optimum duration for therapy is not known.[91] Zidovudine should be considered for all PEP regimens because zidovudine is the only agent for which data supports the efficacy of PEP in a clinical setting.[94] Lamivudine (3TC) should be added to zidovudine for increased antiretroviral activity and activity against many zidovudine-resistant strains. A protease inhibitor (preferably indinavir) should be added as "triple therapy" for high-risk exposures, which include contaminated needle sticks or significant exposure of mucous membranes or broken skin to contaminated blood.[98,99] The risk associated with percutaneous injury through two gloves by a small suture needle used in typical ophthalmic surgery is extremely low and may, to some, call into question the relative benefit of "triple therapy" for these exposures.

The requirements for effective HIV post-exposure prophylaxis may be somewhat different than those for optimum HIV treatment in the chronically ill HIV-positive patient. Ophthalmologists should have an in-depth knowledge of current thinking regarding HIV pathophysiology and treatment. Updated information about HIV PEP may be obtained from the United States Center for Disease Control and Prevention's home page on the Internet at http://www.cdc.gov.

References

1. Broughton W.L., Cupples H.P., Parver L.M. "Bilateral retinal detachment following cytomegalovirus retinitis. *Arch.Ophthalmol.* **96** (1978), 618–619.
2. Meredith T.A., Aaberg T.M., Reeser F.H. "Rhegmatogenous retinal detachment complicating cytomegalovirus retinitis," *Am. J. Ophthalmol.* **87** (1979), 793–796.

3. Jabs D.A., Enger C., Bartlett J.G. "Cytomegalovirus retinitis and acquired immunodeficiency syndrome," *Arch. Ophthalmol.* **107** (1989), 75–80.
4. Gross J.G., Bozzette S.A., Mathews W.C. *et al.* "Longitudinal study of cytomegalovirus retinitis in acquired immune deficiency syndrome," *Ophthalmology.* **97** (1990), 681–686.
5. Freeman W.R., Henderly D.E., Wan W.L. *et al.* "Prevalence, pathophysiology, and treatment of rhegmatogenous retinal detachment in treated cytomegalovirus retinitis," *Am. J. Ophthalmol.* **103** (1987), 527–536.
6. Holland G.N., Sidikaro Y., Kreiger A.E. *et al.* "Treatment of cytomegalovirus retinopathy with ganciclovir," *Ophthalmology.* **94** (1987), 815–823.
7. Roarty J.D., Fisher E.J., Nussbaum J.J. "Long-term visual morbidity of cytomegalovirus retinitis in patients with acquired immune deficiency syndrome," *Ophthalmology.* **100** (1993), 1685–1688.
8. Studies of Ocular Complications of AIDS (SOCA) Research Group in collaboration with the AIDS Clinical Trials Group (ACTG). "Rhegmatogenous retinal detachment in patients with cytomegalovirus retinitis: The Foscarnet-Ganciclovir Cytomegalovirus Retinitis Trial," *Am. J. Ophthalmol.* **124** (1997), 61–70.
9. Jabs D.A., Enger C., Haller J. *et al.* "Retinal detachments in patients with cytomegalovirus retinitis," *Arch. Ophthalmol.* **109** (1991), 794–799.
10. Irvine A.R. "Treatment of retinal detachment due to cytomegalovirus retinitis in patients with AIDS," *Trans. Am. Ophthalmol. Soc.* **89** (1991), 349–363; discussion 363–367.
11. Freeman W.R., Quiceno J.I., Crapotta J.A. *et al.* "Surgical repair of rhegmatogenous retinal detachment in immunosuppressed patients with cytomegalovirus retinitis," *Ophthalmology.* **99** (1992), 466–474.
12. Jabs D.A. "Ocular Manifestations of HIV infection," *Trans. Am. Ophthalmol. Soc.* **97** (1995), 623–683.
13. Freeman W.R., Friedberg D.N., Berry C. *et al.* "Risk factors for development of rhegmatogenous retinal detachment in patients with cytomegalovirus retinitis," *Am. J. Ophthalmol.* **116** (1993), 713–720.
14. Sidikaro Y., Silver L., Holland G.N. *et al.* "Rhegmatogenous retinal detachments in patients with AIDS and necrotizing retinal infections," *Ophthalmology.* **98** (1991), 129–135.
15. Zegans M.E., Tufail A., Holland G.N. *et al.* "Five cases of unusually heavy vitritis in AIDS patients with CMV retinitis and increased CD4 counts on protease inhibitors," *Invest. Ophthalmol. Vis. Sci.* (1997), S739–S739 (Abstract)
16. Karavellas M.P., Lowder C.Y., Macdonald C. *et al.* "Immune recovery vitritis associated with inactive cytomegalovirus retinits," *Arch. Ophthalmol.* **116** (1998) 169–175.
17. Kuppermann B.D., Flores-Aguilar M., Quiceno J.I. *et al.* "A masked prospective evaluation of outcome parameters for cytomegalovirus-related retinal detachment surgery in patients with acquired immune deficiency syndrome," *Ophthalmology.* **101** (1994). 46–55.

18. Martin D.F., Parks D.J., Mellow S.D. *et al.* "Treatment of cytomegalovirus retinitis with an intraocular sustained-release ganciclovir implant. A randomized controlled clinical trial," *Arch. Ophthalmol.* **112** (1994), 1531–1539.

19. Pepose J.S., Holland G.N., Nestor M.S. *et al.* "Acquired immune deficiency syndrome. Pathogenic mechanisms of ocular disease," *Ophthalmology.* **92** (1985), 472–484.

20. Orellana J., Teich S.A., Lieberman R.M. *et al.* "Treatment of retinal detachments in patients with the acquired immune deficiency syndrome," *Ophthalmology.* **98** (1991), 939–943.

21. McCluskey P., Grigg J., Playfair T.J. "Retinal detachments in patients with AIDS and CMV retinopathy: A role for laser photocoagulation," *Br. J. Ophthalmol.* **79** (1995), 153–156.

22. Davis J.L., Hummer J., Feuer W.J. "Laser photocoagulation for retinal detachments and retinal tears in cytomegalovirus retinitis," *Ophthalmology.* **104** (1997), 2053–2060.

23. Vrabec T.R. "Laser photocoagulation repair of macula-sparing cytomegalovirus-related retinal detachment," *Ophthalmology.* **104** (1997), 2062–2067.

24. Regillo C.D., Vander J.F., Duker J.S. *et al.* "Repair of retinitis-related retinal detachments with silicone oil in patients with acquired immunodeficiency syndrome," *Am. J. Ophthalmol.* **113** (1992)m 21–27.

25. Morlet N., Young S., Corneo M.T. "Risk factors for the development of rhegmatogenous retinal detachment in patients with cytomegalovirus retinitis," *Am. J. Ophthalmol.* **118** (1994), 684–686.

26. Stevens G., Palestine A., Rodrigues M.M. *et al.* "Failure of argon laser to halt cytomegalovirus retinitis," *Retina* **6** (1986), 119–122.

27. Chuang E.L., Davis J.L. "Management of retinal detachment associated with CMV retinitis in AIDS patients," *Eye* **6** (1) (1992), 28–34.

28. Davis J.L., Serfass M.S., Lai M.Y. *et al.* "Silicone oil in repair of retinal detachments caused by necrotizing retinitis in HIV infection," *Arch. Ophthalmol.* **113** (1995), 1401–1409.

29. Sandy C.J., Bloom P.A., Graham E.M. *et al.* "Retinal detachment in AIDS-related cytomegalovirus retinitis," *Eye* **9** (3) (1995), 277–281.

30. Hannouche D., Korobelnik J.F., Cochereau I. *et al.* "Management of viral retinitis-associated retinal detachment in AIDS," *Eye* **11** (1) (1997), 33–36.

31. Dugel P.U., Liggett P.E., Lee M.B. *et al.* "Repair of retinal detachment caused by cytomegalovirus retinitis in patients with the acquired immunodeficiency syndrome," *Am. J. Ophthalmol.* **112** (1991), 235–242.

32. Arevalo J.F., Freeman W.R. "Rhegmatogenous retinal detachments in patients with acquired immunodeficiency syndrome," *Semin. Ophthalmol.* **10** (1995), 183–191.

33. Irvine A.R., Lonn L., Schwartz D. *et al.* "Retinal detachment in AIDS: Long-term results after repair with silicone oil," *Br. J. Ophthalmol.* **81** (1997), 180–183.

34. Nasemann J.E., Mutsch A., Wiltfang R. *et al.* "Early pars plana vitrectomy without buckling procedure in cytomegalovirus retinitis-induced retinal detachment," *Retina.* **15** (1995), 111–116.

35. Kao G.W., Peyman G.A., Fiscella R. *et al.* "Retinal toxicity of ganciclovir in vitrectomy infusion solution. *Retina.* **7** (1987), 80–83.

36. Paques M., Massin P., Santiago P. *et al.* "Visual field loss after vitrectomy for full-thickness macular holes," *Am. J. Ophthalmol.* **124** (1997), 88–94.

37. Lim J.I., Enger C., Haller J.A. *et al.* "Improved visual results after surgical repair of cytomegalovirus- related retinal detachments," *Ophthalmology.* **101** (1994), 264–269.

38. Ross W.H., Bryan J.S., Barloon A.S. "Management of retinal detachments secondary to cytomegalovirus retinitis," *Can. J. Ophthalmol.* **29** (1994), 129–133.

39. Garcia R.F., Flores-Aguilar M., Quiceno J.I. *et al.* "Results of rhegmatogenous retinal detachment repair in cytomegalovirus retinitis with and without scleral buckling," *Ophthalmology.* **102** (1995), 236–245.

40. Geier S.A., Klauss V., Bogner J.R *et al.* "Retinal detachment in patients with acquired immunodeficiency syndrome," *Ger. J. Ophthalmol.* **3** (1994), 9–14.

41. Cochereau I., Korobelnik J.F., Petit E. *et al.* "Pronostic du decollement de retine sur retinite a cytomegalovirus, [Prognosis of retinal detachment in cytomegalovirus retinitis] *J. Fr. Ophtalmol.* **18** (1995), 603–607.

42. Holland G.N. "The management of retinal detachments in patients with acquired immunodeficiency syndrome," *Arch.Ophthalmol.* **109** (1991), 791–793.

43. Engstrom R.E.J., Holland G.N., Hardy W.D. *et al.* "Hemorheologic abnormalities in patients with human immunodeficiency virus infection and ophthalmic microvasculopathy," *Am. J. Ophthalmol.* **109** (1990), 153–161.

44. Forster D.J., Dugel P.U., Frangieh G.T. *et al.* "Rapidly progressive outer retinal necrosis in the acquired immunodeficiency syndrome," *Am. J. Ophthalmol.* **110** (1990), 341–348.

45. Engstrom R.E.J., Holland G.N., Margolis T.P. *et al.* "The progressive outer retinal necrosis syndrome," *Ophthalmology* **101** (1994), 1488–1502.

46. Margolis T.P., Lowder C.Y., Holland G.N. *et al.* "Varicella-zoster virus retinitis in patients with the acquired immunodeficiency syndrome," *Am. J. Ophthalmol.* **112** (1991), 119–131.

47. Engstrom R.E.J., Holland G.N., Margolis T.P. *et al.* "The progressive outer retinal necrosis syndrome. A variant of necrotizing herpetic retinopathy in patients with AIDS," *Ophthalmology.* **101** (1994), 1488–1502.

48. Tamesis R.R., Foster C.S. "Ocular syphilis," *Ophthalmology.* **97** (1990), 1281–1287.

49. Williams J.K., Kirsch L.S., Russack V. *et al.* "Rhegmatogenous retinal detachments in HIV-positive patients with ocular syphilis," *Ophthalmic Surg. Lasers.* **27** (1996), 699–705.

50. Passo M.S., Rosenbaum J.T. "Ocular syphilis in patients with human immunodeficiency virus infection," *Am. J. Ophthalmol.* **106** (1988), 1–6.

51. Knox C.M., Chandler D., Short G.A. *et al.* "Polymerase chain reaction-based assays of vitreous samples for the diagnosis of viral retinitis. Use in diagnostic dilemmas," *Ophthalmology.* **105** (1998), 37–44.

52. Mitchell S.M., Fox J.D., Tedder R.S. *et al.* "Vitreous fluid sampling and viral genome detection for the diagnosis of viral retinitis in patients with AIDS," *J. Med. Virol.* **43** (1994), 336–340.

53. Danise A., Cinque P., Vergani S. *et al.* "Use of polymerase chain reaction assays of aqueous humor in the differential diagnosis of retinitis in patients infected with human immunodeficiency virus," *Clin. Infect. Dis.* **24** (1997), 1100–1106.

54. Garweg J., Fenner T., Bohnke M. *et al.* "An improved technique for the diagnosis of viral retinitis from samples of aqueous humor and vitreous," *Graefes. Arch. Clin. Exp. Ophthalmol.* **231** (1993), 508–513.

55. Ussery F.M.3, Gibson S.R., Conklin R.H. *et al.* "Intravitreal ganciclovir in the treatment of AIDS-associated cytomegalovirus retinitis," *Ophthalmology.* **95** (1988), 640–648.

56. Young S.H., Morlet N., Heery S. *et al.* "High dose intravitreal ganciclovir in the treatment of cytomegalovirus retinitis," *Med. J. Aust.* **157** (1992), 370–373.

57. Daikos G.L., Pulido J., Kathpalia S.B. *et al.* "Intravenous and intraocular ganciclovir for CMV retinitis in patients with AIDS or chemotherapeutic immunosuppression," *Br. J. Ophthalmol.* **72** (1988), 521–524.

58. Engstrom R.E.J., Holland G.N. "Local therapy for cytomegalovirus retinopathy," *Am. J. Ophthalmol.* **120** (1995), 376–385.

59. Tufail A., Holland G.N. "Cytomegalovirus retinitis: Are intraocular devices the answer?" *Br. J. Ophthalmol.* **79** (1995), 1066–1067.

60. Cochereau-Massin I., Lehoang P., Lautier-Frau M. *et al.* "Efficacy and tolerance of intravitreal ganciclovir in cytomegalovirus retinitis in acquired immune deficiency syndrome," *Ophthalmology.* **98** (1991), 1348–1353; discussion, 1353–1355.

61. Morlet N., Young S.H. "Prevention of intraocular pressure rise following intravitreal injection," *Br. J. Ophthalmol.* **77** (1993), 572–573.

62. Cantrill H.L., Henry K., Melroe N.H. *et al.* "Treatment of cytomegalovirus retinitis with intravitreal ganciclovir. Long-term results," *Ophthalmology.* **96** (1989), 367–374.

63. Heinemann M.H. "Long-term intravitreal ganciclovir therapy for cytomegalovirus retinopathy," *Arch. Ophthalmol.* **107** (1989), 1767–1772.

64. Heinemann M.H. "Staphylococcus epidermidis endophthalmitis complicating intravitreal antiviral therapy of cytomegalovirus retinitis. Case report," *Arch. Ophthalmol.* **107** (1989), 643–644.

65. Akula S.K., Ma P.E., Peyman G.A. *et al.* "Treatment of cytomegalovirus retinitis with intravitreal injection of liposome encapsulated ganciclovir in a patient with AIDS," *Br. J. Ophthalmol.* **78** (1994), 677–680.

66. Baudouin C., Chassain C., Caujolle C. *et al.* "Treatment of cytomegalovirus retinitis in AIDS patients using intravitreal injections of highly concentrated ganciclovir," *Ophthalmologica* **210** (1996), 329–335.

67. Hodge W.G., Lalonde R.G., Sampalis J. *et al.* "Once-weekly intraocular injections of ganciclovir for maintenance therapy of cytomegalovirus retinitis: clinical and ocular outcome," *J. Infect. Dis.* **174** (1996), 393–396.

68. Tufail A., Weisz J.M., Holland G.N. "Endogenous bacterial endophthalmitis as a complication of intravenous therapy for cytomegalovirus retinopathy," *Arch. Ophthalmol* **114** (1996), 879–880.

69. Kreiger A.E., Foos R.Y., Yoshizumi M.O. "Intravitreous granulation tissue and retinal detachment following pars plana injection for cytomegalovirus retinopathy," *Graefes. Arch. Clin. Exp. Ophthalmol.* **230** (1992), 197–198.

70. Smith T.J. "Intravitreal sustained-release ganciclovir," *Arch. Ophthalmol.* **110** (1992), 255–258.

71. Sanborn G.E., Anand R., Torti R.E. *et al.* "Sustained-release ganciclovir therapy for treatment of cytomegalovirus retinitis. Use of an intravitreal device," *Arch. Ophthalmol.* **110** (1992), 188–195.

72. Charles N.C., Steiner G.C. "Ganciclovir intraocular implant. A clinicopathologic study," *Ophthalmology.* **103** (1996), 416–421.

73. Anand R., Nightingale S.D., Fish R.H. "Control of cytomegalovirus retinitis using sustained release of intraocular ganciclovir," *Arch. Ophthalmol.* **111** (1993), 223–227.

74. Martin D.F., Ferris F.L., Parks D.J. *et al.* "Ganciclovir implant exchange. Timing, surgical procedure, and complications," *Arch. Ophthalmol.* **115** (1997), 1389–1394.

75. Duker J.S., Robinson M., Anand R. *et al.* "Initial experience with an eight-month sustained-release intravitreal ganciclovir implant for the treatment of CMV retinitis associated with AIDS," *Ophthalmic Surg. Lasers* **26** (1995), 442–448.

76. Reed J.B., Schwab I.R., Gordon J. *et al.* "Regression of cytomegalovirus retinitis associated with protease-inhibitor treatment in patients with AIDS," *Am. J. Ophthalmol.* **124** (1997), 199–205.

77. Studies of Ocular Complications of AIDS (SOCA) Research Group in collaboration with the AIDS Clinical Trials Group (ACTG). "Forscarnet-ganciclovir cytomegalovirus retinitis trial: IV. Visual outcomes," *Ophthalmology.* **7** (1994), 1250–1261.

78. Morinelli E.N., Dugel P.U., Lee M. *et al.* "Opportunistic intraocular infections in AIDS," *Trans. Am. Ophthalmol. Soc.* **90** (1992), 97–108.

79. Holland G.N., Sison R.F., Jatulis D.E. *et al.* "Survival of patients with the acquired immune deficiency syndrome after development of cytomegalovirus retinopathy," (UCLA CMV Retinopathy Study Group) *Ophthalmology.* **97** (1990), 204–211.

80. Jacobson M.A., Causey D., Polsky B. *et al.* "A dose-ranging study of daily maintenance intravenous foscarnet therapy for cytomegalovirus retinitis in AIDS," *J. Infect. Dis.* **168** (1993), 444–448.

81. Musch D.C., Martin D.F., Gordon J.F. *et al.* "Treatment of cytomegalovirus retinitis with a sustained-release ganciclovir implant," (The Ganciclovir Implant Study Group) *N. Engl. J. Med.* **337** (1997), 83–90.

82. Marx J.L., Kapusta M.A., Patel S.S. *et al.* "Use of the ganciclovir implant in the treatment of recurrent cytomegalovirus retinitis," *Arch. Ophthalmol.* **114** (1996), 815–820.

83. Raahave D., Bremmelgaard A. "New operative technique to reduce surgeons' risk of HIV infection," *J. Hosp. Infect.* **18** (Suppl A) (1991), 177–183.

84. Rodenbach M., Gumbel H., Makabe R. Lasertherapie von Lid- und Bindehauttumoren, insbesondere bei AIDS-Patienten," [Laser therapy of eyelid and conjunctival tumors, especially in AIDS patients] *Ophthalmologe* **91** (1994), 691–693.

85. Brun S.C., Jakobiec F.A. "Kaposi's sarcoma of the ocular adnexa," *Int. Ophthalmol. Clin.* **37** (1997), 25–38.

86. Dugel P.U., Gill P.S., Frangieh G.T. *et al.* "Treatment of ocular adnexal Kaposi's sarcoma in acquired immune deficiency syndrome," *Ophthalmology.* **99** (1992), 1127–1132.

87. Shuler J.D., Holland G.N., Miles S.A. *et al.* "Kaposi sarcoma of the conjunctiva and eyelids associated with the acquired immunodeficiency syndrome," *Arch. Ophthalmol.* **107** (1989), 858–862.

88. Waddell K.M., Lewallen S., Lucas S.B. *et al.* "Carcinoma of the conjunctiva and HIV infection in Uganda and Malawi," *Br. J. Ophthalmol.* **80** (1996), 503–508.

89. Ateenyi-Agaba C. "Conjunctival squamous-cell carcinoma associated with HIV infection in Kampala, Uganda," *Lancet* **345** (1995), 695–696.

90. Muccioli C., Belfort R.J., Burnier M. *et al.* "Squamous cell carcinoma of the conjunctiva in a patient with the acquired immunodeficiency syndrome. *Am. J. Ophthalmol.* **121** (1996), 94–96.

91. Centers for Disease Control. Case-control study of HIV seroconversion in health-care workers after percutaneous exposure to HIV-infected blood--France, United Kingdom, and United States, January 1988–August 1994. *MMWR* **44** (1995), 929–933.

92. Henderson D.K., Fahey B.J., Willy M. *et al.* "Risk for occupational transmission of human immunodeficiency virus type 1 (HIV-1) associated with clinical exposures. A prospective evaluation," *Ann. Intern. Med.* **113** (1990), 740–746.

93. Pietrabissa A., Merigliano S., Montorsi M. *et al.* "Reducing the occupational risk of infections for the surgeon: multicentric national survey on more than 15,000 surgical procedures," *World J. Surg.* **21** (1997), 573–578.

94. Cardo D.M., Culver D.H., Ciesielski C.A. *et al.* "A case-control study of HIV seroconversion in health care workers after percutaneous exposure," (Centers for Disease Control and Prevention Needlestick Surveillance Group) *N. Engl. J. Med.* **337** (1997), 1485–1490.

95. Gerberding J.L., Quebbeman E.J., Rhodes R.S. "Hand protection," *Surg. Clin. North Am.* **75** (1995), 1133–1139.

96. Schwartz D.M. "Guarded microvitreoretinal blade," *Arch. Ophthalmol.* **114** (1996), 1524–1525.

97. Gerberding J.L., Henderson D.K. "Management of occupational exposures to bloodborne pathogens: Hepatitis B virus, hepatitis C virus, and human immunodeficiency virus," *Clin. Infect. Dis.* **14** (1992), 1179–1185.

98. Centers for Disease Control. "Provisional Public Health Service recommendations for chemoprophylaxis after occupational exposure to HIV," *MMWR* **45** (1996), 468–472.
99. Landers M.B., Fraser V.J. "Antiviral chemoprophylaxis after occupational exposure to human immunodeficiency virus: Why, when, where, and what," *Am. J. Ophthalmol.* **124** (1997), 234–239.

CHAPTER 9

AIDS AND THE EYE IN DEVELOPING COUNTRIES

Phillipe Kestelyn

Introduction

Since the identification of the first AIDS cases in 1991, HIV has spread over the world causing a global pandemic of unprecedented severity. The developing countries are among the hardest hit regions of the world and according to the estimations of UNAIDS (Table 9.1) more than 90% of the 22 million adults with HIV worldwide live in Sub-Saharan Africa, South and South-East Asia, and Latin America. In sub-Saharan Africa alone an estimated 13.3 million adults are HIV infected and 67% of the one million children with HIV infection worldwide live in the same subcontinent. The epidemic in sub-Saharan Africa probably started in the mid 1970s, earlier than in other developing regions of the world, and has reached an intensity quite unlike anything experienced by populations from other regions of the world. Most experience of HIV infection in developing countries was derived from research conducted in the so-called AIDS belt of Africa — a long belt stretching from the Central African Republic and Southern Sudan through Uganda, Rwanda, Burundi, Kenya and Tanzania to Malawi, Zambia, Zimbabwe, Botswana, South Africa, and Namibia, and unless stated otherwise the information contained in this chapter will mainly focus on the situation in sub-Saharan Africa.

HIV Infection in Developing Countries

Epidemiology

Although there is no such thing as "African AIDS" since the etiology and the underlying defect in cellular immunity are the same as in Western countries, the epidemiology, the clinical presentation, and the therapeutic modalities are

Table 9.1 Percentage of total number of adults living with HIV, by subcontinent in mid-1996 (Global total: 21.8 million).

• E. Asia and Pacific	0.2
• E. Europe and Central Asia	0.1
• Australasia	0.1
• N. Africa and Middle East	0.9
• W. Europe	2.2
• S. and S.E. Asia	23.0
• N. America	3.7
• Latin America	6.0
• Caribbean	1.3
• Sub-Saharan Africa	63.0

(Source : UNAIDS)

very different. In 1984, the first reports of AIDS in Central and East Africa were published.[1-3] A striking difference with the epidemiological pattern initially described in the US was the absence in Africa of homosexuality and intravenous drug use as risk factors for the disease. Men and women were equally affected, strongly implying that heterosexual contact is the main mode of HIV transmission in Africa. Risk factors for HIV seropositivity in Africa include having multiple sexual partners, a history of sexually transmitted disease, and higher socio-economic status.[4] Two age-specific peaks of HIV seropositivity corrresponding to the two main modes of transmission, perinatal and heterosexual, are present: one in children under five and another in sexually active adults in the age group 15 to 50 years. In many of the large urban centres, seroprevalence among the latter group is as high as 30%. The prevalence in rural areas is lower, but slowly rising there as well.

There are few studies on the natural history of HIV infection in developing countries, but from the available evidence it seems that both the interval from seroconversion to symptomatic disease and from advanced HIV disease to death are shorter than in Europe or the US. Recent evidence estimates that the latency period in Africans is seven to eight years and the survival period after symptomatic disease eight to nine months.[5] One difficulty in assessing data from developing countries for comparison is the fact that very few studies in Africa use the CDC AIDS case surveillance definition, as this definition requires sophisticated equipment to count CD4 lymphocytes and to diagnose the indicator diseases, which is not readily available in most developing countries. Most epidemiological studies in developing countries are based on a clinical case definition established by WHO in 1986 that does not require laboratory testing.[6] This definition requires the presence of two major signs and one minor sign, as listed in Table 9.2, in the absence of known immunosuppression. Kaposi's sarcoma and cryptococcal meningitis are considered AIDS defining in themselves.

Table 9.2 World Health Organization clinical case definition for AIDS.

Major criteria
- Weight loss (> 10 % of body weight)
- Chronic diarrhoea (> one month)
- Prolonged fever (> one month)

Minor criteria
- Persistent cough (> one month)
- Generalised pruritic dermatitis
- Recurrent herpes zoster
- Oropharyngeal candidiasis
- Chronic progressive and disseminated herpes virus infection
- Generalised lymphadenopathy

Two studies have evaluated the sensitivity, the specificity, and the positive predictive value of the WHO case definition against the CDC definition.[7,8] It seems that the sensitivity is reasonable (79%), the specificity is good (91%), but the positive predictive value is poor (30%) for an HIV seroprevalence in the population of 10%. Including HIV testing in the WHO case definition would certainly improve its value as a surveillance tool, but unfortunately this technology is not always available in developing countries.[9]

Clinical Features

The common signs and symptoms of HIV infection in developing countries include weight loss, night sweats, fever, and diarrhoea. Early manifestations in otherwise apparently healthy patients are skin disorders, especially herpes zoster and pruriginous dermatitis, an itchy, papular rash that leaves pigmented macules as a result of scratching. The best known clinical picture associated with HIV disease in Africa is "slim" disease, the term used in Uganda to denote the wasting syndrome (see Fig. 9.1). Dominant features are profound wasting, fever, chronic diarrhoea, and fever. Both gastrointestinal causes (cryptosporidiosis, microsporidiosis, isosporiasis) and disseminated tuberculosis may play an aetiological role in this entity. Tuberculosis is one of the most common opportunistic infections in African patients, occurring in about one-third at presentation of HIV disease. Bacterial septicaemia with non-typhoidal Salmonella species and pneumonia due to *Streptococcus pneumoniae* are other common manifestations of HIV infection in developing countries.

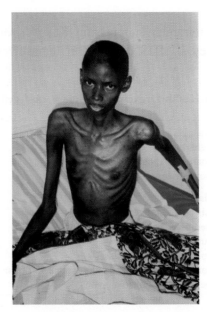

Fig. 9.1 "Slim disease."

Cerebral toxoplasmosis and cryptococcal meningitis are probably more common in African than Western patients. On the other hand, certain opportunistic infections which are common in Western patients are rare in AIDS patients in developing countries. Examples include *Pneumcystis carinii* pneumonia, CMV retinitis, and infections with atypical mycobacteriae.

Treatment

Treatment of HIV infection, associated conditions and opportunistic infections should not be very different from what is done in the Western world, but unfortunately the lack of diagnostic capabilities and therapeutic resources seriously interferes with the correct management of these patients.

Ocular Manifestations of HIV Infection in Developing Countries

HIV infection is associated with a protean range of ocular manifestations. Although new observations will probably be added to this already long list of ocular manifestations of HIV infection in the coming years, it is now clear that the most common ocular lesions in HIV-infected patients are due to herpes zoster ophthalmicus, non-infectious HIV retinopathy, CMV retinitis, and a number of tumours of the eyelids and the conjunctiva (Kaposi's sarcoma and, as far as African patients are concerned, conjunctival neoplasias). In developing countries

HIV-infected patients often present with so-called minor opportunistic infections — diseases that may occur in normal healthy people, but that will occur with greater severity, with greater frequency, or with atypical features in HIV-seropositive patients. The presence of these diseases may alert the clinician to the possibility of an underlying HIV infection in an individual patient and their rising frequency in the community may serve as a "clinical marker" for the seroprevalence of HIV infection in the population. A typical example of a minor opportunistic infection that will come to the attention of the ophthalmogist is herpes zoster ophthalmicus. Other minor opportunistic infections are the viral diseases of the skin of the eyelids, such as molluscum contagiosum and papillomata.

Opportunistic infections of the retina such as CMV retinitis are less common in developing countries than in the industrialised world. Cryptococcal meningitis with its associated ocular findings, papilledema, optic atrophy, and oculomotor disturbances, is very prevalent in Africa. Non-infectious HIV retinopathy, cotton wool spots, small haemorrhages, and microaneurysms, seem to occur with equal frequency in both settings. Kaposi's sarcoma, an opportunistic tumour which may involve the eyelids and the conjunctiva, seems to occur with greater frequency in East Africa than in either West Africa or the Western world. A dramatic increase in the incidence of conjunctival malignancies in HIV patients is reported from several African countries, whereas only isolated case reports are published from Europe and the US. A common complication of treatment with sulfa drugs in black HIV-seropositive patients is a severe form of Stevens-Johnson syndrome. At the present time it is unclear whether the rise in the prevalence of tuberculosis with the advent of the HIV/AIDS epidemic will provoke a similar increase in ocular pathology due to this pathogen.

Herpes Zoster Ophthalmicus

Herpes zoster is a dermatomal skin eruption due to the varicella-zoster virus that occurs in patients who have had varicella previously (see Fig. 9.2). During primary infection the virus migrates centripetally along the nerve fibers to the sensory ganglia where latent infection is established. Virus reactivation at a later date may occur as a result of decreased immune response related to older age or acquired immune deficiency.

Herpes zoster is more common in HIV-seropositive patients than in healthy people of comparable age and it occurs in 10% to 15% of African patients with HIV.[10] The disease may occur at any stage of HIV infection, but it is often the first sign of the disease and thus a marker for HIV seropositivity in otherwise healthy patients.[11-13] The disease tends to run a more severe course in terms of corneal involvement and postzonal neuralgia in HIV-seropositive

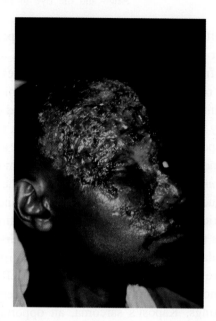

Fig. 9.2 Severe herpes zoster ophthalmicus in a HIV-positive patient.

patients[13] especially in developing countries where adequate antiviral treatment is often unavailable. The particularly destructive nature of the disease in these circumstances is exemplified by the fact that 66% of affected eyes in a series of 27 patients with HZO from Malawi had a final visual acuity of less than 20/60, while four eyes were eviscerated mainly due to severe keratouveitis and corneal perforation.[14] The administration of steroids, often advocated to prevent postherpetic neuralgia, is controversial and should probably be avoided in patients with advanced immunosupression. Several small studies have reported that the topical application of capsaicin, a plant derivative with anesthetic properties, is effective in relieving the postzonal pain.[15]

HIV-Related Microvasculopathy

Cotton wool spots, haemorrhages, microaneurysms, and telangiectasias are the expression of a microvasculopathy that is typical but by no means pathognomonic of HIV infection (see chapter 2). These lesions are much more prevalent in AIDS patients than in asymptomatic HIV-infected persons and their presence is generally associated with more profound immune depression.[16] In general, these lesions do not cause clinically significant visual symptoms. If confluent lesions develop around the fovea, ischaemic maculopathy with serious loss of central vison may ensue (see Fig. 9.3).

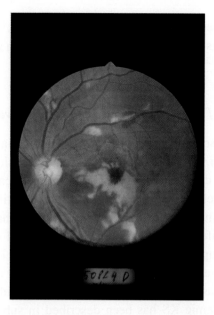

Fig. 9.3 Confluent cotton wool spots leading to macular ischaemia.

The fact that HIV-related microvasculopathy is as common in African AIDS patients as in their Western counterparts supports the idea that the aetiology of this ocular sign is the result of haemoreological and immunological abnormalities associated with progression of HIV infection itself. In the beginning of the AIDS epidemic two opportunistic infections were thought to play a role in the aetiology of cotton wool spots: *Pneumcystis carinii* and CMV. The observation that these two opportunistic infections are rare in African patients, in whom cotton wool spots are common, was one argument among others to invalidate the hypothesis that HIV-related microvasculopathy was associated with opportunistic infections.

Tumours Of The Eye And The Ocular Adnexae In HIV Patients

Three tumours of the periocular structures have been described in association with HIV infection: KS of the eyelids and the conjunctiva, squamous cell carcinoma of the conjunctiva, and lymphoma of the orbit. Both KS and squamous cell carcinoma are of particular relevance in African AIDS patients.

KS has been endemic in parts of Sub-Saharan Africa and it is precisely the appearance of an aggressive form of the disease in young patients that heralded the onset of the AIDS epidemic in Zambia.[18] Several reports from three different African countries emphasise the increased prevalence of aggressive squamous cell carcinomas of the conjunctiva in HIV-infected patients.[19–21] Although childhood Burkitt's lymphoma is endemic in Africa, there has been no association reported with HIV infection.[22]

Kaposi's Sarcoma of the Eyelids and the Conjunctiva

KS is a malignant vascular tumour probably of endothelial vascular or lymphatic endothelial cell origin.[23,24] Although it is classically considered to be a neoplastic disorder, a number of characteristics set it apart from typical tumours. Cytogenetic abnormalities are rarely observed,[25] the disease is multifocal in nature but the lesions at different sites cannot be explained by lymphatic or haematogenous spread, vascular proliferation is a prominent feature, and spontaneous regression may occur[26] (see chapter 4). The classic form of KS is an indolent sarcoma that occurs on the lower extremities, most often in elderly men of Mediterrranean, Middle Eastern, or Eastern European descent.[27] As already mentioned, a similar form of indolent endemic KS has been described in sub-Saharan Africa before the AIDS era.[28] By far, the most common form of Kaposi's sarcoma nowadays is the AIDS-related variant.

KS is the most common neoplasm in AIDS patients. However, the proportion of AIDS patients who develop KS at any point in their illness seems to be steadily declining. In one study the incidence of KS in AIDS patients dropped from 60% to 20% between 1981 and 1987.[29] This decline may reflect the change toward risk-reducing behaviour in homosexual men as KS is probably caused by a sexually transmissible agent. The AIDS-related form of KS coexists in Africa with the indolent endemic form and is then called atypical or epidemic KS. It is estimated that 5% to 15% of African patients with advanced HIV disease (less than 200 CD4 cells/µl) present with KS, but there are considerable geographical variations.[30]

Treatment of KS does not seem to influence survival.[31] Therefore, patients with stable or slowly progressive asymptomatic disease do not require specific anti-Kaposi treatment. The more sophisticated treatment modalities for rapidly progressive or symptomatic disease such as chemotherapy or radiation therapy are not available in most developing countries. However, locally symptomatic and unsightly lesions can be treated with local excision or cryosurgery.

Ocular involvement

Twenty percent of patients with systemic KS have ocular involvement.[31–35] Since 5% to 15% of African AIDS patients have systemic KS, one expects to find ocular KS in about 1% to 3% of them.

KS may develop on the margin and skin of the eyelid, on the conjunctiva, and rarely within the orbit. The clinical presentation of the lesions on the eyelid skin as deep purple-red nodules is identical to the cutaneous lesions elsewhere. The conjunctival lesions are bright red and may resemble sub-conjunctival haemorrhages (see Fig. 9.4(a) and 9.4(b)). Slit-lamp examination shows the difference. The lower fornix is more often involved than the upper fornix. The ocular localisation may be the initial manifestation of AIDS-related KS. The ocular lesions are usually slowly growing and rarely invasive. Indications for treatment include cosmetically disturbing lesions and discomfort or visual obstruction from bulky lesions. Lesions can be treated with excision, cryosurgery, or focal radiation therapy if available.

(a)   (b)

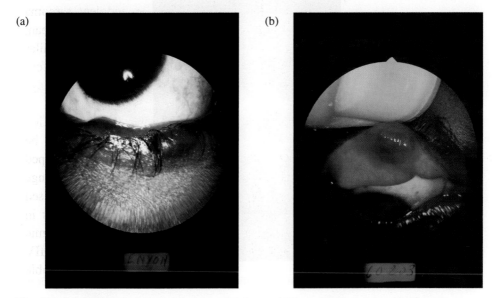

Fig. 9.4 (a) Kaposi's sarcoma of the eyelid in an African AIDS patient; (b) Kaposi's sarcoma of the tarsal conjunctiva.

Conjunctival Squamous Cell Carcinoma

Squamous cell carcinomas of the skin, oral cavity, epiglottis, oesophagus, lung, anorectum, and cervix have been reported in HIV-infected patients. Two case reports of conjunctival squamous cell carcinoma (see Fig. 9.5) in American patients with HIV infection suggested a possible relationship between conjunctival neoplasias and HIV seropositivity.[36,37] In Africa, the disease is probably much more common and a case-control study in Rwanda demonstrated that HIV seropositivity is a significant risk factor for conjunctival malignancy in this continent.[19] Of 11 patients with conjunctival malignancy, nine were HIV seropositive, whereas only six of 22 controls were HIV seropositive (odds ratio for multiple matched control = 13). Striking clinical features in these eleven patients with conjunctival neoplasia were their young age and the short interval between disease onset and excision, suggesting rapid progression. Seven patients of the 11 were symptom free, indicating that conjunctival malignancies in HIV-seropositive patients are not necessarily associated with advanced HIV disease. A similar study from Uganda arrived at essentially the same conclusions.[20] The severity of the condition is underscored by a case report from Malawi.[38]

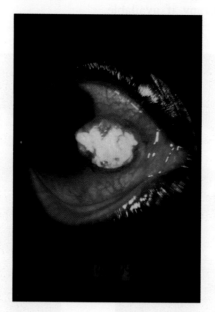

Fig. 9.5 Squamous cell carcinoma of the conjunctiva in an African HIV-positive patient.

The analogy with cervical neoplasias in HIV-infected women is obvious. HIV-infected women are at greater risk of developing cervical neoplasias[39] and therefore the CDC recently amended the AIDS surveillance case definition to include invasive cervical cancer in women with HIV infection among the conditions qualifying for AIDS diagnosis.[40] It seems plausible that the immunodeficiency in HIV-infected women releases the oncogenic potential of the human papilloma virus, a well known co-factor in the pathogenesis of cervical malignancies.[41]

Whether human papillomavirus plays the same role in the pathogenesis of conjunctival malignancies should be the focus of future research. Human papillomavirus 16 has been isolated from conjunctival premalignant and malignant lesions in a substantial number of immunocompetent patients.[42] Human papilloma virus 16 was isolated from a pigmented conjunctival dysplasia in an African HIV-positive woman.[43] However, this virus was not demonstrated in the conjunctiva of three Malawian patients with squamous cell carcinoma.[38] If this negative finding is confirmed, other factors than human papilloma virus infection must be suspected to play a role in the development of conjunctival neoplasias in HIV-infected patients.

Complete surgical excision is the treatment of choice for squamous cell carcinomas. If one doubts whether the entire lesion is removed, cryotherapy with a double freeze-thaw cycle may be applied to the margins.

Infections of the Retina and Choroid

CMV retinitis

Patients with advanced HIV disease are at risk for vast array of chorioretinal infections. By far, the most common opportunistic infection of the retina is CMV[44] (see chapter 6). Whereas CMV (see Fig. 9.6) occurred in 30% to 40% of AIDS patients in the industrialised world before the introduction of protease inhibitors, the prevalence in Africa probably does not exceed 5%. In order to understand the differences in prevalence of CMV retinitis it is worthwile to analyse the risk factors for CMV retinitis, which include the following:

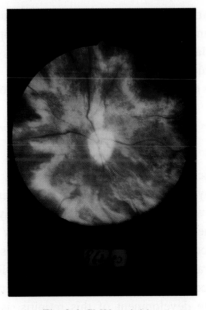

Fig. 9.6 CMV retinitis.

1) CD4 counts lower than 50/μl.[45] CMV retinitis is a disease of the stage of profound immune depression and the major risk factor to develop CMV retinitis is a CD4 count lower than 50 cells/μl. This is true to the point that the diagnosis of CMV retinitis in patients with higher CD4 counts should be carefully reconsidered. The marked geographical differences in the prevalence of CMV retinitis are explained to a large extent by the presence or absence of this risk factor. It is clear that better treatment of opportunistic infections and life-sustaining measures in the industrialised world prolong the stage of advanced immune depression placing more patients at risk of developing CMV retinitis for longer periods. African AIDS patients die from other opportunistic infections (tuberculosis, cryptococcal meningitis) and do not survive long enough once they enter the stage of severe immune depression.

2) Previous exposure to CMV. Serologic evidence of past CMV infection is present in nearly 100% of male homosexuals, but only in 50% of of the adult population in Europe and the US.[46] The seroprevalence in the adult population in developing countries is probably higher than 50% because of crowded living conditions and frequent transmission by breast milk, but does not reach the 100% observed in male homosexuals. This difference could for a small part be responsible for the lower incidence of CMV in developing countries.

Treatment of CMV retinitis in developing countries

In industrialised countries different therapeutic modalities are available for the treatment of CMV retinitis[47,48] (see chapter 6). In developing countries, antiviral drugs are hardly available and are too expensive for systemic treatment. The only acceptable treatment modality for CMV in these circumstances is local treatment (see chapters 6 and 8) of the better eye in cases of bilateral involvement.

The progressive outer retinal necrosis (PORN) syndrome

This is a variant of acute retinal necrosis seen in AIDS patients[49] (see chapter 5). It is characterised by a rapidly progressive, homogeneous necrosis of the outer retinal layers caused by the varicella-zoster virus. It destroys the retina in a matter of weeks and may be bilateral. Early retinal detachment is a common feature. The differential diagnosis with CMV retinitis is based upon the homogeneous aspect of the retinal necrosis, the absence of haemorrhages, and the much faster rate of progression in PORN. PORN is readily observed in African patients (see Fig. 9.7) since a history of dermatomal zoster, which is a risk factor for the development of this retinitis, is very common among

HIV patients in that continent. Moreover, PORN, may occur in patients with CD4 counts higher than 50 cells/μl.

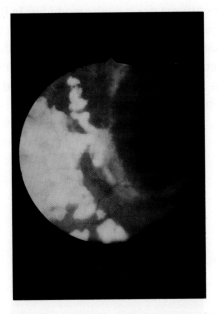

Fig. 9.7 Progressive Outer Retinal Necrosis (PORN).

Toxoplasmosis

The prevalence of toxoplasmic chorioretinitis in AIDS patients probably reflects the basic seroprevalence of antibodies to T. gondii in the population, which is subject to marked geographical differences. In East African countries such as Rwanda and Zimbabwe, for instance, toxoplasmic chorioretinitis both in healthy and in immune depressed patients is rare, whereas it is the most common cause of uveitis in West African Sierra Leone.[50] In Brazil, a 5% incidence of active ocular toxoplasmosis in 445 new HIV-infected patients was detected at the first eye examination.[51]

Tuberculosis

From the public health standpoint it is important to realise that part of the burden of HIV infection will arise from the interaction between HIV and tuberculosis. An alarming rise in the recrudescence of tuberculosis parallels the spread of the HIV epidemic.[52] In developing countries 30% to 50% of the adults have latent tuberculosis that may be reactivated in the presence of HIV infection, and HIV seropositivity is already the single most important risk factor for the development of active tuberculosis in areas where HIV is highly prevalent.[53] At present, it is unclear whether the increased prevalence of tuberculosis will be associated with an significant rise in ocular morbidity. In Rwanda, an examination of 32 HIV-positive patients with tuberculosis revealed that five (15.6%) had ocular involvement due to TB, including disseminated choroidal granulomas, phlyctenulosis, and solitary choroidal granulomas (see Fig. 9.8). In Malawi, however, an examination of 68 HIV-positive TB patients revealed only one with ocular disease that was probably TB related.[54]

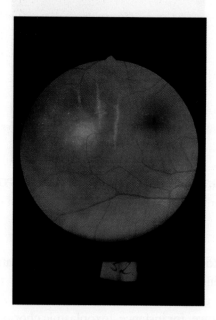

Fig. 9.8 Choroidal granuloma and overlying serous detachment in an HIV-positive patient with tuberculosis.

Syphilis

There is evidence that syphilitic disease may progress more rapidly in HIV-infected patients.[55] Taking into account the high prevalence of sexually transmitted disease in Africa, serological testing for syphilis should be performed on all HIV-seropositve patients with ocular inflammation of unknown origin. Ocular manifestations of syphilis described in HIV-seropositve patients include uveitis, retinitis and neuroretinitis, papillitis, and optic neuritis[56] (see chapter 5). Ocular involvement should be treated as for neurosyphilis in which the standard treatment consists of 12–24 million units of aqueous penicillin G IV for ten to 14 days, followed by intramuscular benzathinepenicillin G 2.4 million units per week for three weeks.

Neurophthalmic Manifestations

HIV may be associated with a large variety of neurophthalmological manifestations, including optic nerve disease (oedema, inflammation, atrophy), retrobulbar neuritis, visual field defects, cortical blindness, pupillary defects, and ocular motor nerve palsies (see chapter 7). Most of these disorders are due to infectious lesions of the central nervous system. In Africa the first pathogens to be suspected in such cases are cryptococcal meningitis and central nervous system toxoplasmosis. Less frequent causes of neurophthalmological manifestations are HIV encephalopathy, intracranial tumours, and neurosyphilis.

Cryptococcus neoformans is the most common life-threatening fungal pathogen and is significantly more common in African patients than in their Western counterparts, probably due to the high prevalence of *Cryptococcus neoformans* in the environment. The combination of low grade papilloedema and headaches in an HIV-positive patient, even in the absence of fever and neck stiffness, should alert the ophthalmologist to the possibility of cryptococcal meningitis (see Fig. 9.9). In a study of 80 HIV-positive patients with cryptococcal infection in Rwanda, papilloedema was observed in 26 (32.5%), visual loss in seven (9%), sixth cranial nerve palsy in seven (9%), and optic atrophy in two (2.5%). Actual invasion of the intraocular structures with *Cryptococcus neoformans* was an uncommon complication in Rwanda.[57]

Cutaneous Hypersensitivity Reactions

Stevens-Johnson syndrome is part of a spectrum of skin and generalised disease due to a hypersensitivity reaction to various drugs or toxins. Sulfa drugs have been strongly implicated. A study in Kenya demonstrated that TB patients infected with HIV have an increased risk of developing hypersensitivity reactions when treated with thiacetazone.[58] The syndrome, which may be fatal in up to 50% of patients, begins with malaise, arthralgia, and fever, followed by a bullous rash including the mucous membranes of mouth, pharynx, and anogenital region. Severe mucopurulent conjunctivitis (often with keratitis) results in raw conjunctival surfaces which stick together, shortening or obliterating the fornices in a matter of days. The mucin-producing goblet cells are destroyed and a severe dry eye results.

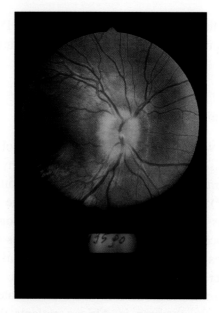

Fig. 9.9 Papilloedema in a patient with cryptococcal meningitis.

In Malawi, about 75% of the patients admitted with SJS to the eye ward were HIV positive.[59] Many of these patients had taken Fansidar (sulfadoxine-pyrimethamine), a widely used antimalarial drug.

The treatment of SJS in the acute stage consists of topical antibiotics and steroids and the prevention of symblepharon formation by manually breaking the synechiae with a glass rod several times a day. After healing of the acute lesions a severe dry eye syndrome with corneal keratinisation, neovascularisation, and trichiasis will often develop. Despite abundant lubrication, mucous membrane grafts and corrective surgery for the lid problems, corneal ulceration, surinfection, and scarring may occur and contribute to the poor prognosis for useful vision in these eyes.

Ocular Manifestations of HIV Infection in Children

Vertically acquired infection from mother to child accounts for the large majority of HIV infection in infants and children. The vertical route of transmission is a relatively efficient mode of transmission as compared to transmission through sexual contact. In industrialised countries the rate of vertical transmission ranges from 15% to 25%, whereas in developing countries it ranges from 25% to 40%.[60] The higher rate in developing countries may be due to the extra risk associated with HIV transmission through breastfeeding, but controlled trials in developing countries are needed to substantiate this suspicion.

Diagnosis of HIV Infection in Children

The diagnosis of HIV infection in infants is not easy. Infants passively acquire maternal antibody *in utero*, which may persist up to age 18 months. Since serum tests for IgG antibodies against HIV do not differentiate between infant or passive maternal antibodies, they are unable to distinguish between infected and uninfected children from HIV-seropositive mothers. The diagnosis of active infection should be based on more sophisticated laboratory methods, e.g. the detection of HIV-specific IgA and IgM or the demonstration of virus or viral antigen. In developing countries with limited resources this technology is rarely available and the WHO has developed a provisional clinical case definition of paediatric AIDS for use in the developing countries.[61] A child is suspected of having AIDS if at least two major signs and at least two minor signs are present in the absence of known immunodeficiency from other causes (see Table 9.3).

Table 9.3. Provisional WHO paediatric clinical case definitions of AIDS.

Major Signs	Minor Signs
• Weight loss or failure to thrive	• Generalised lymphadenopathy
• Chronic diarrhoea for > one month	• Oral thrush
• Chronic fever for > one month	• Repeated common infections (otitis media,
	• pharyngitis, etc.)
	• Persistent cough
	• Generalised dermatitis
	• Confirmed maternal infection

A striking difference between adults and children in the clinical manifestations of HIV infection is the severe degree of B-cell dysfunction in children with perinatal HIV infection. This immunological abnormality explains the severe and recurrent bacterial infections in HIV-infected children.[62] In addition to the AIDS-indicator diseases in adult HIV infection, a pulmonary syndrome called lymphoid interstitial pneumonitis (LIP) is added to the list of CDC-defined AIDS-indicator diseases in children with perinatal HIV infection. The aetiology of this syndrome is poorly understood, but suggested aetiologies include an exaggerated immunologic reaction to inhaled or circulating antigens, or primary infection of the lung with HIV, Epstein-Barr virus or both. Children with LIP have a significant survival advantage over those with other AIDS-defining diseases.[63]

The rate of disease progression in infants is much faster than in adults. Survival models based on data from 838 infected children and from 2910 children with AIDS suggest a bimodal mortality peak.[64-66] A first group of children dies before the age of four years with a median survival of from five to 11 months. A second group lives longer and has a median survival of five years. Typical clinical manifestations in the first group will include *Pneumocystis carinii* pneumonia, cytomegalovirus infection, wasting syndrome, and encephalopathy. In the second group, children will present at an older age with a clinical picture including LIP, lympadenopathy, hepatosplenomegaly, and parotid gland enlargement.

Ophthalmic Manifestations

The literature on the ophthalmic manifestations of HIV in children is limited, but from the available data it seems that the ocular aspects are also different in adults and children.[67-70] In a cross-sectional study of 162 Rwandese HIV-infected children (P. Kestelyn, personal data) the most commmon finding was inflammation or sheathing of the peripheral retinal vessels (see Fig. 9.10). CMV retinitis was present in three children (2%). Cotton wool spots, the most common ocular manifestaton of HIV in adults, were not observed in these children. The most common external findings were multiple mollusca contagiosa on the eyelids and the face, but this is quite common even in healthy African children. In HIV-infected children, however, there was a tendency towards larger lesions with bacterial superinfection. Other external findings included two cases of herpes zoster, two cases of conjunctival xerosis which responded to vitamin A administration, and a single case each of conjunctival telangiectasias and recurrent palpebral abscesses. Diminished tear secretion, present in up to one-third of the children, was a prominent finding in this series.

An important point to keep in mind when analysing the results of this cross-sectional study is the fact that three quarters of the children were older than one year and one quarter older than three years. In other words the findings in this study are probably representative for the second group of children — those who survive the first mortality peak and present more often with LIP than with opportunistic infections. Indeed, as many as 22% of these children had radiological evidence of LIP. It is possible that LIP, parotitis, lacrimal gland involvement (diminished tearing), and perivasculitis in HIV-infected children are in fact the expression of the same immunopathological response at different sites of the body. For example, exactly the same combination of target organs — lung, lacrimal gland, parotid gland and retinal vessels (periphlebitis) — is involved in sarcoidosis.

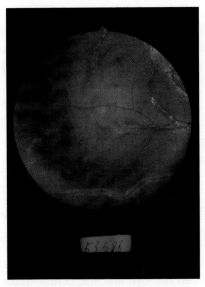

Fig. 9.10 Perivasculitis of the peripheral retinal vessels in a child with LIP.

Furthermore, a series of HIV-infected adults who had a syndrome characterised by diffuse lymphocytic visceral infiltration, especially of the salivary glands and the lungs,[71] has been reported. They found that this syndrome of diffuse infiltrative lymphocytosis syndrome or DILS was associated with a certain subtype of HLA-DR5 which is more common in blacks and they speculated that DILS in adults may be analogous to LIP and parotid gland enlargement in children. The hypothesis that the retinal perivasculitis found in HIV-infected children is part of the LIP-DILS complex, would explain then why this retinal manifestation is observed with greater frequency in blacks (higher prevalence of HLA-DR5), why it is more frequently observed in children (LIP is the most characteristic feature of HIV infection in childen), and why this sign is over-represented in a cross-sectional study in which children with a survival advantage are more likely to be included (LIP is associated with a better survival). Finally, it should be noted that most paediatric HIV patients with LIP in the US are of African-American descent, which also points to the possibility of a genetic predisposing factor.

The finding that cotton wool spots and CMV retinitis are rare in children has been confirmed by other series.[68] In one study cotton wool spots were typically absent in perinatally infected children. They were only observed in children older than eight years of age, who had acquired the infection through transfusion of blood or blood products.[70]

In our series of African HIV-infected children, we did not observe an increased incidence of optic atrophy or strabismus. An increased incidence of optic nerve atrophy has been reported in 18% of children from HIV-infected Italian mothers,[79] but this finding has not been confirmed by other studies. It may well be that maternal drug and alcohol abuse, quite common in HIV-seropositive women in Europe, was the real cause of optic nerve atrophy and acted as a confounding variable in this study. An increased incidence of strabismus has been noted in a cohort of American children with symptomatic HIV infection: 9% of the patients had heterotropia, whereas the incidence in the general population is below 5%.[80] The reason for this is not yet clear.

Implications of the Presence of HIV in the Eye and the Ocular Tissues

HIV has been isolated from the tears,[72] the conjunctiva,[73] the cornea,[74] aqueous humour,[75] vitreous,[76] retinal vascular endothelium, and from iris and retinal tissue.[77] The recovery of HIV from the eye and the ocular tissues and secretions raises the important issue of the nosocomial risk of HIV transmission in the eye care setting, especially in developing countries with a high seroprevalence of HIV infection and often insufficient resources to implement the guidelines issued by the Centers for Disease Control for the protection of health care workers.[78]

Fortunately, the risk of HIV infection in an occupational setting seems extremely small for ophthalmic care providers and to date there are no confirmed cases of HIV transmission resulting from contact during eye examination or surgery. Ophthalmic surgery is different from other specialties in that exposure to blood is limited so that the risk of acquiring HIV through surgical procedures is small (see chapter 8). With the advent of the HIV epidemic, the still common practice in developing countries to perform eye surgery without gloves should be abandoned and double gloving is probably indicated in selected ophthalmic procedures such as exenteration or dacryocystorhinostomy.

Potential transmission from patient to patient in the eye care setting is another problem that is particularly relevant in urban centres of the AIDS belt where up to 30% of the adult patients are HIV positive. The presence of HIV in tears and ocular surface tissues raises the possibility of accidental transmission during tonometry or from touching the ocular surface or the tears with instruments. Contact lens fitting, although another source of concern, is still an uncommon practice in most African countries. Wiping the tonometer tip with an isopropyl alcohol swab provides a ready and efficient means of inactivating HIV. Instruments coming into contact with the ocular surface or tears should be cleaned and then disinfected in between patients by one of the following procedures: five to ten minutes exposure to 3% hydrogen peroxide; a 1:10 dilution of common household bleach; 70% ethanol; or 70% isopropyl alcohol[79].

A special concern is the potential transmission of HIV through corneal transplantation, although to date no such cases have been reported. Despite the fact that donor corneas are routinely screened for HIV, the risk of grafting a cornea from an HIV-infected donor is not zero: recently infected persons in the window period, loss of anti-HIV antibodies or failure to mount an adequate immune response will all contribute to false negative ELISA tests. A simple formula has been derived to calculate the risk for a patient undergoing penetrating keratoplasty of receiving a cornea from an HIV-infected donor despite a negative ELISA.[80] This risk would be 1.2% if the HIV seroprevalence in the donor population is 10%, which is a realistic estimate for the urban population in certain African countries.

Developed Versus Developing Countries

The epidemiology of HIV infection itself varies according to factors such as route of transmission, socio-economic context, and geographical area. Likewise, the ophthalmic manifestations of HIV infection provide several good examples to illustrate that heredity, environmental and socio-economic factors may all influence the clinical epidemiology of these manifestations and partly explain the differences observed between industrialised and developing countries. Perivasculitis of the peripheral retinal vessels in African children is probably linked to the prevalence of a certain HLA type in black patients. Cryptococcal meningitis is a frequent opportunistic infection in African patients, but is much less common in American and European patients. The ubiquitous presence in African households of the causative opportunistic agent, *Cryptococcus neoformans*, is invoked to explain the difference (environment). CMV retinitis, which is a common opportunistic infection of the retina in the Western world, is hardly seen in developing countries where patients probably die from other causes before they reach the stage of advanced immune depression associated with disseminated CMV infection, since they are denied the high-tech medical care needed to reach this stage (socio-economic). Finally, conjunctival squamous cell carcinoma is more frequent in African patients for unknown reasons.

Future research on the ocular manifestations of HIV infection in developing countries will have its own list of priorities, based on the specific problems and opportunities of the region. The major ocular problem in developing countries is herpes zoster ophthalmicus and its complications. Although an effective drug is available, aciclovir is far too expensive for general use and innovative research is needed to come up with other treatment modalities. Since there are much larger numbers of children with HIV infection in Africa, studies on the ocular manifestations in children should be undertaken in this continent. The link between perivasculitis of the retinal vessels and lymphoid interstitial pneumonitis in African HIV-seropositive children should be clarified as well as the potential prognostic value of this retinal sign to predict survival. The intriguing fact that African HIV-seropositive patients are ten times more likely to develop conjunctival neoplasias than HIV-seronegative controls — a feature that is not observed in western patients — should stimulate research on the role of carcinogenic co-factors.

Over the last decades HIV infection has evolved from an obscure disease confined to certain risk groups into a pandemic that represents a major public health problem both in the industrialised countries and the developing world. It causes a great deal of suffering and places a heavy burden on Society in terms of direct and indirect costs. Recently, the introduction of a new generation of antiretroviral drugs, the protease inhibitors, has brought new hope for improved survival in HIV patients, reinforcing the idea that a fatal disease will slowly be converted into a chronic disease with a more or less normal life expectancy. That new hope will unfortunately not be shared by most patients and populations in developing countries where antiretroviral drugs and drugs used to treat opportunistic infections and tumours are rarely available, or can only be purchased at the detriment of other priorities. The indirect costs of HIV disease due to excess morbidity and premature mortality are especially high in those countries since the disease not only strikes young adults at the peak of their economic abilities but also young children.

A vaccine for HIV infection is not yet in sight and the dramatic situation in developing countries is unlikely to change over the next decade. Therefore, most health care workers, including ophthalmologists, working in that area of the world will be concerned with HIV infection for most of their professional lives. In order to provide competent care to his/her patients, the ophthalmologist should be thoroughly familiar with the general and the ocular aspects of the disease as they present in the area where he/she works.

References

1. Van de Perre P., Rouvroy D., Lepage P. et al. "Acquired immunodeficiency syndrome in Rwanda," *The Lancet* (1984).

2. Piot P., Quinn T.C., Taelman H. et al. "Acquired immunodeficiency syndrome in a heterosexual population in Zaire," *Lancet* 2 (1984), 65–69.

3. Bayley A.C. "Agressive Kaposi's sarcoma in Zambia, 1983," *Lancet* 1 (1984), 1318–1320.

4. Dallabetta G.A., Miotti P.G., Chiphangwi Jd. *et al.* "High socioeconomic status is a risk factor for human immunodeficiency virus type 1 (HIV-1) infection but not for sexually transmitted diseases in women in Malawi: implications for HIV-1 control," *J. Infect. Dis.* **167** (1993), 36–42.

5. Caldwell J.C. "The impact of the African AIDS epidemic," *Health Transition Review* 2(Suppl 7) (1997), 169–188.

6. World Health Organization. "Provisional case definition for AIDS," *Wkly. Epidemiol. Rec.* **61** (1986), 72–73.

7. Colebunders R., Mann J.M., Francis H. *et al.* "Evaluation of a clinical case-definition of acquired immunodeficiency syndrome in Africa," *Lancet* 1 (1987), 492–494.

8. Gilks C.F. "What use is a clinical case definition for AIDS in Africa? *Brit. Med. J.* **301** (1993), 1189–1190.

9. De Cock K.M., Selik R.M. Soro B. *et al.* "For debate. AIDS surveillance in Africa: A reappraisal of case definitions," *Brit. Med. J.* **303** (1991), 1185–1188.

10. Colebunders R.L., Latif A.S. "Natural history and clinical presentation of HIV-1 infection in adults," *AIDS* **5** (1991), S103–S112.

11. Cole E.L., Meisler D.M., Calabrese L.H. *et al.* "Herpes Zoster ophthalmicus and acquired immune deficiency syndrome," *Arch. Ophthalmol.* **102** (1984), 1027–1029.

12. Sandor E.V., Millman A., Croxson T.S. *et al.* "Herpes zoster ophthalmicus in patients at risk for the acquired immune deficiency syndrome (AIDS)," *Am. J. Ophthalmol.* **101** (1986), 53–55.

13. Kestelyn P., Stevens A.M., Bakkers E. *et al.* "Severe herpes zoster ophthalmicus in young African adults: A marker for HTLV-III seropositivity," *Br. J. Ophthalmol.* **71** (1987), 806–809.

14. Lewallen S. "Herpes Zoster Ophthalmicus in Malawi," *Ophthalmology* **101** (1994), 1801–1804.

15. Peikert A., Hentrich M., Ochs G. "Topical 0.025 % capsaicin in chronic post-herpetic neuralgia: Efficacy, predictors of response and long term course," *J. Neurol.* (1991), 238–452.

16. Freeman W.R., Chen A., Henderly D.E. *et al.* "Prevalence and significance of acquired immunodeficiency syndrome related retinal microvasculopathy," *Am. J. Ophthalmol.* **107** (1989), 229–235.

17. Kestelyn P., Van de Perre P., Rouvroy D. *et al.* "A prospective study of the ophthalmic findings in the acquired immune deficiency syndrome in Africa," *Am. J. Ophthalmol.* **100** (1985), 230–238.

18. Bayley A.C., Downing R.G., Cheingsong-Popov R. *et al.* "HTLV-III serology distinguishes atypical and endemic Kaposi's sarcoma in Africa," *Lancet* **1** (1985), 359–361.

19. Kestelyn P., Stevens A.M., Ndayambaje A. *et al.* "HIV and conjunctival malignancies," *Lancet* **336** (1990), 51–52.

20. Ateenyi-Agaba C. "Conjunctival squamous cell carcinoma associated with HIV infection in Kampala, Uganda," *Lancet* **345** (1995), 695–696.

21. Waddell K.M., Lewallen S., Lucas S.B. *et al.* "Carcinoma of the conjunctiva and HIV infection in Uganda and Malawi," *Br. J. Ophthalmol.* **80** (1996), 503–508.

22. Lucas S.B., Odida M., Wabinga H. "The pathology of severe morbidity and mortality caused by HIV infection in Africa," *AIDS* **5** (1991), S143–S148.

23. Rutgers J.L., Wieczorek R., Bonetti F. *et al.* "The expression of endothelial cell surface antigens by AIDS-associated Kaposi's sarcoma: Evidence for a vascular endothelial cell origin," *AM. J. Pathol.* **122** (1986), 493–499.

24. Beckstead J.H., Wood G.S., Fletcher V. "Evidence of the origin of Kaposi's sarcoma from lymphatic endothelium," *AM. J. Pathol.* **119** (1985), 294–300.

25. Sanchez M., Ames E.D., Erhardt K. *et al.* "Analysis of DNA distribution in Kaposi's sarcoma in patients with and without the acquired immune deficiency syndrome," *Anal. Quant. Cytol. Histol.* **10** (1988), 16–20.

26. Real F., Krown S.E. "Spontaneous regression of Kaposi's sarcoma in patients with AIDS," *N. Engl. J. Med.* **313** (1985), p.1659.

27. Safai B., Good R.A. "Kaposi's sarcoma : a review and recent developments," *Cancer* **31** (1981), 2–12.

28. Taylor J.F., Templeton A.C., Vogel C.L. *et al.* "Kaposi's sarcoma in Uganda: A clinico-pathological study," *Int. J. Cancer* **8** (1971), 122–135.

29. Rutherford G.W., Schwarcz S.K., Lemp G.F. *et al.* "The epidemiology of AIDS-related Kaposi's sarcoma in San Francisco," *J. Infect. Dis.* **159** (1989), 569–572.

30. Desmond-Hellman S.D., Katongole-Mbidde E. "Kaposi's sarcoma: recent developments," *AIDS* **5** (1991), S135–S142.

31. Volberding P.A., Kusick P., Feigal D.W. "Effect of chemotherapy for HIV associated Kaposi's sarcoma on longterm survival," *Proceedings of the American Society of Clinical Oncology*, San Francisco, (1989), p.11.

32. Centers for Disease Control. "Update: Acquired immunodeficiency syndrome United States," *MMWR.* **35** (1986), 17–21.

33. Shuler J.D., Holland G.N., Miles S.A. *et al.* "Kaposi sarcoma of the conjunctiva and eyelids associated with the acquired immunodeficiency syndrome," *Arch. Ophthalmol.* **107** (1989), 858–862.

34. Deugel P.U., Gill P.S., Frangieh G.T. *et al.* "Treatment of ocular adnexal Kaposi's sarcoma in acquired immune deficiency sydrome," *Ophthalmology* **99** (1992), 1127–1132.

35. Ghabrial R., Quivey J.M., Dunn J.P. *et al.* "Radiation therapy of acquired immunodeficiency syndrome-related Kaposi's sarcoma of the eyelids and conjunctiva," *Arch. Ophthalmol.* **110** (1992), 1423–1426.

36. Winward K.E., Curtin V.T. "Conjunctival squamous cell carcinoma in a patient with human immunodeficiency virus infection," *Am. J. Ophthalmol.* **107** (1989), p.554.

37. Kim R.Y., Seiff S.R., Howes E.L. *et al.* "Necrotizing scleritis secondary to conjunctival squamous cell carcinoma in acquired immunodeficiency syndrome," *Am. J. Ophthalmol.* **109** (1990), 231–233.

38. Lewallen S., Shroyer K.R., Keyser R.B. *et al.* "Aggressive conjunctival squamous cell carcinoma in three young Africans," *Arch. Ophthalmol.* **114** (1996), 215–218.

39. Schrager L.K., Friedland G.H., Maude D. *et al.* "Cervical and vaginal squamous cell abnormalities in women infected with human immunodeficiency virus," *J. Acquir. Immune Defic. Syndr.* **2** (1989), 570–575.

40. Centers for Disease Control. "1993 revised classification system for HIV infection and expanded surveillance case definition for AIDS among adolescents and adults," *NMWR* **41** (1992), 1–19.

41. Feingold A.R., Vermund S.H., Burk R.D. *et al.* "Cervical cytologic abnormalities and papillomavirus in women infected with human immunodeficiency virus," *J. Acquir. Immune Defic. Syndr.* **3** (1990), 896–903.

42. McDonnel J.M., Mayr A.J., Martin J.W. "DNA of human papillomavirus type 16 in dysplastic and malignant lesions of the conjunctiva and cornea," *N. Engl. J. Med.* **320** (1989), 1442–1446.

43. Loeffler K.U., Witschel H., Ikenberg H. *et al.* "Pigmented conjunctival epithelial dysplasia in an HIV positive African: Detection of human papillomavirus type 16," *Br. J. Ophthalmol.* **79** (1995), 1138–1139.

44. Culbertson W.W. "Infections of the retina in AIDS," *Int. Ophthalmol. Clin.* **29** (1989), 108–117.

45. Kupperman B.D., Petty J.G., Richman D.D. *et al.* "Correlation between CD4+ counts and prevalence of cytomegalovirus retinitis and human immunodeficiency virus related noninfectious retinal vasculopathy in patients with acquired immunodeficiency syndrome," *Am. J. Ophthalmol.* **115** (1993), 575–582.

46. A.S. Benenson (Ed.), Control of Communicable Diseases in Man, ed. 14. The American Public Health Association, Washington, (1985), 96–99.

47. Dhillon B. "Perspective: The management of cytomegalovirus retinitis in AIDS," *BJO* **78** (1994), 66–69.

48. Engstrom R.E., Holland G.N. "Local therapy for cytomegalovirus retinopathy," *Am. J. Ophthalmol.* **120** (1995), 376–385.

49. Engstrom R.E. Jr, Holland G.N., Margolis T.P. *et al.* "The progressive outer retinal necrosis syndrome," *Ophthalmology* **101** (1994), 1488–1502.

50. Ronday M.J., Stilma J.S., Barbe R.F. *et al.* "Aetiology of uveitis in Sierra Leona, west Africa," *Br. J. Ophthalmol.* **80** (1996), 1–6.

51. Belfort R., Mucciolo C. "Experience of HIV/AIDS and the eye in Brazil, South America," *Community Eye Health*, **8** (1995), 26–27.

52. Horsburgh C.R., Poznick A. "Epidemiology of tuberculosis in the era of HIV," *AIDS* **7**(suppl 1) (1993), S109–S114.

53. Mertens T.E., Belsey E., Stoneburner R.L. *et al.* "Global estimates and epidemiology of HIV infections and AIDS," *AIDS* **9** (1995), S259–S272.

54. Lewallen S., Kumwenda J., Maher D. *et al.* "Retinal findings in Malawian patients with AIDS," *Br. J. Ophthalmol.* **78** (1994), 757–759.

55. Johns D.R., Tierney M., Felsenstein D. "Alterations in the natural history of neurosyphilis by concurrent infection with the human immunodeficiency virus," *N. Engl. J. Med.* **316** (1987), 1569–1572.

56. Kuo I.C., Kapusta M.A., Narsing A.R. "Vitritis as the primary manifestation of ocular syphilis in patients with HIV infection," *Am. J. Ophthalmol.* **125** (1998), 306–311.

57. Kestelyn P., Taelman H., Bogaerts J. *et al.* "Ophthalmic manifestations of infections with Cryptococcus neoformans in patients with the acquired immunodeficiency syndrome," *Am. J. Ophthalmol.* **116** (1993), 721–727.

58. Nunn P., Kibuga D., Gathua S. *et al.* "Cutaneous hypersensitivity reactions due to thiacetazone in HIV-1 seropositive patients treated for tuberculosis," *Lancet* **337** (1991), 627–630.

59. Kestelyn Ph., Lewallen S. "Ocular problems with HIV infection and AIDS in Africa," *Community Eye Health* **8** (1995), 20–23.

60. Workshop on mother-to child transmission of HIV: Ghent-Belgium, 17–20 February 1992. Brussels: European Economic Community AIDS Task Force, (1992).

61. World Health Organization. "Acquired immunodeficiency syndrome (AIDS)," *Wkly. Epidemiol. Rec.* **62** (1986), 69–73.

62. Bernstein L.J., Krieger B.Z., Novick B. *et al.* "Bacterial infection in the acquired immunodeficiency syndrome of children," *Pediatr. Infect. Dis.* **4** (1985), 472–475.

63. Connor E.M., Andiman W.A. "Lymphoid interstitial pneumonitis, in: *Pediatric AIDS*," Williams & Wilkins (1994), 467–481.

64. Byers B., Caldwell B., Oxtoby M. "Pediatric Spectrum of Disease Project. Survival of children with perinatal HIV infection: Evidence for two distinct populations," (Abstract WS-C10-6) *Ninth International Conference on AIDS*, Berlin, June 1993.

65. Auger I., Thomas P., De Gruttola V. *et al.* "Incubation periods for pediatric AIDS patients," *Nature* **336** (1988), 575–577.

66. Blanche S., Tardieu M., Duliege A. *et al.* "Longitudinal study of 94 symptomatic infants with perinatally acquired human immunodeficiency virus infection: Evidence

for a bimodal expression of clinical and biological symptoms," *Am. J. Dis. Child.* **144** (1990), 1210–1215.

67. Kestelyn P., Lepage P., van de Perre P. "Perivasculitis of the retinal vessels as an important sign in children with the AIDS-related complex," *Am. J. Ophthalmol.* **100** (1985), 614–615.

68. Dennehy P.J., Warman R., Flynn J.T. *et al.* "Ocular manifestations in pediatric patients with acquired immunodeficiency syndrome," *Arch. Ophthalmol.* **107** (1989), 978–982.

69. Blini M., Bertoni H.G., Chiama M. *et al.* "Ocular involvement in children with HIV infection," (Abstracts) *5th International Conference on AIDS*, Montreal (1989), p. 258.

70. de Smet M.D., Butler K.M., Rubin I.B. *et al.* "The ocular complications of HIV in the pediatric population, in: Demouchamps J.P., Verougstraete C., Caspers-Velu L., Tassignon M.J. (Eds.), *Recent Advances in Uveitis*, Kugler, Amsterdam, (1993), 315–320.

71. Itescu S., Brancato L.J., Winchester R. "A sicca syndrome in HIV infection: Association with HLA-DR5 and CD8 lymphocytosis," *Lancet* **2** (1989), 466–469.

72. Fujikawa L.S., Salahuddin S.Z., Palestine A.G. *et al.* "Isolation of human T-lymphotropic virus type III from tears of a patient with the acquired immunodeficiency syndrome," *Lancet* **2** (1985), 529–530.

73. Fujikawa L.S., Salahuddin S.Z., Ablashi D. *et al.* "Human T-cell leukemia/lymphotropic virus type III in the conjunctival epithelium of a patient with AIDS," *Am. J. Ophthalmol.* **100** (1985), 507–509.

74. Doro S., Navia B.A., Kahn A. *et al.* "Confirmation of HTLV-III virus in cornea," *Am. J. Ophthalmol.* **102** (1986), 390–391.

75. Kestelyn P., van de Perre P., Sprecher-Goldberger S. "Isolation of the human T-cell leukemia/lymphotropic virus type III from aqueous humor in two patients with perivasculitis of the retinal vessels," *Int. Ophthalmol.* **9** (1986), 247–251.

76. Cowan W.T., Wahab S., Lucia H.L. "Detection of human immunodeficiency virus antigen in vitreous humor,:" *J. Clin. Microbiol.* **26** (1988), 2421–2422.

77. Cantrill H.I., Henry K., Jackson B. *et al.* "Recovery of human immunodeficiency virus from ocular tissues in patients with acquired immune deficiency syndrome," *Ophthalmology* **95** (1988), 1458–1462.

78. Centers for Disease Control. "Recommendations for prevention of HIV transmission in health-care settings," *MMWR* **36**(suppl.) (1987), 1s–18s.

79. Centers for Disease Control: "Recommendations for preventing possible transmission of human T-lymphotropic virus type III/lymphadenopathy-associated virus from tears," *MMWR* **34** (1985), p.533.

80. Goode S.M., Hertzmark E., Steinert R.F. "Adequacy of the ELISA test for screening corneal transplant donors," *Am. J. Ophthalmol.* **106** (1988), 463–466.

INDEX